RHEUMATISM AND MUSCULOSKELETAL DISORDERS

INTERVERTEBRAL DISC DEGENERATION

PREVALENCE, RISK FACTORS AND TREATMENTS

RHEUMATISM AND MUSCULOSKELETAL DISORDERS

Additional books in this series can be found on Nova's website under the Series tab.

Additional e-books in this series can be found on Nova's website under the e-book tab.

RHEUMATISM AND MUSCULOSKELETAL DISORDERS

INTERVERTEBRAL DISC DEGENERATION

PREVALENCE, RISK FACTORS AND TREATMENTS

ALLEN L. HO AND ATMAN M. DESAI
EDITORS

VINOD RAVIKUMAR, MANAGING EDITOR
JULIAN LIANG, GRAPHICS DESIGNER

NOVA BIOMEDICAL

New York

Library of Congress Cataloging-in-Publication Data

Library of Congress Control Number: 2016946632
ISBN: 978-1-63485-829-8

Published by Nova Science Publishers, Inc. † New York

CONTENTS

PREFACE

Degenerative disc disease is a significant component of spine disorders and lower back pain that now afflicts nearly one third of the adult population. This represents a significant morbidity and cost burden — nearly a tenth of all health-care spending — that is only increasing in prevalence as the elderly population continues to grow. While current treatment modalities, ranging from conservative approaches to surgical interventions, are continually evolving, new therapies for intervertebral disc disease are also in development. Increased research on the cellular mechanisms underlying DDD have led to novel cell-based treatments which aim to delay rates of degeneration. *Intervertebral Disc Degeneration: Prevalence, Risk Factors and Treatments* is a comprehensive text on all facets of the disease process that covers the pathophysiology, biomechanics, as well as the location specific pathology and treatment options for degenerative disc disease. Written by nationally renowned experts in neurosurgery and orthopedic surgery of the spine, each chapter is a thorough, cogent discussion of an essential topic related to intervertebral disc degeneration that includes many original, easy to understand figures and illustrations. Also included are overviews of the most cutting-edge and emerging surgical and biologic management options of disc disease at all levels of the spine.

Chapter 1 - The degeneration of the intervertebral disc results from several multi-factorial pathophysiologic processes. Here, the authors discuss the anatomy of the intervertebral disc along with a presentation of several pathologic processes including vascular insufficiency (possibly due to cigarette exposure and endothelial dysfunction), anatomic variations, poor nutritional status, infections, autoimmune and/or inflammatory processes, genetic predispositions and iatrogenic occurrences as well as exposure to drugs or toxins that lead to degeneration of the disc. This brief overview establishes a necessary starting point for the understanding of these processes as well as a preview into potential therapeutic targets.

Chapter 2 - Lumbar degenerative disc disease is a very common condition with a high socio-economic burden. The etiology is multifactorial and not entirely understood, and some of the main factors implicated include: genetic predisposition, smoking, increased body mass index, weight lifting or impeded nutrient transportation through the endplates.

The presence of some pro-inflammatory cytokines and growth factors are well documented: the interleukin (IL) family, TNFα and PGE2. Alongside these, recently there has been an increased interest in nerve growth factor (NGF) and brain derived growth factor (BDGF). Their expression in a fibrous cartilaginous enviroment, where normally there are no nerve fibers or blood vessels, is of interest.

Neuronal proliferation is normally blocked out in the outer layers of the annulus fibrosus by the presence of Sema3A and aggrecan, with the latter also disrupting the endothelial proliferation. Degenerative changes may create propitious conditions for the invasion of the disc by endothelial and nerve structures.

Although it was assumed that differentiated cells lose the ability to undifferentiate, recent research supports the hypothesis that these cells can suffer a dedifferentiation process. In this respect, neural cells were obtained through transdifferentiation from keratocites and chondrocytes after stimulating these cells with nerve growth factors. Therefore, during the degenerative process, it is possible that the chondrocyte type cells reach a state of dedifferentiation and, due to the stimulation with nerve growth factors, can have characteristics similar to the nervous cells. Hence chondrocyte-like cells have the potential to transdifferentiate making them a possible source of nerve cells inside the intervertebral disc, and of pain.

This chapter deals with the identification of positive NFAP chondrones in degenerated intervertebral discs, suggesting a transdifferentiation of chondrocyte-like cells into nerve cells. It also reports the presence of NFAP-positive chondrones and pain score in patients with mild LDD (Lumbar Disc Disease).

The number and imunohistological characteristics of chondrocyte-like cells and their aggegated form, the chondrones, are correlated with the symptoms of patients with LDD. The identification of NFAP positive cells indicates the presence of nervous structures and the possibility of chondrocyte-like cells transdifferentiating into nerve cells. This finding might explain the different occurrences and characteristics of pain amongst patients with LDD.

Chapter 3 - The biomechanical properties of the spine offer insights into the mechanisms and consequences behind intervertebral disc degeneration. The intervertebral disc is a dynamic structure which serves a critical function in allowing the many components of the bony vertebrae to interface with and work with one another. The biomechanical properties of the intervertebral disc afford it's properties in helping the spine to withstand compressive, shear, bending, and rotational forces. These biomechanical properties are derived from the biochemical and cellular composition of the disc which afford it unique properties such as its viscoelastic behavior. Degeneration of the disc — either due to injury or aging — perturb the biochemical composition of the disc, and subsequently the biomechanical properties. This chapter will explore the composition and the mechanistic properties of the disc which give the disc it's unique characteristics, and how theses parameters change in degenerative states.

Chapter 4 - Cervical stenosis involves the narrowing of the spinal canal in the cervical spinal region. Cervical spondylosis is oftentimes used synonomously with cervical stenosis, but spondylosis implies age-related degeneration of the spine including congenital spinal stenosis, degeneration of intervertebral discs resulting in focal stenosis, and hypertrophy of spinal elements resulting in narrowing of the spinal canal. One of the most debilitating conditions associated with cervical stenosis is cervical spondylotic myelopathy. Multiple treatments including surgical and non-surgical options are available. However, once symptoms of cervical spondylotic myelopathy are severe, surgery becomes necessary to treat the cervical stenosis.

Chapter 5 - Thoracic disc herniations occur less frequently than cervical or lumbar herniations, yet are common enough that surgeons should understand management strategies. Preoperative assessment of the size, location, presence of calcification, and spinal level are all important factors for deciding upon a surgical approach. While some disc herniations will require anterior approaches, these are typically associated with higher levels of morbidity and lengthier hospital stays, suggesting posterior approaches, when feasible, offer better outcomes. In most surgeries, the need for fusion is low but the final decision needs to be tailored for the individual patient.

Chapter 6 - Cervical disc herniation (CDH) occurs with regular frequency and is the most common indication for cervical spine surgery. While conservative treatment is the first line of defense when managing CDH, severe cases may be treated with anterior, posterior, or combined approaches. Choice of an approach is dependent on careful synthesis of symptoms, exam findings, and imaging results by the surgeon. Studies offer conflicting views regarding which approach results in superior outcomes. The eventual decision on surgical approach, if determined to be necessary, must be individually tailored for each patient.

Chapter 7 - Lumbar spinal stenosis (LSS) is a clinical syndrome characterized by buttock and/or lower extremity pain with or without back pain secondary to degenerative spinal canal narrowing and compression of the neurovascular elements. LSS is the most common reason for spinal surgery in patients over 65 years of age. It results in significant pain and disability, compromising the quality of life and everyday activities of the affected patients. Pain is aggravated by certain postures, including walking, standing or lumbar extension and characteristically alleviated by recumbency, sitting and forward flexion. Initial treatment options include conservative management such as lifestyle modification, physiotherapy, epidural injections and medications. Very few randomized controlled clinical trials have assessed the role and the efficacy of non-surgical modalities for the management of patients with LSS and therefore there is a lack of sufficient evidence to suggest a specific method is superior. Surgical intervention is performed when there is failure of conservative management or neurologic emergency. Current techniques include open or minimally invasive approaches that aim at restoring spinal canal diameter and relieving neurovascular compromise.

Chapter 8 - Lumbar disc herniations occur with relatively high frequency such that surgeons should be aware of prevention, management, and treatment strategies. Clinical presentation including assessment of location, morphology, symptoms, and imaging are crucial sources of information in the determination of the necessity for surgery. Conservative management may include one or a combination of medication, physical therapy, and epidural steroid injections. If needed and depending on the surgeon's preference, minimally invasive microdiscectomies or endoscopic procedures may be utilized to treat patients. Ultimately, the ongoing debate between non-interventional and interventional approaches to treatment requires surgeons to make final decisions tailored to each patient.

Chapter 9 - Lumbar Degenerative Spondylolisthesis (LDS) is a common condition affecting the lumbar spine characterized by chronic arthritis and bony remodeling of the facet joints. Epidemiologic studies have revealed that LDS is a relatively common condition among older patients, and may be asymptomatic in many affected individuals. While conservative treatment measures are often utilized initially, the mainstay of management for persistently symptomatic LDS is surgical decompression. Despite a number of recent well-designed randomized clinical trials, there remains no consensus regarding the optimal method of surgical treatment, including whether or not lumbar spinal fusion provides added clinical benefit beyond decompression alone. This chapter reviews the epidemiology and clinical presentation of LDS, as well as the existing evidence for the range of surgical treatments that have been utilized in patients suffering from this condition.

Chapter 10 - Degenerative disc disease (DDD) is a significant component of spine disorders and low back pain, and the prevalence of disc disease is increasing with an aging population. While current treatment modalities, ranging from conservative approaches to surgical interventions, are continually evolving, new therapies for intervertebral disc disease are also in development. Increased research on the cellular mechanisms underlying DDD have led to novel cell-based treatments which aim to delay rates of degeneration [1, 3]. Most of these cellular therapies remain in the research phase. Recent innovations in engineering have also pioneered several types of surgical constructs that improve the durability of treatment, while minimizing device-associated complications. Several examples include hybrid materials for intervertebral cages, zero-profile implants, expandable cages, sagittal correction implants, and disc arthroplasty. Finally, surgical techniques have been refined and adapted to allow less invasive modalities such as endoscopic and percutaneous techniques to reach adequate treatment effect with less risk of adverse event and further degeneration of the incident and adjacent spinal segments. This chapter highlights several emerging non-surgical and surgical treatments for intervertebral disc disease.

In: Intervertebral Disc Degeneration
Editors: A. L. Ho and A. M. Desai

ISBN: 978-1-63485-829-8

Chapter 1

THE PATHOPHYSIOLOGY OF INTERVERTEBRAL DISC DISEASE

Akwasi Ofori Boah, MD, Nancy Abu-Bonsrah, BS, C. Rory Goodwin, MD/PhD and Daniel Sciubba, MD*

The Johns Hopkins University School of Medicine
Departments of Neurosurgery, The Johns Hopkins University School of Medicine, Baltimore, MD, US

ABSTRACT

The degeneration of the intervertebral disc results from several multi-factorial pathophysiologic processes. Here, we discuss the anatomy of the intervertebral disc along with a presentation of several pathologic processes including vascular insufficiency (possibly due to cigarette exposure and endothelial dysfunction), anatomic variations, poor nutritional status, infections, autoimmune and/or inflammatory processes, genetic predispositions and iatrogenic occurrences as well as exposure to drugs or toxins that lead to degeneration of the disc. This brief overview establishes a necessary starting point for the understanding of these processes as well as a preview into potential therapeutic targets.

* Daniel M. Sciubba, M.D. Department of Neurosurgery, Johns Hopkins University School of Medicine, 600 North Wolfe Street, Meyer 7-109, Baltimore, MD 21287, E-mail: dsciubb1@jhmi.edu.

INTRODUCTION

In this chapter we will aim to elucidate the pathophysiology behind the degenerative processes for an intervertebral disc as well as its biomechanical and clinical impact. This is a multifaceted disease process that may take place in several stages throughout our lives [18]. Highlighted will be: disc development, anatomic considerations, plausible but non-exhaustive mechanisms, and key developments in our recent understanding of this phenomenon.

Although pain is the most common symptom, radiculopathy and other symptoms may also ensue with intervertebral disc degeneration. Diagnosis is made with a detailed history, clinical exam findings as well as imaging (MRI/CT/X-ray). Discogenic back pain/neck pain may be under-diagnosed as the quality of discograms and their subjective nature have led to its controversial association. The Derby criteria are one method of interpreting discography, where concordant responses produce pain greater than 6 out of 10 at a pressure of less than 50 psi above the opening pressure of the disc (having a negative control disc) [28]. The modified Dallas discogram scale is another photographic and descriptive form of identifying radial fissure patterns in the disc, which correlate with provocative studies [29].

Intervertebral discs have a complex anatomical configuration, which is a key determinant in the individual mobility of segmental joints (zygapophyseal) as well as overall regional (cervical, thoracic, and lumbar) flexibility. Intervertebral discs not only anchor segments of vertebral bodies to one another but they distribute gravitational forces throughout the spine in order to protect against rapid breakdown. Understanding the inherent complexity of their design allow us to understand their protective qualities.

ANATOMY AND PATHOPHYSIOLOGIC MECHANISMS

Embryonic development:

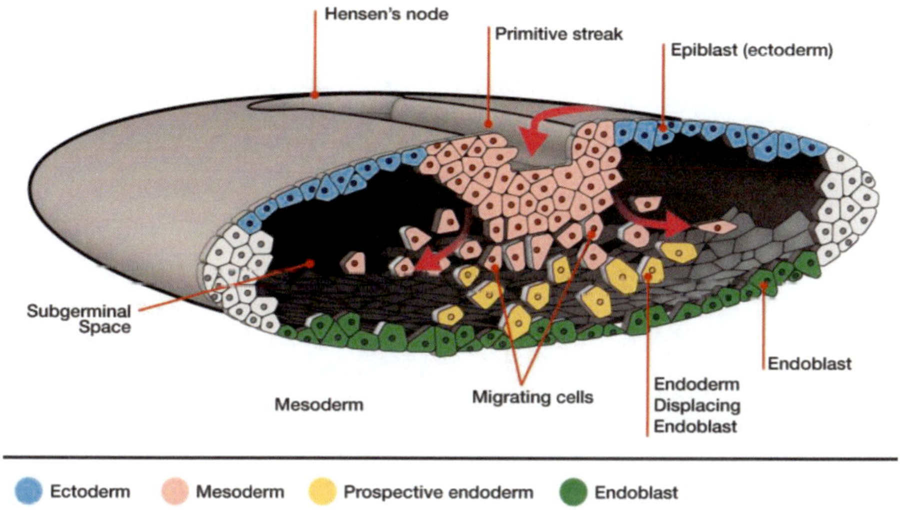

Figure 1. Germ Layers.

In humans, the development of three separate germ layers occurs during gastrulation, which takes place in the third week of gestation. Gastrulation produces ectoderm, mesoderm, and endoderm (Figure 1). Ectodermal precursor epiblast cells invaginate at the primitive node/streak [6]. These epiblast cells will then migrate to the mesodermal layer and eventually form the notochord. Sonic hedgehog growth factor (Shh) along with transforming growth factor - beta (TGF-β) have been established as the necessary stimuli for the development of the eventual nucleus pulposus and annulus fibrosis [5, 10]. These two factors have the ability to orchestrate the migration and apoptosis of cells in the maturing sclerotomes, which will lead to vertebral bodies along with the discs and their subchondral regions along the endplates (Figure 2). Shh factors, Paired box 1 and Paired box 9 (Pax1/9), dictate the vertebral endochondral ossification process and TGF-β helps the endplates form the subsequent fibers of the annulus fibrosis (Sharpey's fibers) [5, 10]. Detailed understanding of the embryology and initial signaling cascades involved in disc formation may provide the basis for future etiologies as well as targeted therapies as we will review later in this chapter.

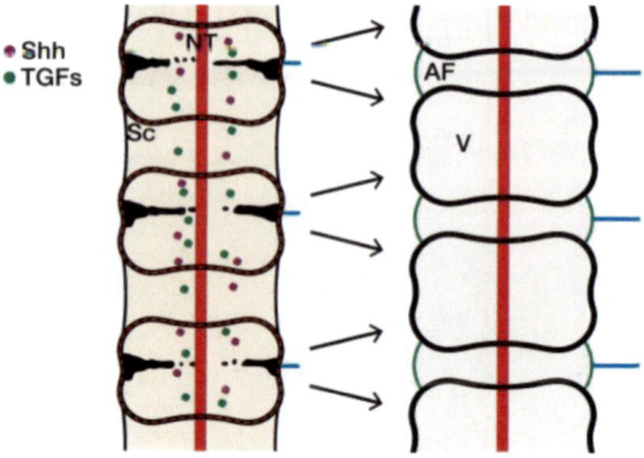

Figure 2. Growth Factors and the Intervertebral Disc.

Anatomy

To deepen our understanding of the intervertebral disc, we will now evaluate the intervertebral disc-endplate complex anatomically. At each intervertebral segment (excluding abnormal ankylosis across the disc space which may or may not be pathologic [33]) the anatomy is preserved and repetitive as a result of the complex differentiation of sclerotomes under the Shh/TGF-β pathways [32]. We must evaluate each structure separately. This includes the nucleus pulposus, annulus fibrosis, and vertebral endplate.

The Annulus Fibrosus

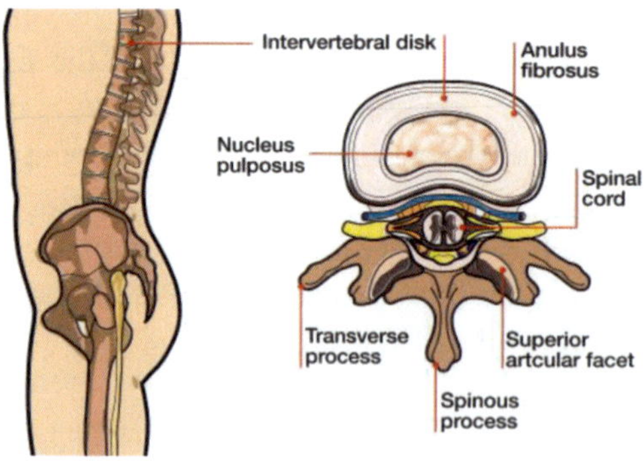

Figure 3. Disc Components.

Named for its shape and texture, the "fibrous ring" which surrounds the nucleus pulposus and is deeply engrained into the subchondral endplate has an inner and an outer layer. (*Figure 3*) It is composed of multiples of concentric lamellae with roughly 9,000 cells per cubic millimeter [10]. The outer layer is composed of fibroblasts and type I collagen, which accounts for the strength we ascribe to it traditionally [26]. Its extracellular matrix is also highly organized which accounts for a very high tensile strength. The inner layer of the annulus contains type II collagen and proteoglycans with a poorly structured extracellular matrix. This is also known as the "transition zone."

The Nucleus Pulposus

Surrounded by the concentric lamellae of the annulus fibrosus, the nucleus pulposus is made of predominantly proteoglycans and water but much less type II collagen. (*Figure 3*) It contains roughly 3,000 cells per cubic millimeter [10]. This provides the nucleus and thus the disc with its elastic mobile properties, which are able to withstand tensile forces. Chondrocyte-type NP cells help to regulate the amount of Hypoxia Inducible Factors (HIF) - 1 and 2 as this is a relatively avascular structure in order to maintain nutrient levels and thus viability.

The Endplates

The vertebral endplates, which themselves are composed of cortical bone, have a subchondral region subjacent to a very thin layer of additional hyaline cartilage where the Sharpey's fibers of the annulus fibrosus insert/anchor themselves. A small microscopic plexus can be found in this region. There are also many negatively charged proteoglycans and type II collagen fibers. Combined with H_20, this loose extracellular matrix allows for diffusion of small positively charged ions from a microscopic vascular network [22]. The vertebral endplates play a key role in the degenerative process with characteristic MRI findings, which would eventually be described by Dr. Michael Modic in 1988 (*Figure 4*) [21]. As our knowledge of the role of the vertebral endplates in degenerative process increases, we are learning that certain conditions which predispose them to decline also compromise the discs themselves [35].

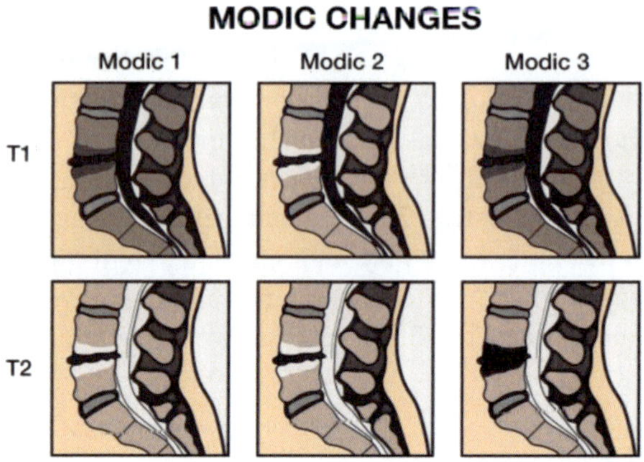

Figure 4. Modic Changes.

Pathophysiologic Mechanisms

The degeneration of an intervertebral disc is a complex process, which typically takes place after skeletal maturity is reached. Many factors will account for its deterioration over time. We will attempt to outline and tie together some of a myriad of reasons that this process occurs as people age, which produces some typical alterations. For example, histologic analysis by Yasuma et al., explained that in cadaveric specimens (the majority of discs from patients in their sixth decade) the orientation of the inner fiber bundles of the annulus fibrosus was reversed, so that they bulged inward [39].

Vascular

As previously mentioned, the intervertebral disc is relatively avascular and has a microscopic vascular supply system. Due to these factors, compromise of the vessels supplying the disc-endplate complex is often seen. Without adequate blood supply, the intervertebral disc will, in theory, degenerate at the rate that its blood supply is unable to keep up with nutritional requirements. Microcirculatory perfusion of the vertebral marrow can be measured with CT-perfusion [23]. The microcirculation develops to maturity by 25 years, remains stable at 35 years, and then begins to decline after 35 years. The age-related decrease of microcirculatory perfusion in the lumbar vertebral marrow precedes the loss of bone mineralization density and the onset of intervertebral disc disease, indicating their possible causal relationship.

Cigarette smoking has deleterious effects throughout the human body. It can play a role in intervertebral disc degeneration via multiple mechanisms, which include vascular insufficiency. In a rabbit model, Iwahashi et al. demonstrated the effects of nicotine on the intervertebral disc [13]. Nicotine treatment caused necrosis and hyalinization of the nucleus pulposus in all rabbits. The micro-analysis of the annulus fibrosus demonstrated a disturbance of the pattern of overlapping lamellae with and without clefts. There was also stenosis of vascular buds with perivascular calcification. Nicotine treatment created hypertrophy of vascular walls, necrotic endothelial cells, and stenotic vascular lumens. Lastly, it also caused a decrease of vascular buds in the vicinity of the vertebral end-plates. Akmal et al. also demonstrated using an in vitro model with nicotine and nicotine-free media (bovine specimens at concentrations simulating the typical serum nicotine concentrations of smokers) the adverse morphologic changes observed on histology [1]. These included reduced cell proliferation, disrupted cell architecture, and the disintegration of cells and extracellular matrix. Immunohistochemistry further revealed the presence of type I collagen in the extracellular matrix rather than the normal type II collagen seen in controls.

Another postulated mechanism with vascular etiology involves endothelial dysfunction. Due to the oxygen poor nature of the intervertebral discs' components, Papalia et al. believed there must be a degree of endothelial dysfunction worthy of further investigation [25]. There appears to be a failure to appropriately activate the vasodilatory nitrous oxide cascade, which eventually dilates vessels using cGMP in order to maintain the appropriate nutrient levels. Repetitive compressive traumatization of the microvasculature is postulated and may explain, in part, the chronic progressive nature of this condition.

Anatomic/Biomechanical

Anatomic variations may produce altered distribution of biomechanical forces. In his evaluation of degenerative intervertebral discs, Boden et al. showed the mean orientation of the lumbar facet angles relative to the coronal plane was more sagittal at all levels in the patients who had degenerative spondylolisthesis [3]. (*Figure 5*) The mean facet angle was 41 degrees in the asymptomatic volunteers versus 60 degrees in the patients who had degenerative spondylolisthesis. Also noted were that the facet joints were more sagittally oriented in the patients who had degenerative spondylolisthesis.

Intervertebral discs must maintain their structural integrity. Brock et al.'s comparison between 242 intradiscal pressure/volume recordings with corresponding discograms (performed at the same occasion) showed a statistically significant relationship between degeneration (radiographic) and compliance [7]. Without appropriate collagenous deposition and reinforcement, a degenerative process can be expected to ensue within the intervertebral disc, which disperses multiple axial and radial forces [11, 19].

Iatridis et al. demonstrated that an increased elastic modulus with degeneration is likely related to an increase in tissue density resulting from the loss of water content within the disc [12]. The significant effects of degeneration reported in this study also were suggestive of a shift in load carriage from fluid pressurization and swelling pressure to deformation of the solid matrix of the annulus fibrosus. Walter et al., in a large ex-vivo animal model, demonstrated asymmetric discal compression has direct deleterious effects on both tissue and cells, which could lead to a degenerative cascade, including apoptosis, the production of inflammatory mediators, and a catabolic shift [36].

Magnetic resonance elastography (MRE) is non-invasive form of imaging which is capable of measuring of the shear modulus of soft tissues including intervertebral discs [38]. This was not able to be performed until twenty years ago. With future advancements in this modality, changes in the shear modulus may provide a reliable way to predict the degenerative process of intervertebral discs.

Nutritional/Metabolic

Poor delivery of nutrients to the disc space can also account for disc degeneration leading to inadequate production of collagen fibers and proteoglycans. Many conditions, including Cystic Fibrosis and marasmus, alter the body's metabolism and thus the delivery of nutrients, such as Vitamin C deficiency (scurvy), to the disc [30]. More in depth studies are required regarding this topic but the inability to appropriately strengthen the annulus fibrosis with further collagen deposition or add elasticity to the nucleus with more proteoglycans and hydration is implicated in the degeneration of intervertebral discs [15].

Infectious

Infections of the disc space as seen in osteomyelitis/discitis lead to a rapidly accelerated degeneration of the intervertebral disc in the setting of a significant inflammatory response. (Figure 6) Once appropriately treated with antimicrobials or surgery (or both), a robust fusion can ensue due to the stimulation of the subchondral endplates by the relative surge in cytokines. Patients who undergo simultaneous instrumentation and decompression were shown by Bydon et al. to not only have a similar reoperation rate (compared to non-instrumented patients) but also have a significantly decreased pseudoarthrosis rate (only 2.4%) [4]. Increased neovascularity in degenerative discs/endplates may represent a robust blood supply that alters the risk profile for an infectious discitis [31]. Discitis is typically spread via hematogenous routes although direct seeding (post-procedural versus local infections) may also be implicated. The rapid reabsorption of the extracellular matrix by pathogens in combination with a severe inflammatory cascade is responsible for the time course of the disease's progression. Discitis may represent the most exaggerated form of degenerative disc disease, which will require further investigation to elucidate.

Genetic

There are significant genetic implications with regards to intervertebral disc degeneration that require further investigation. Programmed cell death and expression of inflammatory cytokines can be altered [20]. It appears that environmental factors influence the variation in disc signal, as monozygotic and dizygotic twins will have separate manifestations of disc degeneration. [2, 27] Ozkanli et al. showed MMP-1 and MMP-3 expressions were significantly higher in patients with recurrent lumbar disc herniations and also had higher magnetic resonance degeneration score (Pfirmann score) [24]. Interestingly, this may be independent of age as Canbay et al. showed that the relationship between Pfirrmann grade, immunohistochemical expression of MMP-3, and the histopathologic signs of intervertebral disc degeneration were not correlated with age [8]. Weber et al. also reminded us that terminal deoxynucleotidyl transferase-mediated dUTP nick-end labeling) which detects breaks in double-stranded DNA that arise through apoptotic endonuclease activity was noted to be higher in patients with degenerative discs versus those without [37]. Also noted was that in comparison to fetal discs (less than 2%), the number of dead cells was significantly increased in the discs of the skeletally mature (50%).

Although many micro RNAs are expressed in degenerative human intervertebral discs, their true impacts are still yet to be elucidated. Thus far, we have been able to ascertain that their expression helps to regulate the intradiscal inflammatory response, extracellular matrix regeneration, and nucleus pulposus cellular apoptosis [14, 34]. Further advancements multi-dimensional genomic analyses applied towards IVD disc disease, particularly involving micro RNAs, are required. There remains potential for a vast array of gene therapies once more is understood regarding the expression of proteins and their potential deleterious effects on disc cells and extracellular matrix.

Iatrogenic

Common iatrogenic causes for disc degeneration are post procedural after injections, discectomies, and fusion procedures. Kim et al. demonstrated that facet joint orientation (relative to the coronal plane) and tropism at the adjacent segment above fusion produces overstress of the adjacent segment in the form of increased anterior shear force [16]. Discectomies and intradiscal injections may also be implicated in an accelerated degenerative process although the etiology surrounding these processes remain poorly understood.

Autoimmune/Inflammatory

Intervertebral disc degeneration is a chronic inflammatory process, which may respond to anti-inflammatory modalities early in its course. Attempts have been made to use systemic and intradiscal anti-inflammatory medications/therapies without success as of yet. Klatwitter et al. measured expression levels of Toll-like receptors (TLR)-1, 2, 4, and 6 and they were found to be elevated with increasing degeneration severity [17]. Walter et al. demonstrated that inflammatory cytokines in NP cells (in vitro model) were shown to produce IL-1β, IL-6, and IL-8 in response to TNF-α at variable rates and magnitudes, which suggests different functions at different times in the disease process overall [37]. Capossela et al. also confirmed that degenerated and post-traumatic discs do in fact contain IgG antibodies against typical extracellular proteins of the nucleus pulposus using immunohistochemical staining on postoperative specimens[9].

Drugs/Toxins

Many substances will affect the systemic microvasculature and thus its ability to deliver nutrients to the disc/subchondral endplate complex. We are yet to characterize the broadly labeled group of exogenous toxins, which may accelerate intervertebral disc degeneration with the exception of nicotine. As the study of the degenerative process continues, other substances will be implicated as we evaluate their deleterious effects on the microphysiology of the disc-endplate complex in each spinal segment.

CONCLUSION

The pathophysiology of intervertebral disc degeneration is a complex multifactorial process that still requires further investigation for a clearer understanding. There are genetic, anatomic, physiologic, and biomechanical factors, which affect its onset, rate of progression, penetrance, and responsiveness to treatment. Continuation of research efforts in field will maximize our therapeutic yield in the future.

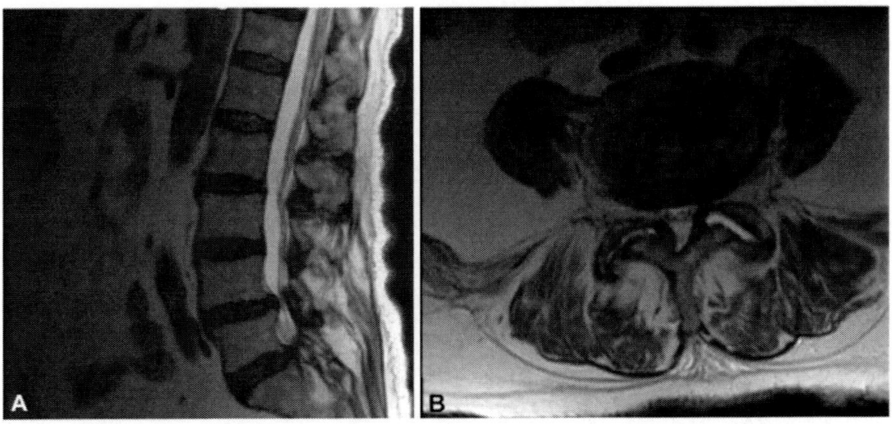

Figure 5. Sagittal (A) and Axial (B) T2 MRI showing degenerative changes in the lumbar spine, worse at the level of L4-L5 with bulging disc and ligamentous hypertrophy. Left-sided synovial cyst and prominence of the dorsal epidural fat contribute to moderate to severe spinal canal narrowing.

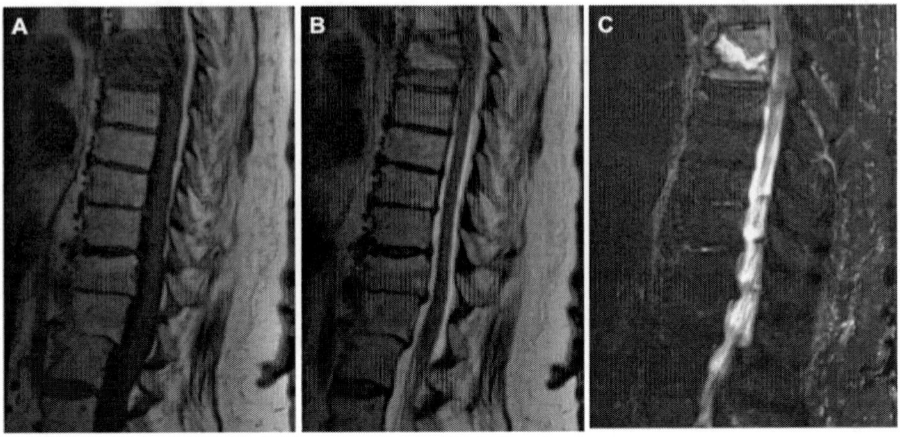

Figure 6. Sagittal T1 (A), T2 (B) and T2 STIR (C) MRI showing discitis/osteomyelitis at the T5-T6 level with associated intravertebral abscess involving the T5 and to a lesser extent T6 vertebral bodies, anterior paraspinal soft tissue phlegmon and right anterior paraspinal abscess.

REFERENCES

[1] Akmal M., Kesani A., Anand B., Singh A., Wiseman M., Goodship A. 2004. "Effect of nicotine on spinal disc cells: a cellular mechanism for disc degeneration." *Spine (Phila Pa 1976)*, 29: 568–575.

[2] Battie M. C., Videman T., Gill K., et al., 1991. "Volvo Award in clinical sciences. Smoking and lumbar intervertebral disc degeneration: an MRI study of identical twins." *Spine (Phila Pa 1976)*, pp. 1015–1021.

[3] Boden S. D., Riew K. D., Yamaguchi K., Branch T. P., Schelliinger D., Wiesel S. W., 1996. "Operation of the lumbar facet joints: association with degenerative disc disease." *Journal of Bone and Joint Surgery. American Volume.* Mar: 78(3):403-11.

[4] Bydon M., De la Garza-Ramos R., Macki M., Naumann M., Sciubba D. M., Wolinsky J. P., Bydon A., Gokaslan Z. L., Witham T. F., 2014. "Spinal instrumentation in patients with primary spinal infections does not lead to greater recurrent infection rates: an analysis of 118 cases." *World Neurosurgery*. 2014 Dec; 82(6): e807-14.

[5] Handbook of Neurosurgery. Greenberg M. S. 2010. 18: 430-431.

[6] Handbook of Spine Surgery. Baaj A. A., Mummaneni P. V., Uribe J. S., Vaccaro A. R., Greenberg M. S. Thieme 2012.

[7] Brock M., Lutze M., 1989. "Lumbar disk compliance and degeneration." *Surgical Neurology*. Jul.; 32(1): 11-5.

[8] Canbay S., Turhan N., Bozkurt M., Arda K., Caglar S., 2013. "Correlation of matrix metalloproteinase-3 expression with patient age, magnetic resonance imaging and histopathological grade in lumbar disc degeneration." *Turkish Neurosurgery*. 2013; 23(4): 427-33.

[9] Capossela S., Schläfli P., Bertolo A., Janner T, Stadler BM, Pötzel T, Baur M, Stoyanov J. V., 2014. Degenerated human intervertebral discs contain autoantibodies against extracellular matrix proteins. *Eur. Cell Mater*. 2014 Apr. 4;27: 251-63.

[10] Colombier P., Clouet J., Hamel O., Lescaudron L., Guicheux J., 2014. "The lumbar intervertebral disc: from embryonic development to degeneration." *Joint Bone Spine*. Mar; 81(2): 125-9.

[11] Henry N., Colombier P., Lescaudron L., Hamel O., Le Bideau J., Guicheux J., Clouet J., 2014. "Regenerative medicine of the intervertebral disc: from pathophysiology to clinical application. "*Medical Science (Paris)*. Dec; 30(12): 1091-100.

[12] Iatridis J. C., Setton L. A., Foster R. J., Rawlins B. A., Weidenbaum M., Mow V. C., 1998. "Degeneration affects the anisotropic and nonlinear behaviors of human annulus fibrosus in compression." *Journal of Biomechanics*. Jun; 31(6): 535-44.

[13] Iwahashi M., Matsuzaki H., Tokuhashi Y., Wakabayashi K., Uematsu Y. 2002. Mechanism of intervertebral disc degeneration caused by nicotine in rabbits to explicate intervertebral disc disorders caused by smoking. Spine (Phila Pa 1976), 27: 1396–1401.

[14] Johnson W. E., Roberts S. 2007."Rumours of my death have been greatly exaggerated": a brief review of cell death in human intervertebral disc disease and implications for cell transplantation therapy." *Biochemical Society Transactions*. Aug: 35(Pt 4): 680-2.

[15] Kambin P., Nixon J.E., Chait A., Schaffer J.L. 1988. "Annular protrusion: pathophysiology and roentgenographic appearance. Spine (Phila Pa 1976) Jun;13(6): 671-5.

[16] Kim H. J., Kang K. T., Son J., Lee C. K., Chang B. S., Yeom J. S. 2015. "The influence of facet joint orientation and tropism on the stress at the adjacent segment after lumbar fusion surgery: a biomechanical analysis." *Spine Journal*. Aug 1; 15(8): 1841-7.

[17] Klawitter M., Hakozaki M., Kobayashi H., Krupkova O., Quero L., Ospelt C., Gay S., Hausmann O., Liebscher T., Meier U., Sekiguchi M., Konno S., Boos N., Ferguson S. J., Wuertz K. 2014. Expression and

regulation of toll-like receptors (TLRs) in human intervertebral disc cells. *European Spine Journal*.Sep; 23(9): 1878-91.
[18] Kramer, J. 1995. "Natural course and prognosis of intervertebral disc diseases. International Society for the Study of the Lumbar Spine Seattle, Washington, June 1994." Spine (Phila Pa 1976). Mar 15:20(6):635-9.
[19] Maidhof R., Alipui D. O., Rafiuddin A., Levine M., Grande D. A., Chahine N. O. 2012. "Emerging trends in biological therapy for intervertebral disc degeneration." 2012. Discovery Medicine. Dec; 14(79): 401-11.
[20] Mayer J. E., Iatridis J. C., Chan D., Qureshi S. A., Gottesman O., Hecht A. C. 2013. "Genetic polymorphisms associated with intervertebral disc degeneration." *Spine Journal*. Mar; 13(3): 299-317.
[21] Modic M. T., Steinberg P. M., Ross J. S., Masaryk T. J., Carter, J. R. 1988. "Degenerative disk disease: assessment of changes in vertebral body marrow with MR imaging." *Radiology*. 1988 Jan; 166(1 Pt 1): 193-9.
[22] Oegema Jr.T. R. 1993. "Biochemistry of the intervertebral disc." *Clinical Sports Medicine*. 12:419–439.
[23] Ou-Yang L., Lu G. M. 2015. "Dysfunctional microcirculation of the lumbar vertebral marrow prior to the bone loss and intervertebral discal degeneration." May 15; 40(10): E593-600.
[24] Ozkanli S., Kaner T., Efendioglu M., Basaran R., Senol M., Zemheri E., Gezen A. F. 2015. "The relation of matrix metalloproteinase 1, 2, 3 expressions with clinical and radiological findings in primary and recurrent lumbar disc herniations." *Turkish Neurosurgery*. 25(1): 111-6.
[25] Papalia R., Albo E., Vadalà G., D'Adamio S., Lanotte A., Di Martino A., Denaro V. 2015. "Is there a role for endothelial dysfunction in the pathogenesis of lumbar disc degeneration? A hypothesis that needs to be tested." *Medical Hypotheses*.Mar; 84(3): 249-51.
[26] Rothman RH. Clinical Neurosurgery. Chapter 12: *The pathophysiology of disc degeneration*. 1973; 20: 174-82.
[27] Sambrook PN, MacGregor AJ, Spector TD. 1999. "Genetic influences on cervical and lumbar disc degeneration: a magnetic resonance imaging study in twins." Arthritis and Rheumatology. Feb: 42(2):366-72.
[28] Scuderi GJ, Brusovanik GV, Golish SR, Demeo R, Hyde J, Hallab N, Vaccaro AR. 2008."A critical evaluation of discography in patients with lumbar intervertebral disc disease."*Spine Journal*. Jul-Aug; 8(4): 624-9.

[29] Simon J., McAuliffe M., Shamim F., Vuong N., Tahaei A. 2014. "Discogenic low back pain." *Physical Medicine and Rehabilitation Clinics of North America*. May; 25(2): 305-17.

[30] Smith, V. H. 2010. "Vitamin C deficiency is an under-diagnosed contributor to degenerative disc disease in the elderly." *Medical Hypotheses*. 2010 Apr; 74(4): 695-7.

[31] Tanaka M., Shimizu H., Yato Y., Asasuma T., Nemoto K. 2010."Acute pyogenic discitis in a degenerative intervertebral disc in an adult." *Internal Medicine Case Reports Journal*. 2010 Aug 4;3: 77-80.

[32] Trumees, E. 2015. "A history of lumbar disc herniation from Hippocrates to the 1990s." *Clinical Orthopedics and Related Research*. Jun: 473(6): 1885-95.

[33] Tsutsumi S., Yasumoto Y., Ito M. 2011. "Idiopathic intervertebral disk calcification in childhood: report and review of the literature." *Child's Nervous System*. Jul: 27(7): 1045-51.

[34] Wang C., Wang W. J., Yan Y.G., Xiang Y.X., Zhang J., Tang Z. H., Jiang Z. S. 2015. "MicroRNAs: New players in intervertebral disc degeneration." *Clinica Chimica Acta*. Oct 23; 450: 333-41.

[35] Wang Y. X., Griffith J. F. 2011. "Menopause causes vertebral endplate degeneration and decrease in nutrient diffusion to the intervertebral discs." *Medical Hypotheses*. Jul: 77(1): 18-20.

[36] Walter BA, Korecki CL, Purmessur D, Roughley P. J., Michalek A. J., Iatridis J. C. 2011. "Complex loading affects intervertebral disc mechanics and biology." *Osteoarthritis Cartilage*." Aug; 19(8): 1011-8.

[37] Walter B. A., Purmessur D., Likhitpanichkul M., Weinberg A., Cho S.K., Qureshi S. A., Hecht A. C., Iatridis J. C. 2015. "Inflammatory Kinetics and Efficacy of Anti-inflammatory Treatments on Human Nucleus Pulposus Cells." *Spine* (Phila Pa 1976). 2015 Jul. 1; 40(13): 955-63.

[38] Weber K. T., Jacobsen T. D., Maidhof R., Virojanapa J., Overby C., Bloom O., Quraishi S., Levine M., Chahine NO. 2015. "Developments in intervertebral disc disease research: pathophysiology, mechanobiology, and therapeutics." Current Reviews in Musculoskeletal Medicine. Mar; 8(1): 18-31.

[39] Yasuma T., Koh S., Okamura T., Yamauchi Y. 1990. "Histological changes in aging lumbar intervertebral discs. Their role in protrusions and prolapses.*" Journal of Bone and Joint Surgery*. American Volume. Feb; 72(2): 220-9.

In: Intervertebral Disc Degeneration
Editors: A. L. Ho and A. M. Desai
ISBN: 978-1-63485-829-8

Chapter 2

NERVE STRUCTURES INSIDE THE INTERVERTEBRAL DISC: A POSSIBLE LINK TO SYMPTOMATIC LUMBAR DISC DISEASE

***Manuel D. Oprea*[1], *Anca Maria Cimpean*[2,*], *Marius Raica*[2] *and Dan V. Poenaru*[1]**

[1]Second Department of Orthopedics, "Victor Babes" University of Medicine and Pharmacy, Timisoara, Romania

[2]Department of Microscopic Morphology/Histology, Angiogenesis Research Center, "Victor Babes" University of Medicine and Pharmacy, Timisoara, Romania

ABSTRACT

Lumbar degenerative disc disease is a very common condition with a high socio-economic burden. The etiology is multifactorial and not entirely understood, and some of the main factors implicated include: genetic predisposition, smoking, increased body mass index, weight lifting or impeded nutrient transportation through the endplates.

The presence of some pro-inflammatory cytokines and growth factors are well documented: the interleukin (IL) family, TNFα and PGE2. Alongside these, recently there has been an increased interest in nerve growth factor (NGF) and brain derived growth factor (BDGF).

* Corresponding Author Email: ancacimpean1972@yahoo.com

Their expression in a fibrous cartilaginous enviroment, where normally there are no nerve fibers or blood vessels, is of interest.

Neuronal proliferation is normally blocked out in the outer layers of the annulus fibrosus by the presence of Sema3A and aggrecan, with the latter also disrupting the endothelial proliferation. Degenerative changes may create propitious conditions for the invasion of the disc by endothelial and nerve structures.

Although it was assumed that differentiated cells lose the ability to undifferentiate, recent research supports the hypothesis that these cells can suffer a dedifferentiation process. In this respect, neural cells were obtained through transdifferentiation from keratocites and chondrocytes after stimulating these cells with nerve growth factors. Therefore, during the degenerative process, it is possible that the chondrocyte type cells reach a state of dedifferentiation and, due to the stimulation with nerve growth factors, can have characteristics similar to the nervous cells. Hence chondrocyte-like cells have the potential to transdifferentiate making them a possible source of nerve cells inside the intervertebral disc, and of pain.

This chapter deals with the identification of positive NFAP chondrones in degenerated intervertebral discs, suggesting a transdifferentiation of chondrocyte-like cells into nerve cells. It also reports the presence of NFAP-positive chondrones and pain score in patients with mild LDD (Lumbar Disc Disease).

The number and imunohistological characteristics of chondrocyte-like cells and their aggegated form, the chondrones, are correlated with the symptoms of patients with LDD. The identification of NFAP positive cells indicates the presence of nervous structures and the possibility of chondrocyte-like cells transdifferentiating into nerve cells. This finding might explain the different occurrences and characteristics of pain amongst patients with LDD.

Keywords: degenerative disc disease, neuronal and endothelial proliferation, cluster type chondrones

INTRODUCTION

The etiology of lumbar degenerative disc disease (LDDD) is multifactorial and poorly understood. The main etiologic factors identified are genetic predisposition, smoking, increased body mass index, heavy weight lifting or an alteration of nutrient transportation pathways through the endplates [1-4]. The exact mechanisms through which these factors induce the degenerative process have not yet been elucidated, but research reveals that they globally lead to a loss of the cell population in the intervertebral disc, to an increased activity of pro-inflammatory cytokines, proteoglycans and collagen degradation, to the disc dehydration and to the cellular phenotype alteration. As the degenerative process continues, these changes lead to intervertebral disc (IVD) height loss resulting in an alteration of normal biomechanics, in structural instability, and may finally cause a disc herniation with root compression or spinal stenosis [5].

A high percentage of patients with degenerated IVD remains asymptomatic, and can be attributed to the normal aging process. As such, in addition to structural changes of normal aging, in degenerative disc disease (DDD) there is a secondary process following either a traumatic event, or a disc herniation that causes acceleration and accentuation of the degenerative processes. The IVD tissue recruits immune cells and triggers pro-inflammatory processes that result in the emergence of different intensities of pain [3, 5]. Thus, intervertebral disc degeneration is thought to be mediated by an abnormal production of pro-inflammatory cytokines secreted by the nucleus pulposus and the annulus fibrosus, but also by macrophages, T cells or neutrophils. In the IVD cells these cytokines can initiate autophagy, cell senescence or apoptosis. The secreted pro-inflammatory mediators are TNF-α, IL-1α, IL-1β, IL-2, IL-4, IL-6, IL-8, IL-10, IL-17, IFN-γ, and PGE 2. Apart from all these cytokines, the most frequently studied ones are IL-1 and TNF-α, which were proven to increase and regulate the activity of genes encoding the degradative enzymes within the extracellular matrix.

In the early stages, the degenerative process involves the intervertebral disc, but afterwards the inflammatory changes also extends to the surrounding tissues. The gelatinous discal material may herniate via cracks and fissures forming inside the nucleus pulposus and annulus fibrosus, and causing the activation and infiltration of the immune cells. Therefore, in addition to blood vessels that may proliferate, different cells like macrophages, neutrophils and T cells can also migrate into the IVD. Following these changes, nociceptive nerve fibers emerge from the dorsal root ganglia [6]. Later studies on chondrocyte type cells from the degenerated nucleus pulposus found the presence of the NGF (nerve growth factor), the neuronal proliferation factors and the BDNF (brain-derived growth factor). These neurotrophins induce the expression of pain associated cation channels within the dorsal root ganglion [5, 7].

Neuronal proliferation inside the intervertebral disc is blocked on the external surface of the annulus fibrosus by the presence of semaphorin, family member of the Class 3 semaphorins (Sema3A). In the nucleus pulposus, aggrecan is also a natural barrier against endothelial and neuronal proliferation [7, 8]. Studies on animal models reported that a gap in the annulus fibrosus triggers an inflammatory process mediated by cytokines, followed by endothelial and neuronal proliferation and also leading to an increase in sensitive nerve-endings within the intervertebral disc [9].

A direct link between the nerve fibers and blood vessels invading the intervertebral disc was reported, meaning that the NGF secreted by endothelial cells is necessary for neuronal survival and growth [6]. The nerve fibers that encroach on the intervertebral disc are considered nociceptive, deriving from the dorsal root ganglion, and they express acetylcholinesterase, substance P, BDNF and neurofilament associated protein (NFAP) [10-12]. IL-1β activity is also increased in the degenerated disc, stimulating NDF and BDNF expression by the nucleus pulposus cells, while TNF-α stimulates the expression of substance P. These players interact to form a link between pro-inflammatory cytokines, neurotrophins and the occurrence of pain.

Chondrocyte-like cells from the nucleus pulposus are derived from the notochord's cells originating from the mesoderm. Formed during embryogenesis, mesodermal cells are multipotent migrating cells, that can differentiate into chondrocytes, melanocytes, endocrine cells, glial cells, neurons and many other mesenchymal-derived cells. Until recently, it was assumed that mesodermal cells, once differentiated into functional cells, lose the ability to become undifferentiated. However recent research demonstrates that dedifferentiation can still occur [13, 14]. This process where differentiated and functional cells can turn into a different type of cells is called transdifferentiation. Transdifferentiation is the result of a certain modification in the expression of regulating genes, responsible for the identification of future developing tissues. Reports of nerve cells being obtained via transdifferentiation from keratocytes and chondrocytes after stimulation with nerve growth factors such as Neurobasal-A, EGF (epidermal growth factor), IGF-1 (insulin growth factor 1) and FGF-2 (fibroblast growth factor 2) are present in the literature [15, 16]. Therefore, during the degenerative process, chondrocyte-like cells may reach a state of dedifferentiation and may acquire characteristics similar to those of neural cells following their stimulation with nerve growth factors. This possible evolution may explain the occurrence of pain in degenerative disc disease, and its different characteristics among patients.

Previous research carried out by the authors of this chapter aimed at investigating the morphology of chondrocyte-like cells within the degenerated intervertebral disc [17]. It shown that chondrocyte-like cells aggregate into bulk structures – cluster chondrones, that form from multiple cells during the degenerative proccesses. The size of these chondrone clusters were correlated with the degenerative changes and were quantified by clinical and radiographic means. It was also noted that endothelial structures were identified. However, endothelial structures alone could not explain the presence and characteristics of pain in these patients; therefore, another hypothesis had to be considered. One of the currently accepted hypothesis regarding the onset of pain in DDD describes the presence of the nervous structures within the degenerated cartilage tissue. This hypothesis was corroborated by our data, since the possibility of neuronal growth occurs at places where endothelial structures might grow. Currently, there are no data to support the existence of other cellular structures within the intervertebral disc that can cause acute pain. This chapter aims to characterize the potential for chondrocytes to express the neurofilament associated protein during disc degeneration, and to identify possible correlations between expression of these factors and the clinical and imaging parameters of disc degeneration. In order to identify the neurofilaments, immunohistochemical marker NFAP was utilized given its high specificity for Class IV intermediate filaments from the neuronal cells cytoskeleton [16, 18].

METHODS

The current research was undertaken in accordance with the local ethics committee, and was approved by the Ethical Board of Timis County Emergency and Clinical Hospital. Written informed consent for the experimental use of surgical samples was obtained from each patient.

The study included 47 patients treated in the IInd Clinic of Orthopedic and Traumatology at the Clinical and Emergency County Hospital Timisoara, from October 2012 to January 2015. All patients were diagnosed with lumbar disc herniation and surgically treated according to standard of care. All patients had recieved conservatory for 6 weeks before consideration for surgery.

The including criteria were:

- Lumbar disc herniation with neurological deficit, where the symptoms did not improve after a minimum 6 weeks of conservatory treatment;
- Signs of lumbar degenerative disc disease on MRI Scan;
- Age between 18 and 65;

- Written consent from patients for participating to the clinical trial and for using the data anonymously only for scientific purposes;

The excluding criteria were:

- Other lumbar spine diseases: fractures, congenital or acquired deformities, infectious or inflammatory disease (spondylodiscitis, spondylitis), segmental instabilities (spondylolisthesis, spondylosis);
- Severe cardiovascular disease: heart failure or angina at rest, myocardial infarction or heart surgery 3 months before the inclusion, uncontrolled high blood pressure, severe peripheric circulatory insufficiency with vascular claudication;
- Severe respiratory disease: uncontrolled asthma, advanced chronic obstructive pulmonary disease
- Endocrine or metabolic disease: poorly controlled diabetes with neuropathy and/or advanced angiopathy, decompensated endocrine diseases;
- Hematological diseases: coagulation disorder with high risk of bleeding;
- Tumors no matter what the evolution or the origin;
- Infectious or febrile diseases: tuberculosis, active hepatitis (HbV, HCV), HIV/AIDS
- Severe psychiatric disease, uncooperative patients, drug and alcohol abuse;
- Pregnancy or breastfeeding;

Patients were evaluated based on the criteria of the Japanese Society of Orthopaedics and Traumatology for evaluating low back pain (JOABPS score) and using the visual analogical scale (VAS) for assessing lumbar pain and sciatalgia. The possible scores of JOABPS vary between a minimum of -6 to a maximum of 29 points.

Following their clinical evaluation, the patients underwent MRI scans, and were afterwards taken to the operating room for a minimally invasive discectomy (endoscopic or microscopic) by the same team of surgeons. Intervertebral discs fragments obtained after surgical decompression of the nervous elements were assessed histologically and morphologically.

MRI Assessment

MRI scans of the lumbar spine were performed using a 1.5 T scanner (Siemens Magnetom Essenza, Siemens AG, Germany) and a spine-dedicated antenna. The imaging protocol included sagittal and axial T1-weighted and T2-weighted sequences. The images were evaluated and the degenerative changes were classified according to Pfirrmann and Modic scales.

Herniated Disc Tissue Fragments

Intervertebral disc specimens were obtained following surgery of the L4-L5 level or L5-S1. Immediately after surgical intervention, the specimens were processed in a sterile manner by being washed in saline solution and fixed in 10% buffered formalin solution.

Immunohistochemistry

The antigen demasking and the methylene bridges destruction were achieved via applying the Novocastra Bond Epitope Retrieval Solution 1 pH6 for 20 minutes (Leica Biosystems, Newcastle uponTyne, UK), followed by blocking of the endogenic peroxidase with 3% hydrogen peroxide for 5 minutes. Incubation with the primary antibody, NF (mouse monoclonal, clone N52.1.7, Leica Biosystems, uponTyne Newcastle, UK) 30 minutes prior to visualization by the Bond Polymer Refine Detection System (Leica Biosystems, uponTyne Newcastle, UK). 3.3 diaminobenzidine, applied for 10 minutes, was used as chromogen and counterstaining was carried out using hematoxylin, applied for 5 minutes. All steps of the immunohistochemical technique were accomplished with the immunohistochemistry automat Leica Biosystems Leica Bond III. At the end of the program, the sections were placed in absolute ethanol for 5 minutes, and then dried and clarified in benzene for 5 minutes. Mounting was performed using an Entellan type permanent mounting medium, Leica CV Mount (Leica Biosystems, UponTyne Newcastle, UK). The sections prepared were fixed and histologically evaluated with a light microscope at magnifications of 100x, 200x, 400x and 1000x (Axio Imager 2, Carl Zeiss AG, Jena, Germany).

Morphometry

The systematic assessment of sections was performed with the light microscope in order to obtain a well-defined surface. Six visual fields were assessed for each section, using the lens with 400x magnification. Chondrones (defined as a group of cells with distinct territorial chondrocytic matrix) were identified and manually counted. The surface area of chondrones was measured (expressed in µm2) using ZEN software (Zeiss Efficient Navigation, Carl Zeiss AG, Jena, Germany).

Statistical Analysis

The data were subjected to standard statistical analysis using SPSS 21.0 software (IBM Corporation, Armonk, NY, USA), with both parametric and non-parametric correlations being carried out. The noted coefficients were r, Kendall tau-b (τ) and Spearman rho (ρ). P values of ≤ 0.05 were considered statistically significant, and ≤ 0.001 very statistically significant.

Results

A total of 47 patients with an average age of 40.54 years (ranging between 21 and 62 years), gender distribution: 21 women (44.68%) and 26 men (55.32%) were evaluated.

With respect to duration of symptoms, 21 patients had a symptoms duration of one year (44.68%) and 26 had a symptoms duration longer of over one year (55.32%). The JOABPS average clinical score was 7.32 (ranging between 1 and 14), with 48.7% of patients having a score less than 7.

The VAS mean for back pain was 7.35 (ranging between 2 and 10), and the average VAS for sciatica was 8.03 (range of 5 to 10).

The degree of degenerative disc disease was graded according to the Modic classification: 15 patients showed no change (31.91%), 7 patients had type I changes (14.89%), 22 patients had type II changes (46.81%) and 3 patients had type III changes (6.39%).

In terms of the Pfirrmann disc degeneration classification, there were 4 cases of type 2 modifications (8.51%), 15 cases of type 3 (31.92%), 20 cases of type 4 (42.55%) and 8 cases of type 5 (17.02%).

Following the evaluation of the herniated disc tissue fragments, regions corresponding to the nucleus pulposus and containing ovoid chondrocyte-like cells surrounded by pericellular matrix, as well as elongated and fusiform fibroblast type cells originating from annulus fibrosus.

Some specimens also contained hyaline cartilage with chondrocyte cells arranged in lacunas. In the quasi-normal nucleus pulposus the chondrones were rare, scattered, and surrounded by rich extracellular matrix. The specimens that displayed a higher degree of degeneration contained either a greater number of chondrones, or multi-cellular cluster-type chondrones, with cells in different stages of evolution.

The extracellular matrix presented a series of discontinuities, with a disorganized appearance. The annulus fibrosus was identifiable due to the characteristic fibroblast-like cells deposited between fibrous bands with alternating orientation. At the interface between the annulus fibrosus and the nucleus pulposus, this specific arrangement of collagen fibers decreased and both fibroblast-like and chondrocyte-like scattered cells were identifiable.

The immunohistochemical analysis was focused on the regions of nucleus pulposus tissue identified using the previously described characteristics. All specimens contained the nucleus pulposus, but there were specimens without hyaline cartilage or annulus fibrosus. The immunohistochemical assessment of the fibrocartilaginous tissue sections revealed the NFAP-positivity of the chondrones, especially in the specimens with severe degenerative changes (Figure 1).

Bands and cords of NFAP-positive extracellular matrix bypassing the chondrones and their pericellular matrix were observed at the interface between the nucleus pulposus and the endplates or the annulus fibrosus (Figure 1). Some sections, especially at the periphery of the analyzed specimens, exhibited small nerve fibres (similar to nerve fibers) that could be pinpointed.

In general, the small chondrones that contained one or two cells, were NFAP-negative, while the larger chondrones were mainly NFAP-positive (Figure 2). There were also cases when the small chondrones were positive and rare cases of medium-large sized chondrones that were NFAP-negative.

A total of 235 fields of view corresponding to a total of 47 specimens were assesed (using x40 magnification). 1,367 chondrocytes were identified and measured. The statistical analysis of the performed measurements performed revealed a mean surface area of 555.89 μm^2 (values between 81.94 and 9923.85 μm^2), with a median of 327.10 μm^2 and a geometric median of 355.44 μm^2 (ranging 337.1 to 374.8 μm^2) (Figure 3).

The average ratio of chondrones/field of view (with the total surface area of a field of view at 40x magnification is 200,000 µm2) was 5.82 chondrones/visual field (with values between 4 to 10 chondrones/field of view). The analysis of the surface area histogram, clearly pointed out that 89.49% of the chondrones had areas smaller than 1100 μm^2 (Figure 4), indicating the presence of large cluster type chondrones as a special feature, and suggesting its association with the degenerated tissue.

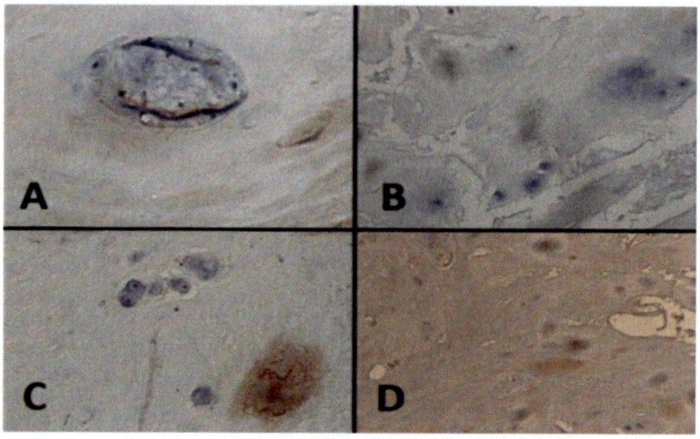

Figure 1. A. Area of fibrocartilaginous tissue with a high degree of degeneration, containing clusters of chondrones positive for NFAP (magnification x10); B. Imunohistological stain of a NFAP-positive cluster-type chondrone (magnification x100) C. Microscopic detail demonstrating a nerve structure at the periphery of a NFAP-positive cluster type chondrone (magnification x40) D. NFAP-positive extracellular matrix zones surrounding chondrones, starting from the endplate and penetrating nucleus pulposus (magnification x10).

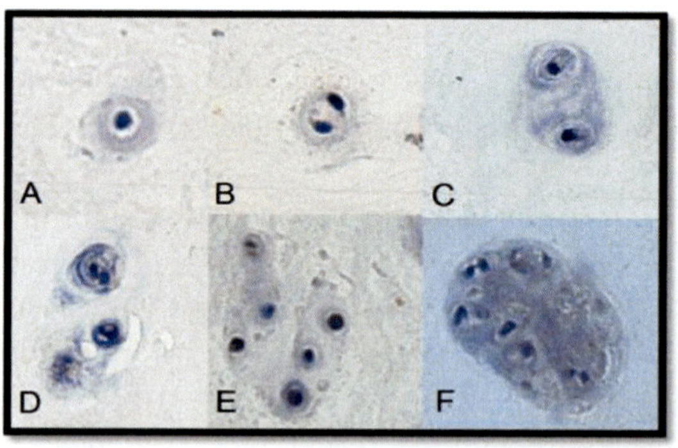

Figure 2. Chondrones in detail during different evolutionary stages. A. Monocellular chondrone B. Hypocellular chondrone that is NFAP-positive C. Chondrone composed of two cells D, E, F. Chondrones containing multiple NFAP-positive cells.

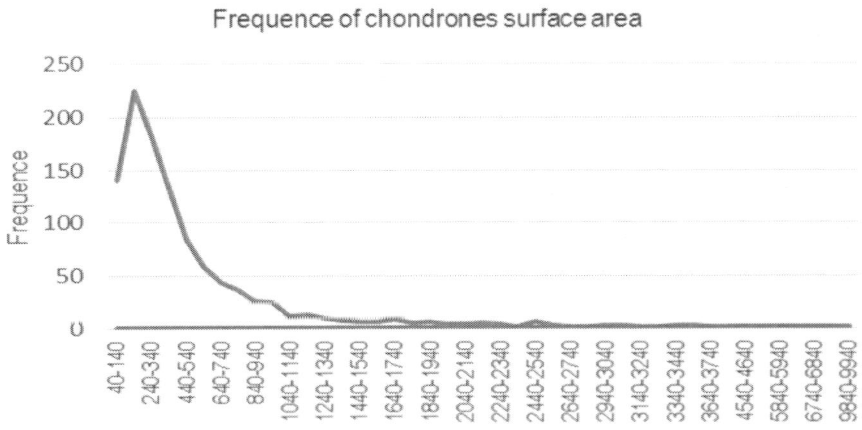

Figure 3. Chondrone areas size distribution.

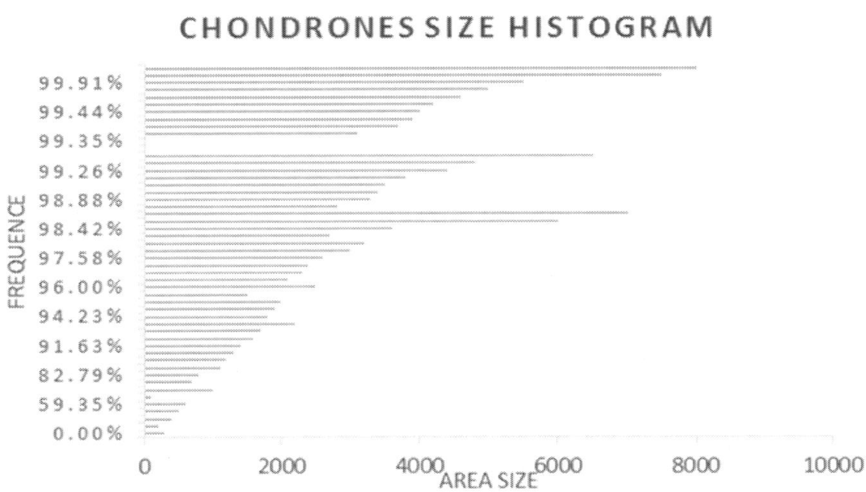

Figure 4. Chondrones size histogram.

Based on these observations, patients were divided into two groups, according to the chondrones area size, 327.10 μm^2 being considered the threshold value. As a result, the patients in group A presented a low degree of degeneration, with a median area lower than 327.10 μm^2. This group consisted of 22 patients representing 46.8% of total. The group B of patients, with a measured median area larger than 327.10 μm^2, consisted of 25 patients, representing 53.2% of the total number of patients. In group A, patients had

NFAP-positive chondrones in 13 cases (59.09%) and NFAP-negative chondrones in 9 cases (40.91%). In group B, there were 18 NFAP-positive cases (72%) and 7 negative cases (28%).

In group A, the average JOABPS score was 8.18 and mean VAS score for back pain was 6.89, while the mean VAS value for sciatica was 7.65. Pfirrmann degenerative changes were mostly type III in a percentage of 41.2%, and 52.9% of the patients had no Modic changes.

In group B, the average JOABS score was 6.6 and VAS for back pain was 7.75 while mean VAS for sciatica was 8.35. Pfirrmann degenerative changes were mostly type IV (in 56% of cases), and 72% of patients had type II Modic changes.

In group A there was a direct correlation between age and median area (r=0.507; p=0.038; tau=0.436; rho=0.506), age and symptom duration over a year (r=0.592; p=0.012; tau=0.475; rho=0.555), and a negative correlation between age and VAS for back pain (r=-0.603; p=0.010; tau=-0.418; rho=0.526). A correlation between the median area and the symptom duration was observed (r=0.571; p=0.017; tau=0.401; rho=0.477), as well as the median area and Pfirrmann degeneration changes (r=0.591; p=0.012; tau=0.364; rho=0.465). Duration of symptoms was correlated with the mean of NFAP-positive chondrones (r=0.560; p=0.019; tau=0.515; rho=0.591), NFAP-positive chondrones (r=0.545; p=0.024; tau=0.545; rho=0.545), Pfirrmann type degenerative changes (r=0.606; p=0.010; tau=0.560; rho=0.601) and VAS for low back pain (r=0.578; p=0.015; tau=0.614; rho=0.683). JOABPS clinical score was correlated with the mean NFAP-positive chondrones (r=-0.509; p=0.037; tau=-0.408; rho=-0.566) and NFAP-positive chondrones (r=-0.497; p=0.042; tau=-0.431; rho=-0.495). The NFAP-positive mean of the chondrones was correlated with the duration of symptoms, JOABPS score, the number of NFAP-positive chondrones (r= 0.830; p=0.000; tau=0.739; rho=0.848) and VAS for back pain (r=0.547; p=0.023; tau=0.453; rho=0.629). The number of NFAP-positive chondrones was correlated with the duration of symptoms, the JOABPS score, the mean of NFAP-positive chondrones and VAS for low back pain (r=0.547; p=0.015; tau=0.486; rho=0.541). Pfirrmann degenerative changes were correlated with the median of the surface area of chondrones, Modic type changes, duration of symptoms and VAS for low back pain (r=0.589; p=0.013; tau=0.466; rho=0.534).

In group B there was a correlation between age and the median surface area of chondrones (r=0.463; p=0.040; tau=0.349; rho=0.456), patients age and duration of symptoms (r=0.624; p=0.003; tau=0.580; rho=0.683), age and the number of NFAP-positive chondrones (r=0.559; p=0.010; tau=0.487;

rho=0.572), age and Pfirrmann type changes (r=0.537; p=0.015; tau=0.434; rho=0.540), and age and Modic type changes (r=0.601; p=0.005; tau=0.555; rho=0.642). The mean of surface area of NFAP-positive chondrones was correlated with VAS for low back pain (r=0.526; p=0.016; tau=0.566; rho=0.650). The number of NFAP-positive chondrones were correlated with the duration of symptoms and VAS for back pain (r=0.619; p=0.004; tau=0.486; rho=0.541). VAS for low back pain correlated with age, the median of the surface area of NFAP-positive chondrones, the number of NFAP-positive chondrones, and VAS for sciatica.

CONCLUSION

The normal intervertebral disc has a very high threshold for mechanical stimuli and does not contain sensitive nerve fibers, which makes it is relatively inert to nociceptive stimuli.

In the early stages of degeneration there was an observed proliferation of the blood vessels accompanied by nerve fibers, along the cracks and tears beginning from the annulus fibrosus, towards the interior of the intervertebral disc, which is normally an avascular, aneural and lymphatic-free organ [5, 19, 20]. This process might be the result of synergistic action of pro-inflammatory cytokines and neurotrophins, and of decreased suppression, due to decreased concentration of aggrecan and decreased expression of Sema3A semaphorin. In a healthy intervertebral disc, aggrecan and other matrix molecules serve as a natural barrier against endothelial and neuronal proliferation. In the degenerative process, cytokines mediate the activity of the ADAMTS 4 and 5 proteolytic enzymes resulting in an increase of the keratan sulphate/chondroitin sulphate ratio, decreasing the concentration of aggrecan and thus creating the optimal conditions for endothelial and neuronal proliferation. Another barrier against neuronal proliferation is the expression on the outer surface of the annulus fibrosus of Sema3A, a member of semaphorins class 3. It was observed that this expression is reduced in patients with advanced stages of disc degeneration, suggesting that it has an inhibitory role towards neural proliferation [21].

The normal innervation of the intervertebral disc is limited to the first 2-3 external layers of the annulus fibrosus. It consists of different types of nerve fibers, including nociceptive peptidergic NGF-dependent fibers, non-peptidergic GDNF-dependent fibers that are morphologically similar to Pacini mechanoreceptors, and Ruffini endings and Golgi complexes [22, 23]. They originate in the small neurons of the dorsal root ganglion, and express TrkA, TrkB and Ret receptors with a high affinity for NGF, BDNF and GDNF [10].

Lee et al. have reported increased levels of NGF in the degenerated discs, using the ELISA technique. Furthermore, Aoki et al. have reported high levels in the herniated discs, which implies that these neurotrophins may be playing an important role in the modulation of disc degeneration [24, 25]. Purmessur et al. reached the same conclusion after using an immunohistochemical method to identify increased levels of NGF. Although these authors detected the same phenomena, the cells responsible for NGF expression were not identified. It is speculated that the cells responsible for the secretion of these neurotrophins might be chondrocyte-like cells, endothelial cells or inflammatory cells [6, 26, 27]. Results detailed in this chapter confirm the presence of the neurofilaments inside chondrocyte-like cells that form cluster type large chondrones frequently identified in the specimens with high grade degenerative changes. Greene et al. managed to induce the transdifferentiation of chondrocytes into neural cells, although they could not assess their functionality [13]. It is possible that some of the chondrocyte-like cells inside the nucleus pulposus are transdifferentiating into neural cells (capable of expressing TrkA, TrkB and Ret receptors), thus explaining the appearance of pain during disc degeneration. Furthermore, inside the degenerated disc there was reported an increased expression of growth factors IGF, FGF, VEGF, NGF, BDNF that could create an ideal environment for chondrocyte-like cells to transdifferentiate into neural cells, as observed by Greene et al., but further research is required to confirm this hypothesis.

Kokubo et al. asssessed of 500 degenerated intervertebral discs and identified NGF-positive free nerve fibers, GAP-43 and substance P in the external layers of herniated disc fragments. However, they did not report any information about the immunopositivity of the chondrocyte-like cells [28]. The research carried out in this chapter, identified both nerve fibers within the extracellular matrix of herniated disc tissue as previously described by Kokubo et al., and NFAP-positive chondrocyte-like cells.

Utilizing a three-dimensional microscopic study of porcine chondrocytes harvested from the femoral condyle, Choi et al. [29] measured the volume of chondrones and found average values of 2,218 ± 832μm^3 (in the average cartilage region where chondrones have a predominantly spherical shape), which corresponds to an approximate area of 206 ± 106 μm^2. The assessed chondrones in this research had an average area of 555.89 μm^2 (values between 81.94 and 9923.81 μm^2). 71.14% of them had values less than 540 μm^2. However, these differences underscore the morphometric differences between normal chondrones and those found in the degenerated fibrocartilaginous tissue.

Another observation resulting from this research is that in the group with more advanced degeneration changes (defined by a mean surface area of chondrones higher than 327.10 μm^2), the intervertebral discs also presented radiographic changes of degenerative disease quantified with Pfirrmann and Modic classifications. At the same time, these patients also recorded clinical pain assessment scores higher than the patients with more mild degenerative changes. NFAP-positive chondrones were frequently found among the larger chondrones.

The correlations between age and the median values of the chondrones surface area, duration of symptoms under one year, and VAS for low back pain suggests the involvement of the senile degenerative changes. Notably, the patients included for this research had herniated discs resulting not from normal disc aging. In group A patients, this may simply reflect the natural history of disc changes over time. This hypothesis is supported by the correlation between age and the NFAP-positive or -negative nature of the chondrones, in that the number of chondrones increases with age. Moreover, the evolving nature of this condition is also supported by the correlation between the median of the chondrones surface area and the symptoms onset, with lower values of chondrone areas being found in patients whose symptoms have occurred for less than one year. The duration of symptoms was correlated with the VAS for low back pain in group A, a correlation not seen in patients with more advanced degenerative changes. Considering that the chondrones dimensions correlate with the symptoms duration, we can hypothesize that once the degenerative process has started, there is an initial phase where the intensity of the symptoms increases in parallel with the size chondrones size, after which the intensity of the symptoms reaches a plateau, then stagnates or regresses, while the chondrones continue to grow in size. Degenerative changes quantified using Modic and Pfirrmann systems were corroborated, and correlated with histological changes; however, they were not an objective of this research [30-34]. However, there was a correlation between the Pfirrmann type changes and both the median of the chondrones surface area and the symptoms duration. These observations emphasize the important role played by the morphometry of chondrones in the pathophysiology of disc degeneration and its clinical expression.

This chapter confirmed the presence inside the degenerated intervertebral disc of nerve structures which are not normally present. Moreover, the results have clinical significance, indicating that the presence of NFAP positive chondrones is correlated with pain scores and with duration of symptoms greater than one year. However, further research is needed to investigate the functionality of these chondrocytes with neural expression and their possible involvement in the generation of pain.

- Degenerated intervertebral discs contain chondrones positive for NFAP, suggesting the possible transdifferentiation of the chondrocyte-like cells into neural cells.
- Within the extracellular matrix of the degenerated fibrocartilaginous tissue, nerve fibers or free nerve endings were identified.
- Patients presenting with larger chondrones had more severe symptoms.
- NFAP-positive chondrones correlate with the clinical and imaging scores in patients with herniated discs with symptoms duration greater than one year.
- NFAP-positive chondrones are correlated with clinical VAS score for low back pain, suggesting that the former are involved in the development and the modulation of pain in patients with degenerative disc changes.

References

[1] Videman, Tapio, Laura E. Gibbons, Jaakko Kaprio, and Michele C. Battié. "Challenging the Cumulative Injury Model: Positive Effects of Greater Body Mass on Disc Degeneration." *The Spine Journal* 10, no. 1 (2010): 26-31.

[2] Vo, Nam, Dong Wang, Gwendolyn Sowa, William Witt, Kevin Ngo, Paulo Coelho, Ronald Bedison, Barbara Byer, Rebecca Studer, Joon Lee, Y. Peter Di, and James Kang. "Differential Effects of Nicotine and Tobacco Smoke Condensate on Human Annulus Fibrosus Cell Metabolism." *Journal of Orthopaedic Research J. Orthop. Res.* 29, no. 10 (2011): 1585-591.

[3] Wang, Yue, and Michele C. Battie. The Intervertebral Disc: Molecular and Structural Studies of the Disc in Health and Disease. Edited by Irving M. Shapiro and Makarand V. Risbud. Wien: *Springer-Verlag,* 2014.

[4] Battié, Michele C., Tapio Videman, Esko Levalahti, Kevin Gill, and Jaakko Kaprio. "Heritability of Low Back Pain and the Role of Disc Degeneration." *Pain* 131, no. 3 (2007): 272-80.

[5] Risbud, Makarand V., and Irving M. Shapiro. "Role of Cytokines in Intervertebral Disc Degeneration: Pain and Disc Content." *Nat Rev Rheumatol Nature Reviews Rheumatology* 10, no. 1 (2013): 44-56.

[6] Freemont, A. J., A. Watkins, C. Le Maitre, P. Baird, M. Jeziorska, M. T. N. Knight, E. R. S. Ross, J. P. O'brien, and J. A. Hoyland. "Nerve Growth Factor Expression and Innervation of the Painful Intervertebral Disc." *J. Pathol. The Journal of Pathology* 197, no. 3 (2002): 286-92.

[7] Ohtori, Seiji, Gen Inoue, Takana Koshi, Toshinori Ito, Hideo Doya, Tomoko Saito, Hideshige Moriya, and Kazuhisa Takahashi. "Up-Regulation of Acid-Sensing Ion Channel 3 in Dorsal Root Ganglion Neurons Following Application of Nucleus Pulposus on Nerve Root in Rats." *Spine* 31, no. 18 (2006): 2048-052.

[8] Battie, Michele C., Tapio Videman, Kevin Gill, Giovanni B. Moneta, Rickard Nyman, Jaakko Kaprio, and Markku Koskenvuo. "1991 Volvo Award in Clinical Sciences." *Spine* 16, no. 9 (1991): 1015-021.

[9] Miyagi, Masayuki, Tetsuhiro Ishikawa, Sumihisa Orita, Yawara Eguchi, Hiroto Kamoda, Gen Arai, Miyako Suzuki, Gen Inoue, Yasuchika Aoki, Tomoaki Toyone, Kazuhisa Takahashi, and Seiji Ohtori. "Disk Injury in Rats Produces Persistent Increases in Pain-Related Neuropeptides in Dorsal Root Ganglia and Spinal Cord Glia but Only Transient Increases in Inflammatory Mediators." *Spine* 36, no. 26 (2011): 2260-266.

[10] García-Cosamalón, José, Miguel E. Del Valle, Marta G. Calavia, Olivia García-Suárez, Alfonso López-Muñiz, Jesús Otero, and José A. Vega. "Intervertebral Disc, Sensory Nerves and Neurotrophins: Who Is Who in Discogenic Pain?" *Journal of Anatomy* 217, no. 1 (2010): 1-15.

[11] Abe, Yumiko, Koji Akeda, Howard S. An, Yasuchika Aoki, Rajeswari Pichika, Carol Muehleman, Tomoatsu Kimura, and Koichi Masuda. "Proinflammatory Cytokines Stimulate the Expression of Nerve Growth Factor by Human Intervertebral Disc Cells." *Spine* 32, no. 6 (2007): 635-42.

[12] Purmessur, Devina, Anthony J. Freemont, and Judith A. Hoyland. "Expression and Regulation of Neurotrophins in the Nondegenerate and Degenerate Human Intervertebral Disc." *Arthritis Res Ther Arthritis Research and Therapy* 10, no. 4 (2008).

[13] Greene, Carol Ann, Colin R. Green, and Trevor Sherwin. "Transdifferentiation of Chondrocytes into Neuron-like Cells Induced by

Neuronal Lineage Specifying Growth Factors." *Cell Biology International Cell Biol Int* 39, no. 2 (2014): 185-91.

[14] Perán, Macarena, Juan Antonio Marchal, Fernando Rodríguez-Serrano, Pablo Álvarez, and Antonia Aránega. "Transdifferentiation: Why and How?" *Cell. Biol. Int. Cell Biology International* 35, no. 4 (2011): 373-79.

[15] Greene, Carol Ann, Chuan-Yuan Chang, Cameron J. Fraser, Dasha E. Nelidova, Jing A. Chen, Angela Lim, Alex Brebner, Jennifer Mcghee, Trevor Sherwin, and Colin R. Green. "Cells from the Adult Corneal Stroma Can Be Reprogrammed to a Neuron-like Cell Using Exogenous Growth Factors." *Experimental Cell Research* 322, no. 1 (2014): 122-32.

[16] Orita, Sumihisa, Tetsuhiro Ishikawa, Masayuki Miyagi, Nobuyasu Ochiai, Gen Inoue, Yawara Eguchi, Hiroto Kamoda, Gen Arai, Tomoaki Toyone, Yasuchika Aoki, Takekazu Kubo, Kazuhisa Takahashi, and Seiji Ohtori. "Pain-related Sensory Innervation in Monoiodoacetate-induced Osteoarthritis in Rat Knees That Gradually Develops Neuronal Injury in Addition to Inflammatory Pain." *BMC Musculoskeletal Disorders BMC Musculoskelet Disord* 12, no. 1 (2011): 134.

[17] Oprea, Manuel D., Iulian Popa, Anca Maria Cimpean, Marius Raica, and Dan V. Poenaru. "Microscopic Assessment of Degenerated Intervertebral Disc: Clinical Implications and Possible Therapeutic Challenge." *In Vivo* 29, no. 1 (Jan-Feb 2105): 95-102.

[18] Ferreira-Gomes, Joana, Sara Adães, Jana Sarkander, and José M. Castro-Lopes. "Phenotypic Alterations of Neurons That Innervate Osteoarthritic Joints in Rats." *Arthritis and Rheumatism* 62, no. 12 (2010): 3677-685.

[19] Oprea, Manuel D. Optimization of Therapeutic Management of Low Back Pain Pacients through the Correlation of the Degree of Histologic Degeneration, Pelvic Sagittal Balance and Mri Characteristics. Master's thesis, Timisoara/University of Medicine and Pharmacy "Victor Babes", 2015. Timisoara: Editura Victor Babes, 2015.

[20] Hadjipavlou, A. G., M. N. Tzermiadianos, N. Bogduk, and M. R. Zindrick. "The Pathophysiology of Disc Degeneration: A CRITICAL REVIEW." *Journal of Bone and Joint Surgery - British Volume* 90-B, no. 10 (2008): 1261-270.

[21] Tolofari, Sotonye K., Stephen M. Richardson, Anthony J. Freemont, and Judith A. Hoyland. "Expression of Semaphorin 3A and Its Receptors in the Human Intervertebral Disc: Potential Role in Regulating Neural Ingrowth in the Degenerate Intervertebral Disc." *Arthritis Res Ther Arthritis Research and Therapy* 12, no. 1 (2010).

[22] Johnson, William E. B., Bruce Caterson, Stephen M. Eisenstein, and Sally Roberts. "Human Intervertebral Disc Aggrecan Inhibits Endothelial Cell Adhesion and Cell Migration In Vitro." *Spine* 30, no. 10 (2005): 1139-147.

[23] Mwale, Fackson. "Molecular Therapy for Disk Degeneration and Pain." *Global Spine J Global Spine Journal* 03, no. 03 (2013): 185-92.

[24] Aoki, Yasuchika, Arata Nakajima, Seiji Ohtori, Hiroshi Takahashi, Fusako Watanabe, Masato Sonobe, Fumiaki Terajima, Masahiko Saito, Kazuhisa Takahashi, Tomoaki Toyone, Atsuya Watanabe, Takayuki Nakajima, Makoto Takazawa, and Koichi Nakagawa. "Increase of Nerve Growth Factor Levels in the Human Herniated Intervertebral Disc: Can Annular Rupture Trigger Discogenic Back Pain?" *Arthritis Res Ther Arthritis Research and Therapy* 16, no. 4 (2014).

[25] Lee, Seungcheol, Chan Sam Moon, Donggeun Sul, Jiyoung Lee, Minyoung Bae, Youngki Hong, Min Lee, Seonyoung Choi, Richard Derby, Byung-Jo Kim, Juhan Kim, Joon-Sik Yoon, Lee Wolfer, Jaemin Kim, Joonho Wang, Sun-Wook Hwang, and Sang-Heon Lee. "Comparison of Growth Factor and Cytokine Expression in Patients with Degenerated Disc Disease and Herniated Nucleus Pulposus." *Clinical Biochemistry* 42, no. 15 (2009): 1504-511.

[26] Lee, Jae Man, Ji Ye Song, Minjung Baek, Hye-Young Jung, Haeyoun Kang, In Bo Han, Young Do Kwon, and Dong Eun Shin. "Interleukin-1β Induces Angiogenesis and Innervation in Human Intervertebral Disc Degeneration." *Journal of Orthopaedic Research J. Orthop. Res.* 29, no. 2 (2010): 265-69.

[27] Akyol, Sibel, Berna Senel Eraslan, Hakan Etyemez, Taner Tanriverdi, and Murat Hanci. "Catabolic Cytokine Expressions in Patients with Degenerative Disc Disease." *Turkish Neurosurgery*, 2010.

[28] Kokubo, Yasuo, Kenzo Uchida, Shigeru Kobayashi, Takafumi Yayama, Ryuichiro Sato, Hideaki Nakajima, Takaharu Takamura, Erisa Mwaka, Norbert Orwotho, Alexander Bangirana, and Hisatoshi Baba. "Herniated and Spondylotic Intervertebral Discs of the Human Cervical Spine: Histological and Immunohistological Findings in 500 En Bloc Surgical Samples." *Journal of Neurosurgery: Spine* 9, no. 3 (2008): 285-95.

[29] Choi, Kyung-Suk, Martin J. Cohn, and Brian D. Harfe. "Identification of Nucleus Pulposus Precursor Cells and Notochordal Remnants in the Mouse: Implications for Disk Degeneration and Chordoma Formation." *Dev. Dyn. Developmental Dynamics* 237, no. 12 (2008): 3953-958.

[30] Pfirrmann, Christian W. A., Alexander Metzdorf, Marco Zanetti, Juerg Hodler, and Norbert Boos. "Magnetic Resonance Classification of Lumbar Intervertebral Disc Degeneration." *Spine* 26, no. 17 (2001): 1873-878.

[31] Modic, M. T., P. M. Steinberg, J. S. Ross, T. J. Masaryk, and J. R. Carter. "Degenerative Disk Disease: Assessment of Changes in Vertebral Body Marrow with MR Imaging." *Radiology* 166, no. 1 (1988): 193-99.

[32] Griffith, James F., Yi-Xiang J. Wang, Gregory E. Antonio, Kai Chow Choi, Alfred Yu, Anil T. Ahuja, and Ping Chung Leung. "Modified Pfirrmann Grading System for Lumbar Intervertebral Disc Degeneration." *Spine* 32, no. 24 (2007).

[33] Jensen, Tue Secher, Per Kjaer, Lars Korsholm, Tom Bendix, Joan S. Sorensen, Claus Manniche, and Charlotte Leboeuf-Yde. "Predictors of New Vertebral Endplate Signal (Modic) Changes in the General Population." *European Spine Journal Eur Spine J* 19, no. 1 (2009): 129-35.

[34] Rahme, R., and R. Moussa. "The Modic Vertebral Endplate and Marrow Changes: Pathologic Significance and Relation to Low Back Pain and Segmental Instability of the Lumbar Spine." *American Journal of Neuroradiology* 29, no. 5 (2008): 838-42.

In: Intervertebral Disc Degeneration
Editors: A. L. Ho and A. M. Desai

ISBN: 978-1-63485-829-8

Chapter 3

SPINAL BIOMECHANICS

James Pan, BS, Arjun V. Pendharkar, MD and Jongsoo Park*, MD

Department of Neurological Surgery, Stanford University School of Medicine, Stanford, California, US

ABSTRACT

The biomechanical properties of the spine offer insights into the mechanisms and consequences behind intervertebral disc degeneration. The intervertebral disc is a dynamic structure which serves a critical function in allowing the many components of the bony vertebrae to interface with and work with one another. The biomechanical properties of the intervertebral disc afford it's properties in helping the spine to withstand compressive, shear, bending, and rotational forces. These biomechanical properties are derived from the biochemical and cellular composition of the disc which afford it unique properties such as its viscoelastic behavior. Degeneration of the disc — either due to injury or aging — perturb the biochemical composition of the disc, and subsequently the biomechanical properties. This chapter will explore the composition and the mechanistic properties of the disc which give the disc it's unique characteristics, and how theses parameters change in degenerative states.

* Corresponding author: Jongsoo Park (jonpark1@stanford.edu), Department of Neurosurgery, Stanford University School of Medicine, 300 Pasteur Drive, R281, Stanford, CA 94303-5327.

Introduction

The vertebral column is the hallmark feature of vertebrates and serves to house the spinal canal, which encloses the spinal cord. Rigid vertebral bodies work in concert with the intervertebral disc to allow for large, complex, three dimensional motions of the spine. Intervertebral discs also perform the function of absorbing large loads sustained by normal motion of the body and stabilizes the spine to prevent it from injury. Though the primary function of the intervertebral disc is mechanical, these properties are derived from the unique cellular and biochemical composition of the disc. A crucial balance of cell types, extracellular matrix components, and water give rise to the biomechanical properties of the disc and explain regional differences in mechanics and mechanisms of injury. Injury and degeneration of the disc occurs due to a perturbation in the biochemistry of disc components which translates into distinct biomechanical failures which make the disc more susceptible to tears, fissures, herniations, and pain. Therefore, an appreciation of the biomechanical properties of the spine is crucial to understanding the pathophysiology of degenerative disc disease and the consequences of treatment and rehabilitation.

General Anatomy of the Spine

Bony Vertebrae

The spine is composed of 33 vertebrae, which are divided into five distinct regions — cervical, thoracic, lumbar, sacral, and coccygeal. Adjacent vertebrae in the cervical, thoracic, and lumbar regions are connected by the intervertebral disc anteriorly and by the facet joint ligaments and other connective tissues laterally and posteriorly. One noticeable difference is that the sacral and coccygeal regions contain three to five fused vertebrae. All the vertebrae have a similar general structure with sight variations in size and anatomy. The increasing size of vertebrae from top to bottom is reflective of the increasing weight and axial load sustained by each successive vertebra.

Each vertebra is comprised of an anterior body, and a posterior arch composed of two pedicles and two laminae. The laminae are joined posteriorly in the midline to form the spinous process. On the lateral aspects of the vertebra, the posterior arch also supports a transverse process and superior and inferior articular processes. The transverse and spinous processes provide levels for muscles which attach to them. The articular processes are part of synovial joints that are posterior contact points for adjacent vertebral segments.

The cervical spine consists of seven vertebrae in a lordotic shape and is generally the most flexible portion and most susceptible to injury. The craniocervical junction is comprised of the occiput and the first two bony vertebrae: C1 (atlas) and C2 (axis). Atlas has only a bony ring with no vertebral body, encircles the dens of axis at the point where it protrudes rostrally from C2, and articulates with the occiput of the skull via a pair of bilateral synovial condylar joints. The complex bony and ligamentous articulations of the craniocervical junction gives its unique biomechanical properties which accounts for 25% of the flexion and extension, and 50% of rotation of the neck. Subaxial cervical vertebrae (C3-C7) are distinct anatomically from the atlas and axis and are generally the smallest in size compared to other regions of the spine. The end plates of the subaxial cervical vertebrae are concave superiorly and convex inferiorly, and they articulate to form the uncovertebral joints (of Luschka). The pedicles associated with this region are short and are derived from the midpoint of the vertebral bodies.

The thoracic spine consists of 12 vertebrae and is kyphotic. In general, the thoracic spine is quite rigid due to its association with the chest wall. As it is the transition zone between the cervical and lumbar sections of the cord, the first thoracic vertebrae share cervical features, and the last four maintain some lumbar features. Notable landmarks include the superior vertebral notch in T1, and the lateral direction and inferior articular processes of T12. The inferior and superior faces of the vertebral body are generally flatter and the transverse processes are located more posteriorly and appear to be more elongated than in the cervical spine. The thoracic vertebrae laminae overlap and are broader compared to that of the cervical region. The transverse processes also increase in size as the thoracic spine descends (Berry et al. 1987). Finally, ribs articulate with the lateral processes in the thoracic spine.

The lumbar spine consists of five vertebrae and is lordotic. The largest vertebral bodies of the spine, each lumbar vertebra increase in diameter when approaching the sacrum and are larger in transverse width relative to anteroposterior diameter. The lateral processes are the longest and are located at the junction between the lamina and the vertebral body. That articular pillars are located more posteriorly compared to the cervical vertebrae and are integrated within the laminae in the thoracic and lumbar regions. Pedicles in the lumbar region are derived from the rostral aspect of the vertebral body.

Intervertebral Disc

The intervertebral disc (IVD) is a structure found between adjacent vertebrae and acts as a ligament to hold the vertebrae together. This separates the bony vertebral bodies and allows for complex three-dimensional motion of the spine. Accounting for roughly 20-33% of the height of the entire vertebral column, it is the largest avascular and aneural structure in the body and connects adjacent vertebral bodies via a cartilaginous endplate form which nutrients are received by diffusion. There are twenty three discs in the vertebral column starting between C2 and C3 and extending distally to L5-S1. The diameter and shapes of the disc vary according to the region of the spine — they are generally ellipsoid in the cervical and lumbar regions, and more triangular shaped in the thoracic region. Each disc is comprised of four concentrically arranged layers: the outer annulus fibrosus, the fibrocartilaginous inner annulus fibrosus, the transition zone, and the nucleus pulposus (Figure 1) (Buckwalter 1995). The superior and inferior aspects of the IVD are associated with the cartilage end plates (Figure X). These components are intricately linked to one another such that the pathology of one can affect the ability of the others to carry out their normal functions. Furthermore, the discs remain in an intricate balance of having to be rigid enough to support the vertebral bodies, but soft enough to allow spinal motions of axial compression, flexion–extension, lateral bending, and axial rotation (Figure 2).

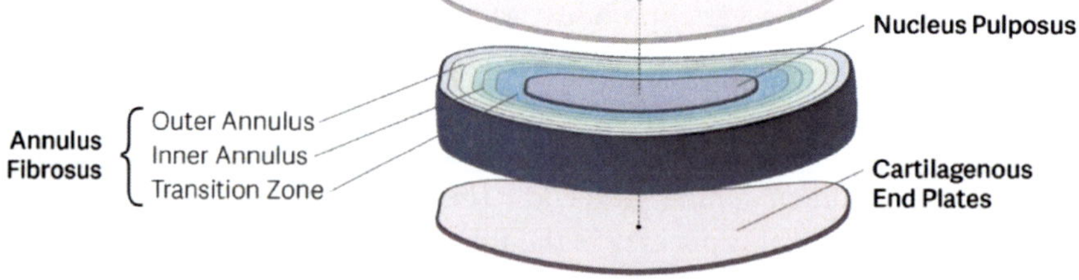

Figure 1. Anatomy of the Intervertebral Disc.

The outer annulus consists of approximately 90 collagen sheets bonded together in concentric laminated bands, within which the fibers are arranged in a helicoid manner (Doers and Kang 1999). The sheets are found 30° to the disc plane and 120° to each other in alternate bands. This orientation allows the annulus to resist the high pressure of the nucleus and also to withstand rotational forces. The inner annulus fibrosus is softer, less dense, and has a larger fibrocartilagenous component, composed mostly of type II collagen fibers. The fibers of the outer annulus attach directly to the vertebral body as Sharpey fibers while the fibers of the inner annulus attach to the cartilaginous endplate. Additionally, due to the dense collagen network, the outer annulus is less permeable than the inner annulus (Figure 1) (Houben et al. 1997; Poole 1997).

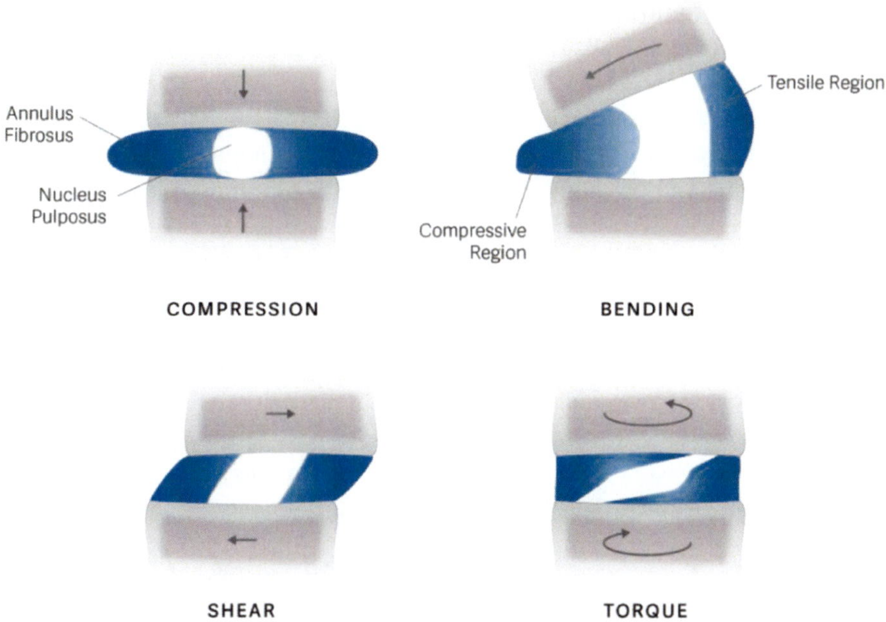

Figure 2. Spinal Loading Configurations.

The nucleus pulposus (NP) comprises the central core of the intervertebral disc. It's embryological origin is distinct from that of the other components of the intervertebral disc- it is derived from the notochord (or endodermal origin) which contrasts with the mesodermal origin of the other components of the disc (Roberts et al. 2006). Biochemically, the NP is made from a soft gelatinous material comprised of proteoglycans surrounded by the annulus fibrosus. The high proteoglycan content allows for the NP to maintain an increased hydration state, which allows for its viscoelastic properties leading to its load-bearing properties in the spine (Iatridis, Setton, Weidenbaum, and Mow 1997b). The NP is also rich in type II collagens, which comprises 80% of the collagen content in the NP. Elastin fibers are also present, and are arranged in both a radial distribution from the center to the periphery and a vertical orientation anchoring the NP to the end plates (Yu et al. 2002). This orientation is thought to be important for the maintenance of the structure of the NP within the annulus fibrosus by restoring the NP to its original form following load bearing, in addition to facilitating load transmission to the surrounding annulus fibrosus.

The cartilaginous end plates are composed of a thin layer of hyaline cartilage which interfaces between the bony vertebral body and the IVD. Their composition is similar to that of the disc itself, being comprised of proteoglycans, type II collagen, and water (Raj 2008). The thickness of the endplate ranges from 0.5 to 1.5 mm and is thinnest at the points there they interface with the NP (Grignon et al. 2000). The plate is attached to the vertebral body by a thin layer of calcium and is discontinuous in regions where perforations exists throughout the endplates. These perforations exist to allow the passage of vascular channels which traverse from the adjacent vertebral body into the disc which are usually obliterated by the second decade of life (Conventry, Ghormley, and Kernohan 1945). The stiff but porous nature of the endplate serves as a site of diffusion of nutrients and fluid into and out of the disc and to prevent herniation of the disc material into the adjacent vertebral body. Weakness of the endplates can lead to herniation of disc into bone resulting in Schmorl nodes and can be attributed to a perturbation in endplate composition such as a significantly decreased proteoglycan concentration (Roberts, Menage, and Urban 1989).

FUNCTIONAL BIOMECHANICS

Physiology of the Intervertebral Disc

The IVD is primarily a load-bearing structure that absorbs axial loads and redistributes them across the entire disc. The characteristics and capacity of load distribution is partly determined by the molecular and biochemical composition of the disc. The extracellular matrix of the outer annulus is comprised of approximately 80% of type I collagen and 3% of type V collagen. On the interior of the outer annulus, a concentration gradient exists whereas type II collagen proteoglycan increases towards the center of the disc, whereas type I collagen decreases. The concentration of type II collagen can reach 80% inside the nucleus, while type I collagen is typically absent (Buckwalter 1995).

These differences in composition in different areas of the disc are thought to be responsible for the dynamic structural properties that allows it to bear and distribute loads across the entire structure. Furthermore, the mix of type I and II collagen in the annulus fibrosus gives it tensile strength. Other molecules such as type V and XI collagen are also found which interlink collagen fibrils, leading to the overall strong fibrillar collagen meshwork (Setton and Chen 2006). Specifically, when the disc is subjected to axial loads, the NP and inner annulus absorbs the weight to generate hydrostatic pressure which is then distributed evenly to the adjacent outer annulus. The tensile strength of the outer annulus is derived from the lamellar structure of the type I collagen network.

In addition to collagen, proteoglycans are also a significant molecular component of the IVD as they can be found to constitute up to 50% of the cells in the NP. Many types of proteoglycans exist in the extracellular matrix including aggrecan, versican, decorin, biglycan, fibromodulin, lumican, and perlecan. These molecules are characterized by a central core protein with side chains composed of keratin sulfate and chondroiton sulfate. At their N-terminus, proteoglycans such as aggrecans attach to hyaluronic acid, and their C-terminus attaches to components of the extracellular matrix such as collagen (Antoniou et al. 1996; Feng et al. 2006). Because the proteoglycans attach to hyaluronic acid through linkage proteins, they can also form aggregates (Buckwalter, Einhorn, and Simon 2000). Proteoglycans also have a net negative surface charge and is therefore hydrophilic — thus affording the NP's propensity to retain hydration. Proteoglycans are implicated in age-related disc degeneration as breakdown of aggrecans are replaced by non-aggregated proteoglycans, which have a decreased ability to retain water.

The disc matrix is maintained by cells, which comprise only 1% of the disc volume. Histologically, the disc is comprised of at least three distinct cell populations: the chondrocyte-like cells in the NP, fibrocartilaginous cells in the inner annulus, and fibroblast-like cells in the outer annulus (Bibby et al. 2001). The shape and cytoskeletal organization of these cells seems to influence the type of matrix components synthesized (Figure 3) (Horner et al. 2002). These cells respond to a variety of stimuli, and studies how suggested that mechanical stress, nutrient supply, cytokines, and the osmotic and ionic environment have the most profound effects on cellular activity (Bruehlmann et al. 2002).

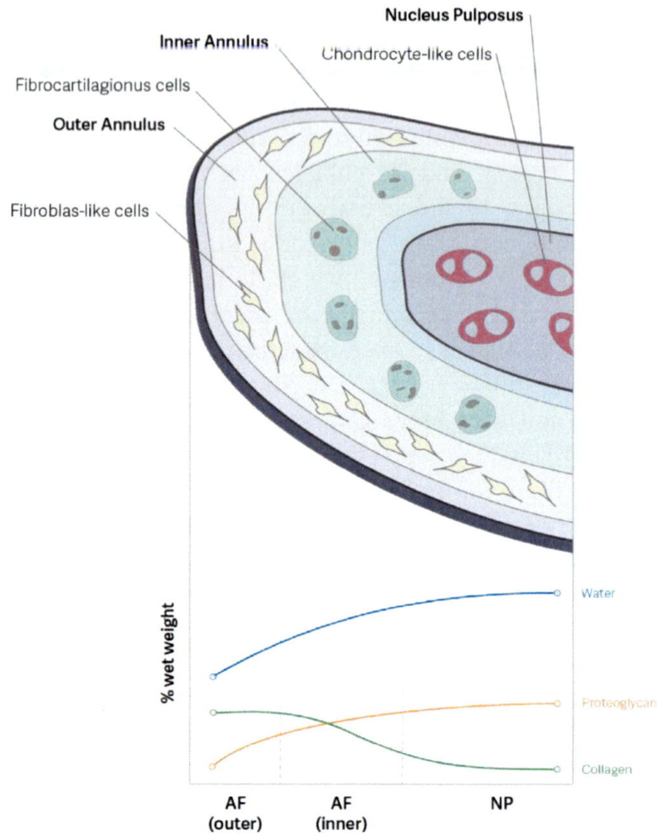

Figure 3. Disc Components.

Table 1. Biomechanical characteristics of the NP

Parameter	Description	Normal NP	Degenerate NP
Shear modulus	Slope of the shear stress versus angle of displacement	0.2 kPa	0.6-0.8 kPa
Dynamic shear modulus	Ratio of stress to strain under vibratory conditions	5-60 kPa	Increased
Compression modulus	Ratio of compressive stress applied to the resulting compression	0.5 MPa	N/A
Viscoelastic behavior	Tendency of a material to exhibit both viscous and elastic characteristics when subjected to deformation	$3\times10^{\wedge-16}$ m^4/Ns	N/A

The mechanism in which the chondrocytes of the NP respond to mechanical stress is not fully understood. However, it is known that the cells are surrounded by a pericellular matrix (PCM), which is characterized by the presence of type VI and III collagen, not found elsewhere in normal cartilage (Hessle and Engvall 1984; Rombers et al. 1991; Söder et al. 2002). *In-vitro* experiments on isolated cells have suggested that the PCM is a protective layer for chrondrocytes during axial loading through an adaptive water loss from PCM proteoglycans (Poole, Flint, and Beaumont 1988). Additionally, the PCM may also have mechanical transduction properties (Poole 1997).

Nucleus Pulposus

The three components of the IVD — the annulus, NP, and endplates — work together to give the disc its unique load absorption abilities. In healthy discs, each component works in concert to provide a balance between stability and mobility of the disc. This is enabled by the viscoelastic properties of the disc, which is secondary to the high concentrations of proteoglycans in the NP. These proteoglycans allow the NP to retain water, thus allowing it to weight-bear compressive loads by conforming its shape to redistribute axial loads to the adjacent AF by transmitting hydrostatic forces. Bulk fluid flow from the disc also contributes to its viscoelastic properties in addition to nutrient transport. The hydrostatic forces transmitted to the annulus is contained by the tensile strength of the collagen meshwork. This allows the annulus to share the compressive load without being directly exposed to external forces.

The NP's highly hydrated mix of proteoglycans and collagens afford it its swelling pressure, compression modulus, permeability, and shear modulus properties. The hydrophilic nature of the NP can be demonstrated by submerging it in water and observing it to swell to at least twice its original volume. This swelling pressure can be measured *in vivo* and in cadaveric spines under mechanical loading. The swelling pressure of a healthy nucleus is 0.1-0.2 MPa in a recumbent position, and 1-3 MPa under axial load (e.g., standing or lifting) (Wilke et al. 1999). These values are also consistent in cadaveric motion segments under external loads (Castagnera and Lavignolle 1989; McNally and Adams 1992). Osmometry methods have also been used to measure swelling pressure, which produces values consistent with *in vivo* measurements (Urban and McMullin 1988). Finally, the swelling pressure has also been shown to be influenced with the glycosaminoglycans content of the NP (Johannessen and Elliott 2005).

Recent studies have also provided insights into specific tissue properties of the NP and their changes with degeneration. These findings are summarized in Table 1.

Annulus Fibrosus

The annulus fibrosus, like the NP, also undergoes axial loading as a result of bending and torsional loading. In addition to axial loading due to body weight, the annulus receives forces radially from swelling of the NP. The swelling pressure, which represents the pressure generated when the annulus is held at the in-situ displacement, is derived from the biochemical properties of glycosaminoglycans when they balance their negative charges. Because glycosaminoglycans are found in the NP and the annulus, the swelling pressure is a similarly important biomechanical property. Studies have shown that the compressive modulus and permeability of the annulus to be 0.6 MPa and 2×10^{-16} m^4/Ns (Iatridis et al. 1998; Yao et al. 2002).

Compression behavior in the annulus is nonlinear and not homogenous. Non-linearity is ascribed to the increase in compressive modulus and the decrease in permeability as a function of increasing compressive forces (Iatridis et al. 1998). Studies have shown that non-linearity is more pronounced for compressive stiffness than for permeability (Best et al. 1994). Non-homogeneity is due to regional and radial variations in both biomechanical properties and biochemical composition (Iatridis et al. 1998; Best et al. 1994). Compression properties are also not very anisotropic as very little anisotropy is observed for samples oriented in the axial and radial direction, which suggests that the alignment of the collagen fibers in the annulus does not strongly affect its behavior during compression (Iatridis et al. 1998). Therefore, loading configuration is primarily influenced by fluid pressurization. Permeability in the annulus is dependent on direction, with the highest permeability in the radial direction (Gu et al. 1999). Swelling is also observed to be more prominent in the radial direction rather than the axial direction (Urban and Maroudas 1980).

Tensile forces applied to the disc is primarily resisted by the annulus. When the NP undergoes axial compression, this force is transmitted to the annulus by tensile forces. Tensile loads are also generated directly on the annulus itself. The nature of the stress-strain curve observed for the annulus under tensile stress is nonlinear and is similar to the material properties of other soft collagenous tissues such as articular cartilage, tendon, and ligament.

Under axial deformation, the annulus exhibits a nonlinear portion of the stress-strain curve known as the "toe region" which represents a lower force observed for small tensile strains. This nonlinear region is then followed by a linear region, and then failure of the tissue at the highest strains. For example, the modulus in the toe region was found to be 2 MPa and in the linear region to be 20 MPa, which demonstrates a nonlinear relationship between modulus and increasing strain (Acaroglu et al. 1995; Ebara et al. 1996; Elliott and Setton 2001).

Anisotropy is another important property of the annulus since it allows it to support large and complex loads. This is evident by the near 1000-fold increase in tensile modulus when loads are applied along the fibril as supposed to across the fibrils. A single layer of the annulus, when loaded parallel to the collagen fibres, has a modulus of 136 MPa at the anterior outer site (Skaggs et al. 1994). Furthermore, the circumferential modulus is 20 MPa, the axial modulus is 0.8 MPa, and the radial modulus is 0.2 MPa (Elliott and Setton 2001; Fujita, Duncan, and Lotz 1997) which illustrates that the anisotropic properties of the annulus is due in part to the structural contributions of aligned collagen fibers.

The annulus is also known to have spatial variation in structure and composition due to its non-homogenous nature. Water, collagen, and proteoglycan content has been found to vary significantly from the outer to inner sites and from the anterior to posterior sites (Eyre and Muir 1976). Despite biochemical non-homogenity, little variation is observed in both radial and axial tensile properties, possibly due to the small contributions of the collagen fibers in these orientations (Yin and Elliott 2005). However, in the circumferential direction, the anterior annulus is stiffer than the posterior annulus, and the outer annulus is stiffer than the inner (Acaroglu et al. 1995; Ebara et al. 1996; Elliott and Setton 2001). The relative lack of structural integrity in the posterolateral region can be due to incomplete lamellar layers, increased fiber interlacing angles, and loose interconnections of fibers (Marchand and Ahmed 1990). Regional variations in composition and biomechanical properties of the posterolateral annulus can point to regions of weaker structural integrity, and can be predisposed to tears, fissures, and herniations (Figure 4).

Shear loading of the annulus has been shown to be nonlinear, viscoelastic, and aniostropic. The shear modulus of the annulus at equilibrium was measured to be 0.1 MPa; however, modeling studies have predicted the shear modulus to be as large as 20 MPa (Yin and Elliott 2005; Spilker, Jakobs, and Schultz 1986; Elliott and Sarver 2004). Although there have been studies showing that the shear modulus increases slightly with degeneration (Iatridis, Kumar, et al. 1999; Iatridis, Mente, et al. 1999), more studies regarding this biomechanical parameter is needed.

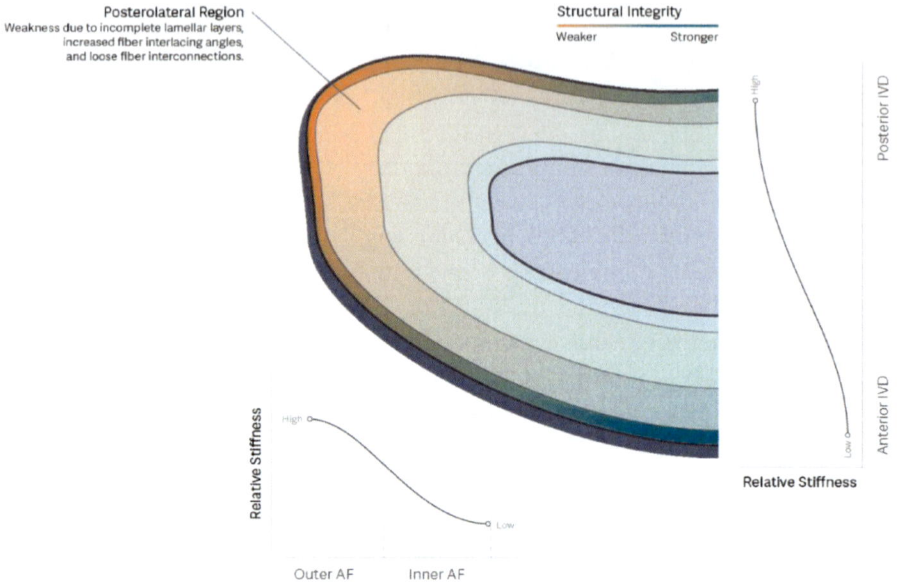

Figure 4. Relative Stiffness and Structural Integrity of the IVD.

Endplate

The cartilaginous endplates, which are thin layers of hyaline cartilage between the IVD and the bony vertebra, play an important role in supporting and distributing the load from the disc to the vertebra (Broberg 1983). For example, as the hydrostatic pressure in the NP increases, this load is transmitted to the endplate, which tends to bulge into the vertebra. For very large axial loads, the endplate is usually the structure that fails first (Brinckmann et al. 1983). Damage to the endplate can result in reduced swelling pressure in the NP and increased stresses in the annulus fibrosus. Another important feature of the endplate is the facilitation of diffusion of nutrients into the IVD (Maroudas et al. 1975; Roberts, Menage, and Urban 1989).

Quantitative biomechanics regarding the endplate is lacking compared to the NP and annulus fibrosus. For example, studies on the compressive properties of the cartilaginous endplates have been limited to the baboon lumbar spine (Setton et al. 1993). This particular study found that the endplate has a hydraulic permeability associated with rapid transport and pressurization of the interstitial fluid in response to loading and an increased emphasis on flow-independent viscoelastic effects.

DEGENERATIVE DISC DISEASE

Characteristics of Injury

Generally, IVD failure occurs when it is exposed to loads and stresses that exceed the strength of the tissue. Stresses to the IVD can be tensile, compressive, or shear. Pure axial compression, even at high loads, does not usually cause herniation of the nucleus pulposus. However, the end plate of the vertebra is usually the first structure to fail (LIU et al. 1983).

At rest, the axial loads on the lumbar spine *in vivo* is 500 newtons (N) when standing, and 700 N when sitting. These loads can increase to 3000-6000 N with moderate weights. Disc prolapse can be observed when axial overloading is combined with bending. Although disc prolapse does not usually occur with pure compression, cyclic overloading can cause tears in the annulus which can lead to disc herniation (Liu et al. 1985). The IVD can also show creep, relaxation, and hysteresis (Twomey and Taylor 1982; Kazarian 1975; Koeller, Meier, and Hartmann 1984). Hysteresis was shown to positively correlate with load, and negatively correlate with age. Non-degenerated discs also creep less slowly than degenerated discs which may indicate decreased viscoelasticity in degenerating discs. It has not been demonstrated however, that mechanical forces alone *in vitro* is sufficient enough to cause disc herniation.

The functional spinal unit (FSU) has also been examined and modeled by finite element analysis (Shiraz-Adl 1989). These studies have shown that during compression, the load is transferred from one vertebra to another through the end plates via the NP and the annulus fibrosus. Specifically, axial forces causes pressure to develop within the disc, pushing structures away and out from the center of the disc. Progressively increasing the load caused rupture of the annular fibers posterolaterally in the innermost layer. Another model showed that under axial compression, disc failure originated at the end plates and not in the annulus (Natarajan, Ke, and Andersson 1994). This suggested that annular injuries were unlikely to be produced purely by compressive loads, and that the presence of discrete peripheral tears may lead to the development of concentric tears and possible acceleration of the degenerative process.

More recently, the FSU in the context of IVD degeneration was investigated in the presence of a compressive follower load. The results of this study indicated that IVD degeneration led to a statistically significant changes in segmental stiffness, range of motion (ROM), and hysteresis area in axial rotation and lateral bending and statistically significant changes in ROM and normalized hysteresis in flexion-extension (Zirbel et al. 2013).

Nucleus Pulposus

The molecular process of IVD degeneration is thought to start in the nucleus pulposus which involves a decreasing concentration of proteoglycans and a gradual change of collagen into fibrotic tissue (Haefeli et al. 2006). These changes in effect dehydrate the NP, with water levels decreasing from approximately 20-30% (Bibby et al. 2001). Desmoplasia of the disc results in a stiffer NP and the shock-absorption properties of the normally hydrated nucleus becomes severely limited. Specifically, the NP loses its hydrostatic pressure feature as a fibrotic nucleus will not behave in the same way as a fluid or hydrogel (Haefeli et al. 2006; Buckwalter 1995) (Figure X). The fibrotic process is associated from a gradual loss of proteoglycan and a transition of collagens from Type II to Type I (Roughley 2004; Buckwalter 1995). This leads to a fibrous and solid tissue mass (Iatridis, Setton, Weidenbaum, and Mow 1997a; Stokes and Iatridis 2004) which amalgamates into one solid phase with the anulus fibrosus in up to 75% of cases shown in one cadaveric study (Haefeli et al. 2006). The loss of proteoglycans decreases the swelling pressure in the NP, which is the main load-bearing mechanism in the normal NP (Urban and McMullin 1988).

Fibrotic causes in the NP causes the shear stiffness to increase, the pressure to decrease, the compression stiffness to increase, and the permeability to decrease (Iatridis et al. 1996; Urban and McMullin 1988). Swelling pressure can decrease to 0.03 MPa or less which represents 15-30% of normal pressures (Nachemson and Morris 1964; Wilke et al. 1999; Sato, Kikuchi, and Yonezawa 1999). Despite the fact that fibrosis increases with degeneration and that the behavior of the NP becomes more solid-like, osmometry and mechanical compression tests still suggest that even in the context of degeneration, the swelling component still remains the dominant property in the overall function of the NP (Urban and McMullin 1985) (Figure 5).

Annulus Fibrosus

Degeneration of the annulus fibrosus is characterized by disorganization of collagen fibers, and perturbations in the elastic response (Schollum, Robertson, and Broom 2010; Wagner and Lotz 2004). Defective annulus tissue also exhibits a two-fold increase in the toe-region modulus in tensile testing and fiber realignment towards the loading region, the prior of which was positively correlated with age (H. A. L. Guerin and Elliott 2006; O'Connell, Guerin, and Elliott 2009). Dynamic viscoelastic testing has also revealed that the dynamic modulus of the annulus increases with degeneration at tensile strains greater than 6% (Sen et al. 2008). Other studies have also shown that degeneration has a strong effect on other elastic properties such as Poisson's ratio, failure stress, and strain energy density of the annulus (Acaroglu et al. 1995; Galante 1967). Permeability of the annulus has also shown to be affected by generation, age, and water content in the disc and these properties have been incorporated in a finite element simulation (Gu et al. 1999; Natarajan, Williams, and Andersson 2006).

Similar to NP degeneration, the swelling pressure of the annulus also decreases dramatically from 0.13 MPa to 0.05 MPa (Iatridis et al. 1998; Best et al. 1994). The permeability of the annulus is also affected by degeneration as the radial permeability decreases and the axial and circumferential permeabilities increase (Gu et al. 1999). This combination of decreased swelling pressure and altered permeabilities results in transfer of a compressive load onto the solid matrix, which is likely to accelerate degeneration due to mechanical wear-and-tear and an altered cellular response. The compromised swelling pressure is compensated in part by an increase in the stiffness of the solid matrix from 0.5 MPa to 1.1 MPa (Iatridis et al. 1998; Best et al. 1994), which can be due to an increase in density after dehydration, increased collagen cross linking, and cellular remodeling in response to the perturbations in loading mechanics.

Although the lamellar structure of the annulus makes it somewhat resistant to mechanical failure, fatigue loading, or extremely high loads can compromise the structural integrity of the annulus (Green, Adams, and Dolan

1993; Iatridis and ap Gwynn 2004). The tensile properties of the annulus also change with aging and degeneration, however, it is not as significant when compared to gross anatomical perturbations. In the degenerate annulus, failure stress, strain energy density, and Poisson's ratio are significantly lower (Acaroglu et al. 1995). The toe region in the stress-strain curve is also perturbed with degeneration (H. A. L. Guerin and Elliott 2006). Overall, these changes causes the annulus to fail at lower stresses and can contribute to IVD injury.

Endplate

The endplates show three major failure patterns: central, peripheral, and the complete endplate (Perey 1957). Central failure in non-degenerate discs is associated with excessive loading caused by forces transmitted by the NP under compressive loads. Peripheral failure is observed in degenerate discs when the NP loses its hydrostatic pressure and most of the compressive load is transmitted through the annulus fibrosus. This causes peripheral loading of the endplate and can result in fracture. In general, the central portion and superior aspect of the endplate is weaker than the peripheral regions and the inferior endplate (Grant, Oxland, and Dvorak 2001). More degeneration is seen with decreased failure properties in the bony endplate, but stiffness is not affected (Grant et al. 2002).

Degeneration Cascade

The degeneration of the aging spine has been categorized into three stages by Yong-Hin and Kirkaldy-Willis (Yong-Hing and Kirkaldy-Willis 1983). The first stage is known as the dysfunction stage which is associated with synovial reaction in the dorsal joints and small tears in the IVD. These changes are a result of natural age-related load bearing and wear-and-tear degeneration of the disc. This eventually progress to the destabilization stage, which is characterized by a loss of disc high and load-bearing capacity of the disc, resulting in an increased load to the zygapophyseal joints. This increase in transmitted load can lead to joint capsule laxity and the subluxation of the joints. Anterior translation of the rostral vertebral body with the caudal vertebral body can occur as a result of this instability. These movements of the vertebral body can result in narrowing of the neural foramina and the weakened joints result in an ever increasing load applied to already damaged discs, thus accelerating the process.

The restabilization stage occurs as a result of joint instability and bony movement. Osteophyte formation is observed between vertebral segments which combined with further degeneration and calcification can lead to fusion of the intervertebral level and loss of joint function. Although the motion segment becomes stabilized, the IVD essentially loses its functional characteristics, and represents the endpoint of the degenerative process.

Relationship to Back Pain

The lumbar intervertebral discs are supplied by a variety of nerves, notably receiving contributions from the sinuvertebral nerves, the ventral primary rami, and the recurrent branches of the rami communicantes (Bogduk, Tynan, and Wilson 1981). In the normal disc, only the superficial layers of the annulus fibrosus have sensory nerve endings, which achieve a depth of 3 mm and only involve the outer three lamellae (Roberts et al. 1995; Palmgren et al. 1999). However, in degenerative discs, nerve fibers have been observed to extend deeper — extension up to the inner third of the disc has been seen in 50% of painful degenerative discs (McCarthy et al. 1991). The ectopic nerve growth has been observed growing in a perivascular pattern, suggesting that they were induced by granulation tissue growing into the degenerative disc. Moreover, it is also thought that nerve fibers cannot withstand the high pressure environment of the normal disc, however, with the loss of pressure in degenerative discs, nerve fibers and capillaries are allowed to proliferate (Adams 2004).

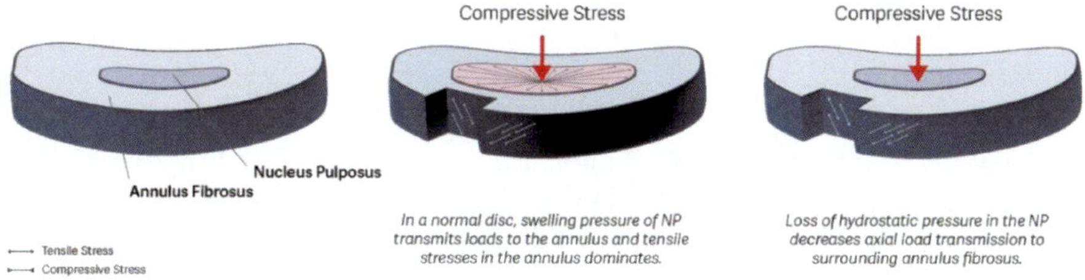

Figure 5. Loss of Swelling Pressure Alters the Biomechanical Properties of IVD.

Histological analysis of the degenerate disc showed substance-P and vasoactive intestinal polypeptide associated with granulation tissue which extended deep into the disc (Peng et al. 2005). Nerve histology was consistent with fibers associated with nociceptive function, and in one study, mechanoreceptors were found in 50% of patients with degenerative discs and back pain (Roberts et al. 1995). This suggests that in the presence of degeneration, the neural microenvironment is perturbed towards proliferation of sensory receptors such as Golgi tendon organs and Ruffini endings. Furthermore, exposed nuclear material is known to irritate the spinal nerve roots and possibly the sinuvertebral nerve, and inflammatory processes associated with degeneration can further cause granulation tissue accumulation, neovascularization, and nerve invasion (Kuslich, Ulstrom, and Michael 1991; Olmarker et al. 1995).

Conclusion

The intervertebral disc is a dynamic structure which plays an essential role in mitigating compressive loads sustained during upright posture and weight bearing activities. It is a complex structure with each unique component contributing to the overall function of the disc. Degenerative disc disease, either from normal aging, or from exposure to excessive loads cause changes both on the microscopic and anatomical level. These changes perturb the biomechanical properties of the IVD and because each part of the disc is intricately linked, failure of one component can lead to a degenerative cascade which cause gross functional and anatomical changes to the spine.

References

Acaroglu, E R, J C Iatridis, L A Setton, R J Foster, V C Mow, and M Weidenbaum. 1995. "Degeneration and Aging Affect the Tensile Behavior of Human Lumbar Anulus Fibrosus." *Spine* 20 (24): 2690–2701.

Adams, Michael A. 2004. "Biomechanics of Back Pain." *Acupuncture in Medicine* 22 (4). BMJ Publishing Group Ltd: 178–88. doi:10.1136/aim.22.4.178.

Antoniou, J, T Steffen, F Nelson, N Winterbottom, A P Hollander, R A Poole, M Aebi, and M Alini. 1996. "The Human Lumbar Intervertebral

Disc: Evidence for Changes in the Biosynthesis and Denaturation of the Extracellular Matrix with Growth, Maturation, Ageing, and Degeneration." *The Journal of Clinical Investigation* 98 (4). American Society for Clinical Investigation: 996–1003. doi:10.1172/JCI118884.

Berry, J L, J M Moran, W S Berg, and A D Steffee. 1987. "A Morphometric Study of Human Lumbar and Selected Thoracic Vertebrae." *Spine* 12 (4): 362–67.

Best, Barbara A, Farhid Guilak, Lori A Setton, Wenbo Zhu, Fatemeh Saed-Nejad, Anthony Ratcliffe, Mark Weidenbaum, and Van C Mow. 1994. "Compressive Mechanical Properties of the Human Anulus Fibrosus and Their Relationship to Biochemical Composition." *Spine* 19 (2): 212.

Bibby, Susan R S, Deborah A Jones, Robert B Lee, Jing Yu, and Jill P G Urban. 2001. "The Pathophysiology of the Intervertebral Disc." *Joint Bone Spine* 68 (6): 537–42. doi:10. 1016/S1297-319X(01)00332-3.

Bogduk, N, W Tynan, and A S Wilson. 1981. "The Nerve Supply to the Human Lumbar Intervertebral Discs." *Journal of Anatomy* 132 (Pt 1). Wiley-Blackwell: 39–56. doi:10. 1111/(ISSN)1469-7580.

Brinckmann, P, W Frobin, E Hierholzer, and M Horst. 1983. "Deformation of the Vertebral End-Plate Under Axial Loading of the Spine." *Spine* 8 (8): 851–56.

Broberg, K B. 1983. "On the Mechanical Behaviour of Intervertebral Discs." *Spine* 8 (2): 151.

Bruehlmann, Sabina B, Jerome B Rattner, John R Matyas, and Neil A Duncan. 2002. "Regional Variations in the Cellular Matrix of the Annulus Fibrosus of the Intervertebral Disc." *Journal of Anatomy* 201 (2). Blackwell Science Ltd: 159–71. doi:10.1046/j.1469-7580.2002.00080.x.

Buckwalter, J A. 1995. "Aging and Degeneration of the Human Intervertebral Disc." *Spine* 20 (11): 1307–14.

Buckwalter, J A, T A Einhorn, and S R Simon. 2000. *Orthopaedic Basic Science: Biology and Biomechanics of the Musculoskeletal System.*

Castagnera, L, and B Lavignolle. 1989. "Intrinsic Disc Pressure as a Measure of Integrity of the Lumbar Spine." *Spine* 14 (7): 777.

Conventry, M S, R K Ghormley, and J W Kernohan. 1945. The Intervertebral Disc: Its Microscopic Anatomy and Pathology: II Changes in the Intervertebral Disc Concomitant with Age. *J. Bone Joint Surg.*

Doers, Thomas M, and James D Kang. 1999. "The Biomechanics and Biochemistry of Disc Degeneration." *Current Opinion in Orthopedics* 10 (2): 117–21. doi:10.1097/00001433-199904000-00006.

Ebara, S, J C Iatridis, L A Setton, R J Foster, V C Mow, and M Weidenbaum. 1996. "Tensile Properties of Nondegenerate Human Lumbar Anulus Fibrosus." *Spine* 21 (4): 452–61.

Elliott, Dawn M, and Joseph J Sarver. 2004. "Young Investigator Award Winner: Validation of the Mouse and Rat Disc as Mechanical Models of the Human Lumbar Disc." *Spine* 29 (7): 713–22. doi:10.1097/01.BRS.0000116982.19331.EA.

Elliott, Dawn M, and Lori A Setton. 2001. "Anisotropic and Inhomogeneous Tensile Behavior of the Human Anulus Fibrosus: Experimental Measurement and Material Model Predictions." *Journal of Biomechanical Engineering* 123 (3). American Society of Mechanical Engineers: 256–63. doi:10.1115/1.1374202.

Eyre, D R, and H Muir. 1976. "Types I and II Collagens in Intervertebral Disc. Interchanging Radial Distributions in Annulus Fibrosus." *Biochemical Journal* 157 (1). Portland Press Limited: 267–70. doi:10.1042/bj1570267.

Feng, Haoyu, Mikael Danfelter, Björn Strömqvist, and Dick Heinegård. 2006. "Extracellular Matrix in Disc Degeneration." *J. Bone Joint Surg. Am.* 88 (suppl. 2). The American Orthopedic Association: 25–29. doi:10.2106/JBJS.E.01341.

Fujita, Yoshi, Neil A Duncan, and Jeffrey C Lotz. 1997. "Radial Tensile Properties of the Lumbar Annulus Fibrosus Are Site and Degeneration Dependent." *Journal of Orthopaedic Research: Official Publication of the Orthopaedic Research Society* 15 (6). Wiley Subscription Services, Inc., A Wiley Company: 814–19. doi:10.1002/jor.11001506 05.

Galante, J O. 1967. "Tensile Properties of the Human Lumbar Annulus Fibrosus." *Acta Orthopaedica Scandinavica*, Suppl. 100:1 Suppl. 100:91.

Grant, J P, Thomas R Oxland, Marcel F Dvorak, and Charles G Fisher. 2002. "The Effects of Bone Density and Disc Degeneration on the Structural Property Distributions in the Lower Lumbar Vertebral Endplates." *Journal of Orthopaedic Research: Official Publication of the Orthopaedic Research Society* 20 (5). Wiley Subscription Services, Inc., A Wiley Company: 1115–20. doi:10.1016/S0736-0266(02)00039-6.

Grant, J Pamela, Thomas R Oxland, and Marcel F Dvorak. 2001. "Mapping the Structural Properties of the Lumbosacral Vertebral Endplates." *Spine* 26 (8): 889.

Green, T P, M A Adams, and P Dolan. 1993. "Tensile Properties of the Annulus Fibrosus." *European Spine Journal* 2 (4). Springer-Verlag: 209–14. doi:10.1007/BF00299448.

Grignon, B, Y Grignon, D Mainard, M Braun, P Netter, and J Roland. 2000. "The Structure of the Cartilaginous End-Plates in Elder People." *Surgical and Radiologic Anatomy* 22 (1). Springer-Verlag: 13–19. doi:10.1007/s00276-000-0013-7.

Gu, W Y, X G Mao, R J Foster, M Weidenbaum, V C Mow, and B A Rawlins. 1999. "The Anisotropic Hydraulic Permeability of Human Lumbar Anulus Fibrosus. Influence of Age, Degeneration, Direction, and Water Content." *Spine* 24 (23): 2449–55.

Guerin, Heather Anne L, and Dawn M Elliott. 2006. "Degeneration Affects the Fiber Reorientation of Human Annulus Fibrosus Under Tensile Load." *Journal of Biomechanics* 39 (8): 1410–18. doi:10.1016/j.jbiomech.2005.04.007.

Haefeli, Mathias, Fabian Kalberer, Daniel Saegesser, Andreas G Nerlich, Norbert Boos, and Günther Paesold. 2006. "The Course of Macroscopic Degeneration in the Human Lumbar Intervertebral Disc." *Spine* 31 (14): 1522–31. doi:10.1097/01.brs.0000222032.52336.8e.

Hessle, H, and E Engvall. 1984. "Type VI Collagen. Studies on Its Localization, Structure, and Biosynthetic Form with Monoclonal Antibodies." *Journal of Biological Chemistry* 259 (6). American Society for Biochemistry and Molecular Biology: 3955–61.

Horner, Heather A, Sally Roberts, Robert C Bielby, Janis Menage, Helen Evans, and Jill P G Urban. 2002. "Cells From Different Regions of the Intervertebral Disc: Effect of Culture System on Matrix Expression and Cell Phenotype." *Spine* 27 (10): 1018.

Houben, Gerard B, Maarten R Drost, Jacques M Huyghe, Jan D Janssen, and Anthony Huson. 1997. "Nonhomogeneous Permeability of Canine Anulus Fibrosus." *Spine* 22 (1): 7.

Iatridis, J C, P L Mente, I A Stokes, D D Aronsson, and M Alini. 1999. "Compression-Induced Changes in Intervertebral Disc Properties in a Rat Tail Model." *Spine* 24 (10): 996–1002.

Iatridis, J C, S Kumar, R J Foster, M Weidenbaum, and V C Mow. 1999. "Shear Mechanical Properties of Human Lumbar Annulus Fibrosus." *Journal of Orthopaedic Research: Official Publication of the Orthopaedic Research Society* 17 (5). Wiley Subscription Services, Inc., A Wiley Company: 732–37. doi:10.1002/jor.1100170517.

Iatridis, James C, and Iolo ap Gwynn. 2004. "Mechanisms for Mechanical Damage in the Intervertebral Disc Annulus Fibrosus." *Journal of Biomechanics* 37 (8): 1165–75. doi:10. 1016/j.jbiomech.2003.12.026.

Iatridis, James C, Lori A Setton, Mark Weidenbaum, and Van C Mow. 1997a. "Alterations in the Mechanical Behavior of the Human Lumbar Nucleus Pulposus with Degeneration and Aging." *Journal of Orthopaedic Research: Official Publication of the Orthopaedic Research Society* 15 (2). Wiley Subscription Services, Inc., A Wiley Company: 318–22. doi:10.1002/jor.1100150224.

Iatridis, James C, Lori A Setton, Mark Weidenbaum, and Van C Mow. 1997b. "The Viscoelastic Behavior of the Non-Degenerate Human Lumbar Nucleus Pulposus in Shear." *Journal of Biomechanics* 30 (10): 1005–13. doi:10.1016/S0021-9290(97)00069-9.

Iatridis, James C, Lori A Setton, Robert J Foster, Bernard A Rawlins, Mark Weidenbaum, and Van C Mow. 1998. "Degeneration Affects the Anisotropic and Nonlinear Behaviors of Human Anulus Fibrosus in Compression." *Journal of Biomechanics* 31 (6): 535–44. doi:10.1016/S0021-9290(98)00046-3.

Iatridis, James C, Mark Weidenbaum, Lori A Setton, and Van C Mow. 1996. "Is the Nucleus Pulposus a Solid or a Fluid? Mechanical Behaviors of the Nucleus Pulposus of the Human Intervertebral Disc." *Spine* 21 (10): 1174.

Johannessen, Wade, and Dawn M Elliott. 2005. "Effects of Degeneration on the Biphasic Material Properties of Human Nucleus Pulposus in Confined Compression." *Spine* 30 (24): E724.

Kazarian, L E. 1975. "Creep Characteristics of the Human Spinal Column." *The Orthopedic Clinics of North America* 6 (1): 3–18.

Koeller, W, W Meier, and F Hartmann. 1984. "Biomechanical Properties of Human Intervertebral Discs Subjected to Axial Dynamic Compression: a Comparison of Lumbar and Thoracic Discs." *Spine* 9 (7): 725.

Kuslich, S D, C L Ulstrom, and C J Michael. 1991. "The Tissue Origin of Low Back Pain and Sciatica: a Report of Pain Response to Tissue Stimulation During Operations on the Lumbar Spine Using Local Anesthesia." *The Orthopedic Clinics of North America* 22 (2): 181–87.

Liu, Y K, V K Goel, Alf Dejong, G Njus, K Nishiyama, and J Buckwalter. 1985. "Torsional Fatigue of the Lumbar Intervertebral Joints." *Spine* 10 (10): 894.

Liu, Y King, Glen Njus, Joseph Buckwalter, and Koichi Wakano. 1983. "Fatigue Response of Lumbar Intervertebral Joints Under Axial Cyclic Loading." *Spine* 8 (8): 857.

Marchand, Francoise, and Abdul M Ahmed. 1990. "Investigation of the Laminate Structure of Lumbar Disc Anulus Fibrosus." *Spine* 15 (5): 402.

Maroudas, A, R A Stockwell, A Nachemson, and J Urban. 1975. "Factors Involved in the Nutrition of the Human Lumbar Intervertebral Disc: Cellularity and Diffusion of Glucose *in Vitro*." *Journal of Anatomy* 120 (Pt 1). Wiley-Blackwell: 113–30.

McCarthy, P W, B Carruthers, D Martin, and P Films Petts. 1991. "Immunohistochemical Demonstration of Sensory Nerve Fibers and Endings in Lumbar Intervertebral Discs of the Rat." *Spine* 16 (6): 653.

McNally, D S, and M A Adams. 1992. "Internal Intervertebral Disc Mechanics as Revealed by Stress Profilometry." *Spine* 17 (1): 66–73.

Nachemson, A, and J M Morris. 1964. "*In Vivo* Measurements of Intradiscal Pressure. Discometry, a Method for the Determination of Pressure in the Lower Lumbar Discs." *J. Bone Joint Surg. Am.* 46 (5). The American Orthopedic Association: 1077–92.

Natarajan, R N, J H Ke, and G B J Andersson. 1994. "A Model to Study the Disc Degeneration Process." *Spine* 19 (3): 259.

Natarajan, Raghu N, Jamie R Williams, and Gunnar B J Andersson. 2006. "Modeling Changes in Intervertebral Disc Mechanics with Degeneration." *J. Bone Joint Surg. Am.* 88 Suppl. 2 (suppl. 2). The American Orthopedic Association: 36–40. doi:10.2106/JBJS. F.00002.

O'Connell, Grace D, Heather L Guerin, and Dawn M Elliott. 2009. "Theoretical and Uniaxial Experimental Evaluation of Human Annulus Fibrosus Degeneration." *Journal of Biomechanical Engineering* 131 (11). American Society of Mechanical Engineers: 111007. doi:10.1115/ 1.3212104.

Olmarker, K, J Blomquist, J Strömberg, U Nannmark, P Thomsen, and B Rydevik. 1995. "Inflammatogenic Properties of Nucleus Pulposus." *Spine* 20 (6): 665.

Palmgren, Tove, Mats Grönblad, Johanna Virri, Eeva Kääpä, and Erkki Karaharju. 1999. "An Immunohistochemical Study of Nerve Structures in the Anulus Fibrosus of Human Normal Lumbar Intervertebral Discs." *Spine* 24 (20): 2075.

Peng, B, W Wu, S Hou, P Li, C Zhang, and Y Yang. 2005. "The Pathogenesis of Discogenic Low Back Pain." *The Journal of Bone and Joint Surgery. British Volume* 87 (1). Bone and Joint Journal: 62–67. doi:10.1302/0301-620X.87B1.15708.

Perey, O. 1957. "Fracture of the Vertebral End-Plate in the Lumbar Spine: an Experimental Biomechanical Investigation." *Acta Orthopaedica Scandinavica*.

Poole, C Anthony. 1997. "Review. Articular Cartilage Chondrons: Form, Function and Failure." *Journal of Anatomy* 191 (1). Blackwell Science Ltd: 1–13. doi:10.1046/j.1469-7580.1997.19110001.x.

Poole, C Anthony, Michael H Flint, and Brent W Beaumont. 1988. "Chondrons Extracted From Canine Tibial Cartilage: Preliminary Report on Their Isolation and Structure." *Journal of Orthopaedic Research : Official Publication of the Orthopaedic Research Society* 6 (3). Wiley Subscription Services, Inc., A Wiley Company: 408–19. doi:10.1002/jor.1100060312.

Raj, P Prithvi. 2008. "Intervertebral Disc: Anatomy-Physiology-Pathophysiology-Treatment." *Pain Practice* 8 (1). Blackwell Publishing Inc: 18–44. doi:10.1111/j.1533-2500.2007.00171.x.

Roberts, S, J Menage, and J P G URBAN. 1989. "Biochemical and Structural Properties of the Cartilage End-Plate and Its Relation to the Intervertebral Disc." *Spine* 14 (2): 166.

Roberts, S, S M Eisenstein, J Menage, E H Evans, and I K Ashton. 1995. "Mechanoreceptors in Intervertebral Discs. Morphology, Distribution, and Neuropeptides." *Spine* 20 (24): 2645–51.

Roberts, Sally, Helena Evans, Jayesh Trivedi, and Janis Menage. 2006. "Histology and Pathology of the Human Intervertebral Disc." *J. Bone Joint Surg. Am.* 88 (suppl. 2). The American Orthopedic Association: 10–14. doi:10.2106/JBJS.F.00019.

Rombers, S, J Menage, V Duance, S Wotton, and S Ayad. 1991. Collagen Types Around the Cells of the Intervertebral Disc and Cartilage End Plate: an Immunolocalization Study. *Spine*.

Roughley, Peter J. 2004. "Biology of Intervertebral Disc Aging and Degeneration: Involvement of the Extracellular Matrix." *Spine* 29 (23): 2691–99. doi:10.1097/01.brs. 0000146101.53784.b1.

Sato, Katsuhiko, Shinichi Kikuchi, and Takumi Yonezawa. 1999. "*In Vivo* Intradiscal Pressure Measurement in Healthy Individuals and in Patients with Ongoing Back Problems." *Spine* 24 (23): 2468.

Schollum, Meredith L, Peter A Robertson, and Neil D Broom. 2010. "How Age Influences Unravelling Morphology of Annular Lamellae – a Study of Interfibre Cohesivity in the Lumbar Disc." *Journal of Anatomy* 216 (3). Blackwell Publishing Ltd: 310–19. doi:10. 1111/j.1469-7580. 2009.01197.x.

Sen, Sounok, John I Boxberger, Yvonne Schroeder, Alejandro Espinoza Orias, and Dawn M Elliott. 2008. "Effect of Degeneration on the Dynamic Viscoelastic Properties of Human Annulus Fibrosus in Tension." *ASME*

2008 Summer Bioengineering Conference, June. American Society of Mechanical Engineers, 609–10. doi:10.1115/SBC2008-193057.

Setton, Lori A, and Jun Chen. 2006. "Mechanobiology of the Intervertebral Disc and Relevance to Disc Degeneration." *J. Bone Joint Surg. Am.* 88 Suppl. 2 (suppl. 2). *The Journal of Bone and Joint Surgery*, Inc.: 52–57. doi:10.2106/JBJS.F.00001.

Setton, Lori A, Wenbo Zhu, Mark Weidenbaum, Anthony Ratcliffe, and Van C Mow. 1993. "Compressive Properties of the Cartilaginous End-Plate of the Baboon Lumbar Spine." *Journal of Orthopaedic Research: Official Publication of the Orthopaedic Research Society* 11 (2). Wiley Subscription Services, Inc., A Wiley Company: 228–39. doi:10.1002/jor.1100110210.

Shiraz-Adl, A. 1989. "Strain in Fibers of a Lumbar Disc: Analysis of the Role of Lifting in Producing Disc Prolapse." *Spine* 14 (1): 96.

Skaggs, D L, M Weidenbaum, J C Iatridis, A Ratcliffe, and V C Mow. 1994. "Regional Variation in Tensile Properties and Biochemical Composition of the Human Lumbar Anulus Fibrosus." *Spine* 19 (12): 1310–19.

Söder, S, L Hambach, R Lissner, T Kirchner, and T Aigner. 2002. "Ultrastructural Localization of Type VI Collagen in Normal Adult and Osteoarthritic Human Articular Cartilage." *Osteoarthritis and Cartilage* 10 (6): 464–70. doi:10.1053/joca.2002.0512.

Spilker, R L, D M Jakobs, and A B Schultz. 1986. "Material Constants for a Finite Element Model of the Intervertebral Disk with a Fiber Composite Annulus." *Journal of Biomechanical Engineering* 108 (1). American Society of Mechanical Engineers: 1–11. doi:10.1115/1.3138575.

Stokes, Ian A F, and James C Iatridis. 2004. "Mechanical Conditions That Accelerate Intervertebral Disc Degeneration: Overload Versus Immobilization." *Spine* 29 (23): 2724–32. doi:10.1097/01.brs.0000146049.52152.da.

Twomey, L, and J Taylor. 1982. "Flexion Creep Deformation and Hysteresis in the Lumbar Vertebral Column." *Spine* 7 (2): 116.

Urban, J P G, and J F McMullin. 1988. "Swelling Pressure of the Lumbar Intervertebral Discs: Influence of Age, Spinal Level, Composition, and Degeneration." *Spine* 13 (2): 179.

Urban, J P, and J F McMullin. 1985. "Swelling Pressure of the Inervertebral Disc: Influence of Proteoglycan and Collagen Contents." *Biorheology* 22 (2): 145–57.

Urban, J, and A Maroudas. 1980. The Chemistry of the Intervertebral-Disk in Relation to Its Physiological-Function and Requirements. *Clinics in ...*

Wagner, Diane R, and Jeffrey C Lotz. 2004. "Theoretical Model and Experimental Results for the Nonlinear Elastic Behavior of Human Annulus Fibrosus." *Journal of Orthopaedic Research: Official Publication of the Orthopaedic Research Society* 22 (4). Wiley Subscription Services, Inc., A Wiley Company: 901–9. doi:10.1016/j.orthres.2003.12. 012.

Wilke, Hans-Joachim, Peter Neef, Marco Caimi, Thomas Hoogland, and Lutz E Claes. 1999. "New *in Vivo* Measurements of Pressures in the Intervertebral Disc in Daily Life." *Spine* 24 (8): 755.

Yao, Hai, Marc-Antoine Justiz, Daniel Flagler, and Wei Yong Gu. 2002. "Effects of Swelling Pressure and Hydraulic Permeability on Dynamic Compressive Behavior of Lumbar Annulus Fibrosus." *Annals of Biomedical Engineering* 30 (10). Kluwer Academic Publishers-Plenum Publishers: 1234–41. doi:10.1114/1.1523920.

Yin, Luzhong, and Dawn M Elliott. 2005. "A Homogenization Model of the Annulus Fibrosus." *Journal of Biomechanics* 38 (8): 1674–84. doi:10.1016/j.jbiomech.2004.07. 017.

Yong-Hing, K, and W H Kirkaldy-Willis. 1983. "The Pathophysiology of Degenerative Disease of the Lumbar Spine." *The Orthopedic Clinics of North America* 14 (3): 491–504.

Yu, Jing, Peter C Winlove, Sally Roberts, and Jill P G Urban. 2002. "Elastic Fibre Organization in the Intervertebral Discs of the Bovine Tail." *Journal of Anatomy* 201 (6). Wiley-Blackwell: 465–75. doi:10.1046/j.1469-7580.2002.00111.x.

Zirbel, Shannon A, Dean K Stolworthy, Larry L Howell, and Anton E Bowden. 2013. "Intervertebral Disc Degeneration Alters Lumbar Spine Segmental Stiffness in All Modes of Loading Under a Compressive Follower Load." *The Spine Journal* 13 (9): 1134–47. doi:10.1016/j.spinee.2013.02.010.

In: Intervertebral Disc Degeneration
Editors: A. L. Ho and A. M. Desai
ISBN: 978-1-63485-829-8

Chapter 4

CERVICAL STENOSIS

Thomas Kosztowski[1], MD, Adetokunbo Oyelese[2], MD, PhD and Ziya Gokaslan[2,*], MD

[1]Department of Neurosurgery, Johns Hopkins University School of Medicine, Baltimore, Maryland, US

[2]Department of Neurosurgery, Warren Alpert Medical School of Brown University, Providence, Rhode Island, US

ABSTRACT

Cervical stenosis involves the narrowing of the spinal canal in the cervical spinal region. Cervical spondylosis is oftentimes used synonomously with cervical stenosis, but spondylosis implies age-related degeneration of the spine including congenital spinal stenosis, degeneration of intervertebral discs resulting in focal stenosis, and hypertrophy of spinal elements resulting in narrowing of the spinal canal. One of the most debilitating conditions associated with cervical stenosis is cervical spondylotic myelopathy. Multiple treatments including surgical and non-surgical options are available. However, once symptoms of cervical spondylotic myelopathy are severe, surgery becomes necessary to treat the cervical stenosis.

* Corresponding author: Ziya Gokaslan (ziya_gokaslan@brown.edu), Department of Neurosurgery, Warren Alpert Medical School, Brown University, Providence, Rhode Island.

Keywords: cervical spondylotic myelopathy, cervical stenosis, cervical spondylosis, anterior cervical disketomy and fusion, posterior cervical decompression and fusion

Introduction

Cervical stenosis results from a narrowing of the spinal canal. This can occur secondary to a multitude of conditions, but most commonly, it is related to degenerative diseases of the spine. Cervical spondylosis is used interchageably with the term cervical stenosis, but it is important to understand that spondylosis implies widespread age-related degeneration of the spine. This chapter will focus on cervical stenosis related to degenerative processes. Cervical spondylosis can ultimately lead to cervical spondylotic myelopathy (CSM) and it is the most common cause of myelopathy and spinal cord dysfunction in patients older than 55 years [10].

Causes

Multiple different degenerative conditions lead to cervical spondylosis and subsequent stenosis. Some patients are born with congenital stenosis of the cervical spine predisposing them to cervical spondylotic myelopathy. But for most, cervical stenosis results from the accumulation of degenerative changes. Degeneration of the intervertebral discs can lead to protrusion or herniation of disc material resulting in focal stenosis. Hypertrophy of the articular facets, ligaments, lamina, or even dura can also result in stenosis (Figure 1). With regards to the ligaments, hypertrophy of the ligamentum flavum can lead to worsened stenosis in neck extension due to the buckling of the ligament. This has been demonstrated on cadaveric and MRI studies [37]. Anterior to the spinal cord, ossification of the posterior longitudinal ligament (OPLL) may also contribute to stenosis often times involving multiple levels. Herniated disc material may often times be seen in combination with osteophytic spurs. Subluxation secondary to facet joint and disc degeneration may also result in cervical stenosis. Severely spondylotic levels can eventually lead to autofusion, which can result in hypermobility at adjacent spinal segments and subsequent narrowing of the spinal canal. If the vertebral bodies lose height, this can result in telescoping of the spine and shingling of the laminae.

Loss of cervical lordosis is also a significant contributor to cervical stenosis and cervical spondylotic myelopathy. Thus, as the cervical spine straightens out or even becomes kyphotic, the spinal cord is forced against the vertebral bodies inducing anterior cord pathology and increasing the longitudinal cord tension on the spinal cord, which is tethered by the dentate ligaments and cervical nerve roots. Over time, as the curve of the spinal canal deviates further away from its natural lordotic curvature, the anterior and posterior margins of the cord compress, and the lateral margins expand (Figure 2) [2].

PATHOPHYSIOLOGY

Musculoskeletal structures that bear weight, such as the cervical spine, can develop spondylitic (osteoarthritic) changes. These spondylytic changes result in hypertrophy of osteophytes, articular facets, and ligaments, which narrow the spinal canal. Cervical stenosis can be accompanied by axial neck pain and radiculopathy. However, myelopathy is the most important and potentially most dangerous complication of cervical stenosis that the physician must be aware of.

Cervical myelopathy that results from cervical stenosis in the cervical spine is known as cervical spondylotic myelopathy (CSM). Myelomalacia demonstrating cord signal changes on MRI is the radiographic counterpart of myelopathy. The primary pathophysiological mechanism resulting in myelopathy is static mechanical compression of the spinal cord resulting in increased spinal cord tension and reduced vascular supply [40]. There is also a dynamic component involved from repeated microtrauma from segmental instability. Patients with cervical spinal stenosis are also at higher risk of developing myelopathy or deterioration of already existing myelopathy in the event of hyperextension of the neck [57].

CLINICAL PRESENTATION

The majority of people greater than 50 years of age will have radiologic evidence of degenerative disease of the spine, however, only a small number actually experience pain and/or neurologic symptoms. The signs and symptoms related to cervical stenosis may be characterized as nerve root compression, spinal cord compression, and idiopathic pain of the head, neck and shoulders.

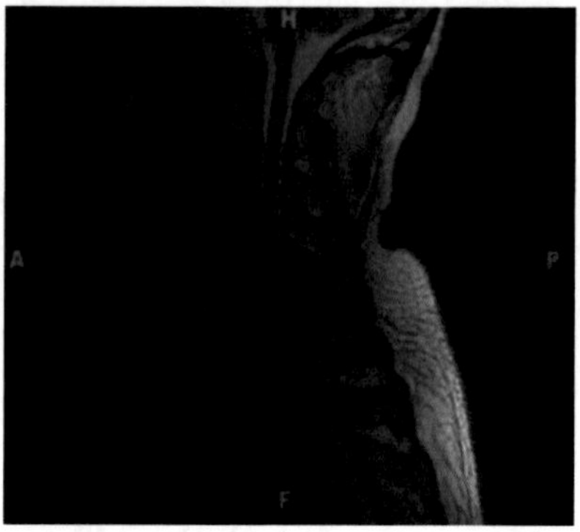

Figure 1. Cervical Stenosis.

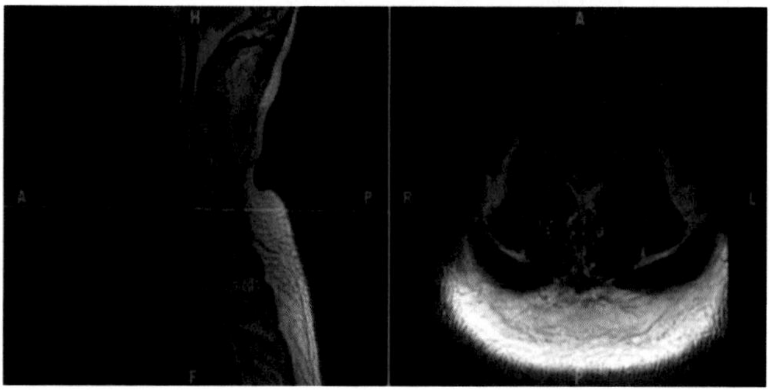

Figure 2. Spinal Cord Changes.

Nerve root compression may be related to cervical stenosis, and the offending element (e.g., herniated intervertebral disc) causes stenosis of both the spinal canal as well as the neural foramen. This may result in weakness of the muscles of the arms (C5-T1 innervation) in the affected myotomes. It may also result in paresthesia or hyperesthesia in the affected dermatomes. In fact, sensory involvement is more common than motor or reflex changes.

Patients with cervical myelopathy often present with paresthesias, dyskinesias, or weakness of the upper or lower extremities. Other symptoms of cervical myelopathy include upper motor neuron involvement, including hyperreflexia, gait problems, balance difficulty, bladder dysfunction, and loss of dexterity. The Nurick classification scheme is an important score for evaluating the severity of cervical spondylotic myelopathy ranging from zero to five: grade 0, for only nerve root symptoms or normal; grade 1, for evidence of spinal cord compression but no gait problems; grade 2, for gait difficulty but able to fulfill activities of daily living (ADL's) and employment; grade 3, for gait difficulties affecting employment but the patient not requiring any assistance with ambulation; grade 4, if the patient requires assisted ambulation; and grade 5, if wheelchair bound (Table 1) [41]. The Ranawat clinical grading system is a similar score for assessing cervical myelopathy, but it is used in rheumatoid arthritis patients [43]. The Japanese Orthopedic Association proposed a scale for cervical myelopathy that has been utilized heavily in clinical studies because it is able to assess the four functions that are most commonly affected in cervical myelopathy: motor strength in the upper extremities (including dexterity), motor strength in the lower extremities (including ambulatory status), sensation, and bladder function [21]. The JOA scale is based on a seventeen point scale, with seventeen indicating normal. However, a limitation of the scale in its application to Western cultures was that it assesses manual dexterity with use of chopsticks. Thus, modified versions have been proposed so that the scale is more applicable to Western cultures. A very important scale that is heavily used today is the modified Japanese Orthopedic Association scale (mJOA) [3]. There are a few versions of the mJOA. One version was proposed by Benzel et al. (Table 2), whereas another was proposed by Chiles et al. [8]. In the version proposed by Benzel et al., the ability to button a shirt is used to substitute for chopstick handling, whereas the version proposed by Chiles assesses the ability to handle a knife and fork.

There is variation in regards to the progression of CSM [9, 30]. In almost 75% cases, patients experience exacerbations interrupted by periods of stable neurologic function, which can last years in some cases. Another 20% of patients experience a steady disease progression. Only 5% of patients suffer from a rapid progression of CSM.

Table 1. Nurick Disability Classification for Cervical Spondylotic Myelopathy [41]

Grade	Description
0	Root signs and symptoms, but no spinal cord involvement
1	Normal gait, signs of spinal cord involvement
2	Mild gait involvement, able to work employed still
3	Gait abnormality that prevents employment
4	Able to ambulate only with assistance
5	Wheelchair-bound or bedridden

Table 2. Modified Japanese Orthopedic Association Scale (Benzel version) for Cervical Spondylotic Myelopathy Functional Assessment [3]

Score	Definition
Motor dysfunction score of the upper extremities	
0	Inability to more the hands
1	Inability to eat with a spoon, but able to move hands
2	Inability to button shirt, but able to eat with spoon
3	Able to button shirt with great difficulty
4	Able to button shirt with slight difficulty
5	No dysfunction
Motor dysfunction of the lower extremities	
0	Complete loss of motor and sensory function
1	Sensory preservation without the ability to move the legs
2	Able to move the legs but unable to walk
3	Able to walk on flat floor with a walking aid (e.g., crutch or cane)
4	Able to walk up and/or down stairs with hand rail
5	Moderate to significant lack of stability, but able to walk up and/or down stairs without hand rail
6	Mild lack of stability but walks with smooth reciprocation unaided
7	No dysfunction
Sensory dysfunction score of the upper extremities	
0	Complete loss of hand sensation
1	Severe sensory loss or pain
2	Mild sensory loss
3	No sensory loss
Sphincter dysfunction score	
0	Inability to micturate voluntarily
1	Marked difficulty with micturition
2	Mild to moderate difficulty with micturition
3	Normal micturition

RADIOGRAPHIC EVALUATION

Although cervical x-rays were performed in the past, they serve little utility in the diagnosis and evaluation of cervical stenosis today. The primary imaging modalities in the evaluation of cervical stenosis are magnetic resonance imaging (MRI) and computed tomography (CT) imaging.

MRI is the most helpful diagnostic modality in the evaluation of stenosis. It is able to capture many of the pathologies that contribute to canal stenosis, especially soft tissue pathology. It also can rule out other pathologies such as tumor or Chiari malformation. When assessing for degenerative changes, the MRI should be evaluated for herniated discs encroaching on the spinal canal or the neural foramina. MRI can identify hypertrophic ligamentum flavum or PLL causing compression on the spinal cord. In the case of OPLL, a hypertrophic PLL may be seen, but CT is helpful in visualizing the calcification in the ligament and making the diagnosis. MRI is able to provide essential information about the spinal cord including signs of edema, spinal cord atrophy, demyelination, and syringomyelia. It can be used to evaluate the degree of spinal cord compression by assessing the cord ratio, CSF effacement, and the degree and extent of myelomalacia. Hyperintense signals on MRI may be indicative of spinal cord edema and neuronal death. These signal changes are known as myelomalacia. Myelomalacia findings on MRI have been found to be associated with a higher degree of clinical disability and are a poor prognostic factor that the patient will experience neurologic recovery following surgery [34, 36]. Spinal cord signal changes should be scrutinized as this will influence whether a patient will need surgery and how soon. Furthermore, MRI allows the evaluation of extent of compression (how many levels are involved) and whether the pathology is primarily anterior, posterior, or both in relation to the spinal cord. Studies have shown that normal mid-sagittal spinal canal diameter measures about 17 mm in depth whereas the normal average spinal cord diameter is 8-13 mm in the anteroposterior plane [12, 39]. Soft tissue structures, including the anterior and posterior longitudinal ligaments and the ligamentum flavum, can add an additional 2-3 mm to the spinal canal contents [5]. Relative stenosis is narrowing of the canal to 13 mm, whereas absolute stenosis is classifies as narrowing of the spinal canal to 10 mm [13]. If there is a contraindication to obtaining an MRI, then a CT myelogram can be performed.

CT myelography may be very useful in situations that a patient cannot undergo an MRI. This study can find if there are focal areas of stenosis and if there are levels of myelographic block. CT may also be useful in the evaluation of cervical stenosis in regards to the bone elements. It is able to provide spinal canal dimensions and suggest spinal canal or neural canal stenosis based on the measurements of the boney structures but it is not helpful in evaluating the extent that neural structures are affected by the stenosis. CT can also be very helpful in differentiating osteophytes from herniated discs, both of which may look alike on MRI. Like MRI, CT can also evaluate the coronal and sagittal alignment of the cervical spine, although standing plain films are most appropriate for evaluating global spinal balance.

TREATMENT OPTIONS

The physician must carefully consider both the clinical presentation as well as the radiographic imaging to determine whether a patient can be managed conservatively or requires surgery. Radiographic findings may not always correlate with the clinical picture, and, thus, a patient may have very concerning radiographic findings without severe clinical symptoms or signs. Furthermore, spondylotic changes may be present in up to 60% of asymptomatic individuals depending on age [4, 54].

Non-Surgical Options

Non-operative treatment options are reserved for patients primarily complaining of neck or radicular pain without any neurologic deficits or radiographic signs of myelopathy. There have been many studies that have studied the role of surgery or conservative management in the setting of asymptomatic cervical spondylotic myelopathy despite radiographic evidence of severe stenosis [23, 48]. Kadanka et al. performed a prospective, randomized and blinded clinical study of patients with non-progressing or very slowly progressing mild and moderate forms of CSM (mJOA score C 12 points). Patients were randomized into two treatment arms: 1) conservative and 2) surgical. At 10-year follow, the authors suggested that conservative and surgical treatment in mild and moderate forms of CSM had not shown, on average, a significant difference in outcomes such as modified Japanese Orthopedic Scale (mJOA) and in subjective evaluation of the patients themselves [23].

Prolonged immobilization with rigid cervical bracing is occasionally utilized to reduce neck movement with the hope of reducing trauma to the cervical spine. Patients may also be recommended to reduce their activity and eliminate “high risk” activities. Lastly, patient may also try anti-inflammatory medications to see if there is any benefit to the neck pain. In formulating a management strategy, patient factors such as level of activity, age, and risk of injury should be considered in formulating a management plan.

Surgical Options

Surgical intervention is the appropriate treatment for advanced cases of CSM with severe symptoms. Patients who develop moderate to severe symptoms of CSM are unlikely to experience regression of their myelopathy. Surgical intervention is considered to alter the natural progression of the disease and prevent further neurologic deterioration. Progression of symptoms, presence of myelopathy for more than 6 months, transverse area of the spinal cord less than 40 mm^2, and compression ratio approaching 0.4 are all poor prognostic factors that conservative treatment will be successful [29]. These factors are indicators for surgical management [29]. The goals of surgery are to decompress the spinal cord, stabilize the spinal column, and re-establish normal sagittal alignment. Preoperative findings that have been found to be associated with successful surgical outcome include younger age at presentation, presence of Lhermitte sign, presence of unilateral symptoms, duration of symptoms less than a year, and pathological involvement limited to fewer levels [35]. Surgical decompression helps to alleviate preoperative pain and paresthesia associated with CSM [15]. Anterior and posterior surgical approaches may be used depending on the pathology and its association to the spinal cord [14]. Other factors that influence whether an anterior and/or posterior approach is appropriate include the number of levels involved, the patient's overall medical status, and the overall alignment and mobility of the spine.

Anterior Surgical Options

Anterior pathologies such as herniated discs, spondylotic bars, and uncovertebral osteophytes can contribute to spinal stenosis in the cervical spine. The anterior approach can be used to directly ventrally decompress the spinal cord and nerve roots. In regards to anterior approaches, anterior cervical discectomy and fusion (ACDF) is commonly the procedure of choice especially when the source of stenosis is discogenic and restricted to one or two levels (Figure 3) [27, 56]. Some argue that ACDF should be restricted to the treatment of cervical spondylosis of no more than 3 levels. With more extensive compression, posterior procedures should be used [56]. Furthermore, sagittal alignment abnormalities resulting in loss of normal cervical lordosis or kypothic deformity are indications for an anterior approach [50, 52]. Anterior cervical corpectomy and fusion (ACCF) may be considered in cases of more extensive compression to the spinal cord along with focal kyphosis in that segment of the cervical spine (Figure 4). Thus, the anterior approach allows direct decompression of ventral compressive pathology, fusion of instable segments, and possible restoration of the cervical lordosis.

The literature suggests that ACDF is associated with good outcomes for patients with CSM. As high as 90% improvement in overall neurologic outcome and functional status have been observed [55, 59]. In regards to long-term outcomes, Irvine and Strachan retrospectively evaluated patients who had undergone ACDF for CSM with an average of ten years follow-up and found that at last follow-up, 78% of the patients had improved ambulation. Only 9% of patients experienced progression of symptoms [22]. In regards to fusion, autologous bone graft remains the gold standard for fusion in ACDF. An 85% fusion rate was observed when autogenous bone graft was used, whereas a 50% fusion rate when allograft was used [59]. However, autologous bone graft harvest has been associated with a significant morbidity rate of 20% including hip fracture, hematoma, seroma, infection, and meralgia paresthetica [51]. This has resulted in the preferred use of allogeneic bone graft.

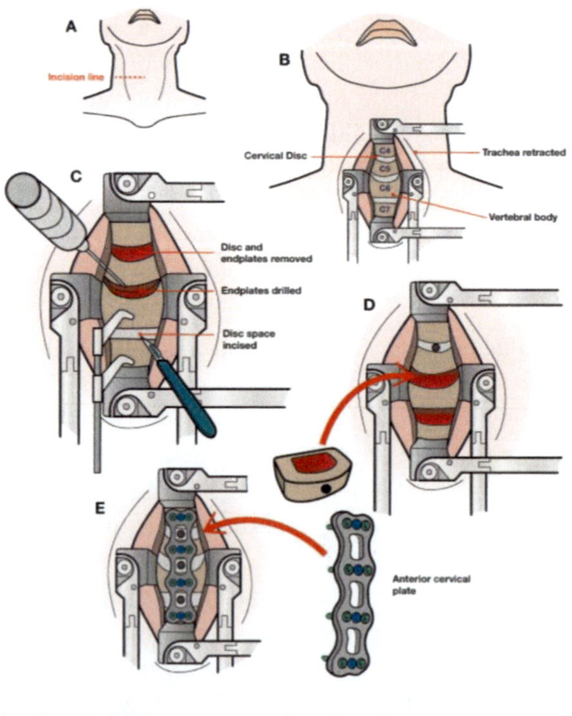

Figure 3. Anterior Cervical Discectomy and Fusion (ACDF).

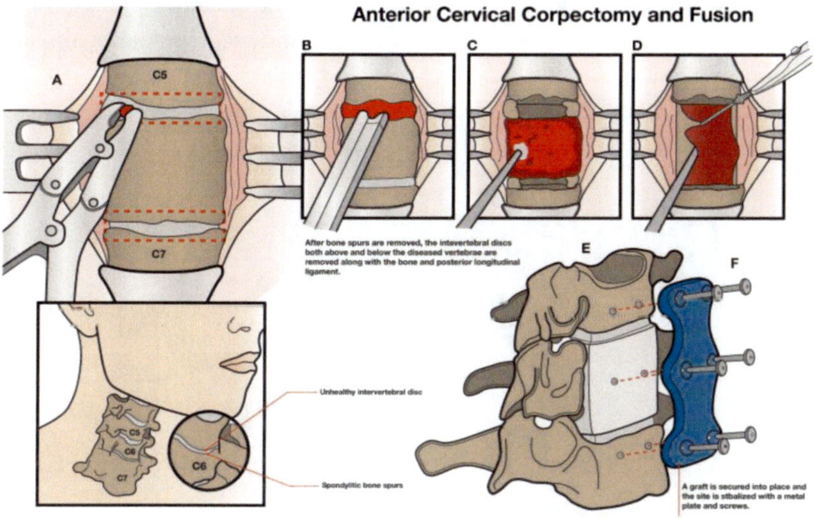

Figure 4. Anterior Cervical Corpectomy and Fusion (ACCF).

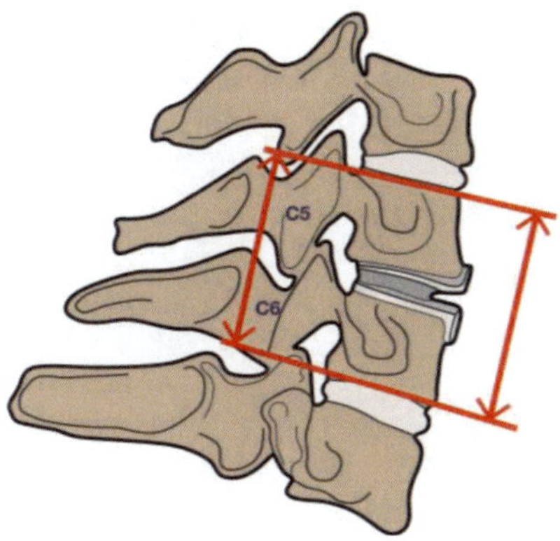

Figure 5. Anterior Cervical Disc Arthroplasty (ACDA).

Another option with increasing popularity is anterior cervical disc arthroplasty (ACDA) (Figure 5). ACDA has been demonstrated to improve clinical outcomes and segmental motion with long-term follow-up [6]. ACDA efficacy has been demonstrated in clinical outcomes, stability, and preservation of index level motion [16, 38]. It has been suggested that anterior fusion may increase the stresses at adjacent levels and thus accelerate adjacent segment disease, whereas total disc replacement (TDR) better preserves motion at the index level [11, 47]. However, thus far, studies comparing ACDF to ACDA have not found any significant difference in adjacent segment disease after surgery [6, 33]. Problems like heterotopic ossification, implant migration, device wear and failure, and segmental kyphosis are potential complications [31, 42].

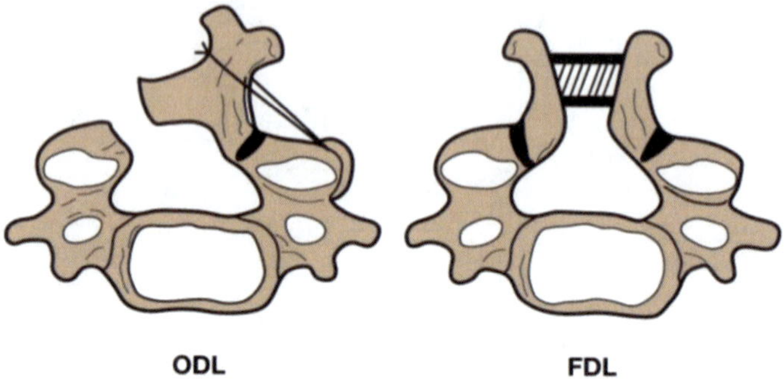

Figure 6. Open Door Laminoplasty (ODL) and French Door Laminoplasty (FDL).

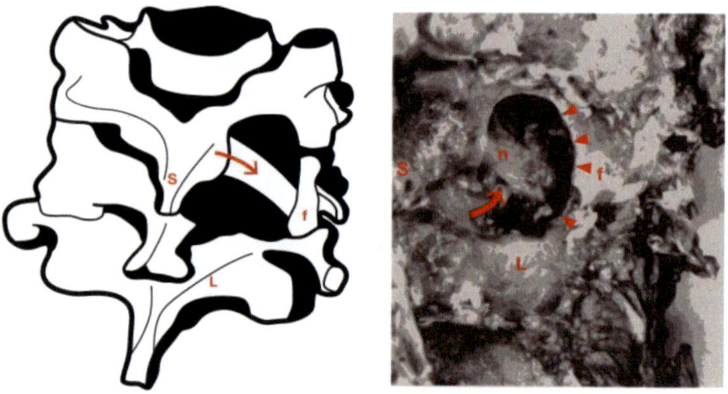

Figure 7. Facet Resection Over Twenty Five Percent.

Posterior Cervical Approaches

The posterior approach has proven to be a safe and effective option in the surgical treatment of CSM (Figures 10, 11, 12). It is indicated for congenital OPLL, ossification of the ligamentum flavum, congenital cervical stenosis, multilevel spondylosis, and posterior compression by a hypertrophied and in-folding ligamentum flavum. The posterior approach provides for direct and indirect compression of the neural elements. If the elements contributing to CSM are ventral to the spinal cord, a posterior decompression indirectly decompresses the spinal cord. In other situations where myelopathy is a consequence of congenital stenosis or posterior compression from redundant ligamentum flavum, the posterior approach allows the surgeon to directly decompress the spinal cord. In order to decompress posteriorly, it is important that the preoperative cervical spinal alignment be neutral or lordotic to allow for posterior translation of the spinal cord after decompression [1]. Some argue that a cervical lordosis of at least ten degrees should be present if posterior decompression is to be considered [17].

Laminectomy is the most common means of decompressing the spinal cord from a posterior approach. It is indicated in cases of multi-level compression in elderly patients or patients with multiple comorbidities. Patients must also have some cervical lordosis as instrumentation can only correct alignment to a certain degree. Laminectomies are performed with decompression to the extent of the junction between the lamina and the lateral mass. Decompression should include all levels that exhibit stenosis on imaging. It has been reported that there is no benefit to limiting the number of levels decompressed when it comes to development of post-laminectomy kyphosis or instability [24]. There are increased rates of recurrent symptoms resulting from disease progression at adjacent segments not involved in the initial decompression [25]. Instrumentation may be necessary after laminectomy. Factors that influence the need for posterior cervical instrumentation include focal and/or iatrogenic instability and flexible kyphosis. Instrumentation is used to stabilize the spine until a mature bony fusion mass forms. Posterior instrumentation helps maintain cervical lordosis and decreases the chances of post-laminectomy kyphosis [19, 28].

Studies have demonstrated that laminectomy is an effective procedure in the treatment of elderly myelopathic patients found to have multilevel cervical spondylosis and lordotic cervical alignment. In one study by Snow and Weiner, of 90 patients who were treated with laminectomy, 77% had neurologic improvement, 13% remained unchanged, and 10% had neurologic deterioration [49]. In another study of 32 patients treated with multi-level cervical laminectomies and instrumented fusion, Huang et al. found a post-operative improvement in Nurick score of at least one grade in 71% of patients [20]. In the study, the other 29% experienced no improvement in Nurick score, and no patients experienced deterioration in the Nurick score.

Laminoplasty is another option of attaining decompression posteriorly, while maintaining cervical alignment and stability through preservation of the posterior spinal elements. Laminoplasty may avoid the potential complications related to instrumented fusion including implant malposition and/or failure and adjacent segment accelerated degeneration. Laminoplasty is indicated in congenital stenosis, OPLL, multi-level disc herniations, and spondylosis. However, the spine should be in a neutral or lordotic cervical alignment. Numerous laminoplasty techniques have been described, including French-door [53] and open-door laminoplasty techniques (Figure 6) [18]. All these techniques involve decompression of spinal canal stenosis through the expansion of the posterior arch with preservation of the posterior elements and of segmental motion. With preservation of the posterior tension band, laminoplasty is rarely associated with iatrogenic instability. Studies have demonstrated a 54% improvement in the JOA scores of patients who underwent laminoplasty. However, with this technique, one must be mindful of closure of the laminoplasty [46], continued thickening of the ligamentum flavum [46] and of an ossified OPLL [26] that may lead to neurologic deficits from root or cord irritation/injury [45].

If the patient has nerve root symptoms, selective foraminotomies may be performed. In cases of selective nerve root compression from lateral herniated disc without any spinal cord compression, foraminotomies may be considered. However, selective posterior foraminotomies had been reported to have reoperation rates of 18.3% and 24.3% at 2 and 10 years, respectively [7]. Studies suggest that when ACDF and posterior cervical foraminotomy are compared, the reoperation rates are statistically equivalent [32]. It must also be noted that if too aggressive of a facet resection is performed that foraminotomy may result in post-operative instability eventually and require fusion [58]. Thus, it is imperative to try to limit facet resection to no more than 25% of the joint to preserve stability (Figure 7) [44].

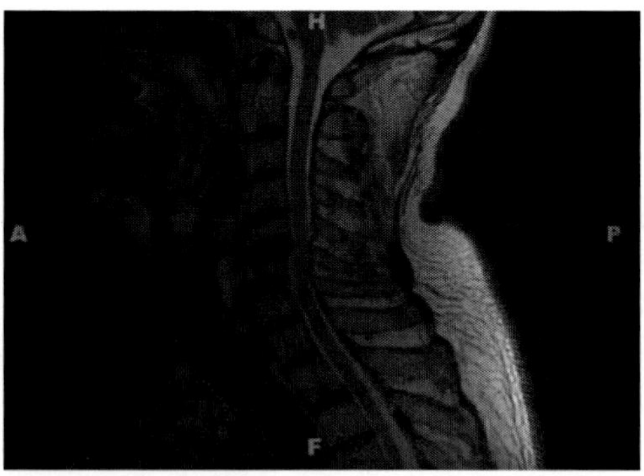

Figure 8. C5-6 Foraminal Narrowing, A-P view.

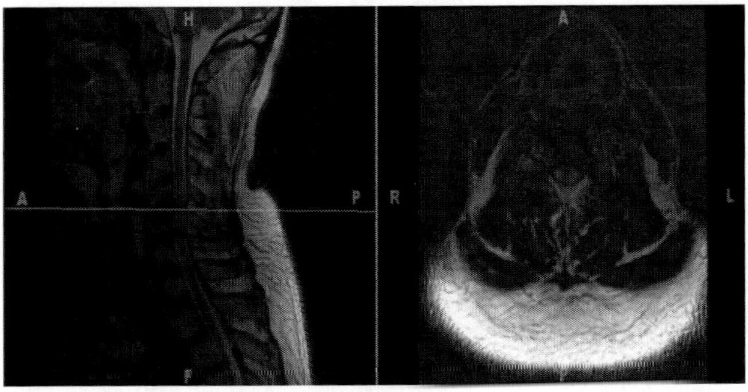

Figure 9. C5-6 Foraminal Narrowing, R-L view.

CONCLUSION

Cervical stenosis may eventually lead to spondylotic cervical myelopathy. Once patients develop severe enough symptoms and signs, operative management is necessary. Several options exist with the anterior and posterior surgical approaches. The chosen procedure should be tailored to the individual patient's pathology targeting the areas of spinal cord and nerve root compression. The goal of surgery should be to halt further neurologic deterioration while preserving the sagittal balance of the spinal column. Further research is necessary to better understand and treat cervical spondylotic myelopathy as a result of cervical stenosis.

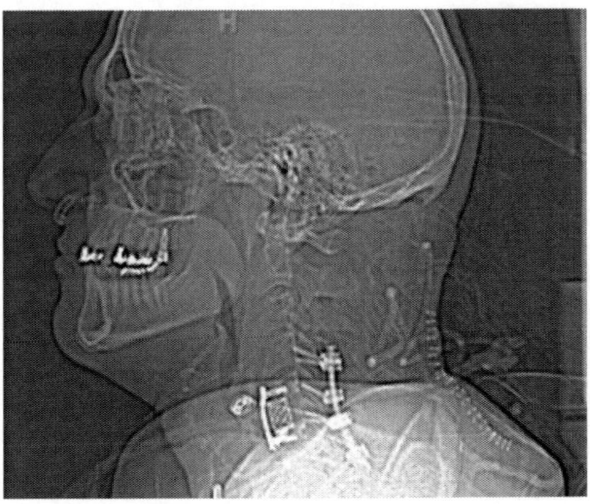

Figure 10. Posterior cervical-thoracic segmental fixation.

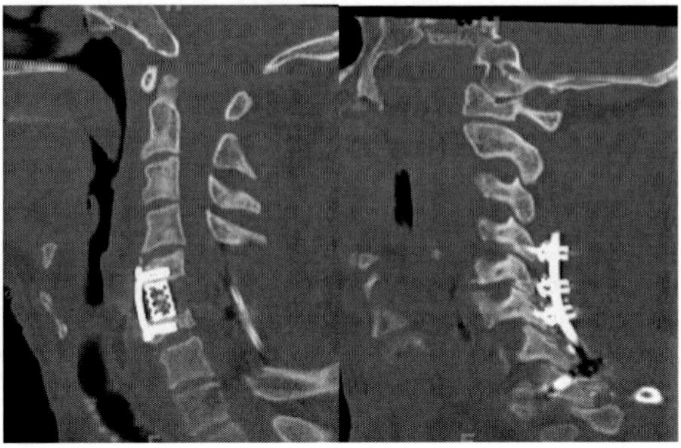

Figure 11. Posterior cervical-thoracic segmental fixation.

A 44 year-old man originally presented with acute onset left-sided upper extremity numbness and weakness. The patient's clinical picture appeared consistent with cervical myelopathy and a left-sided C6 radiculopathy. Imaging studies reportedly demonstrated large disk herniation with significant compression of the spinal cord. The patient had an anterior cervical discectomy and implantation of an artificial disk device at the C5/6 level at another hospital. Following the surgical procedure, the patient felt better for a week, but afterwards, the patient's symptoms recurred.

He presented to our clinic with worsening symptoms, not only on the left, but also on the right side. He also had some paresthesias in both upper extremities as well. The patient exam demonstrated left-sided upper extremity weakness with 4/5 strength in the biceps and dorsiflexion of the wrist consistent with left-sided C6 radiculopathy. The patient also had exaggerated reflexes except for the left knee jerk, which was absent. The clinical picture was consistent with myelopathy.

The patient's MRI of the cervical spine demonstrated myelomalacia on the left side of the spinal cord, as well as significant left-sided C5-C6 foraminal narrowing (Figures 8, 9). Imaging studies demonstrated evidence of osteophyte formation immediately behind the artificial disk at the C5-C6 level, with ventral compression of the spinal cord as well as dorsal compression of the spinal cord at the C6-C7 levels posteriorly.

We recommended a surgical procedure, involving a two-stage anterior-posterior 360 degrees operation. The patient underwent a two-stage surgery. The first stage was performed through an anterior approach. The motion-preserving spacer at C5/6 was removed. Partial corpectomies of C5 caudally and of C6 rostrally were done to aid in the removal of the motion-preserving spacer. The spinal cord and the bilateral nerve roots of C6 were decompressed bilaterally. Anterior reconstruction was performed using a cage with demineralized bone matrix, and a variable angle plate was placed. The second stage was performed through a posterior approach. Laminectomies were completed at C5, 6, and 7. A left-sided laminoforaminotomy was performed to decompress the tight C6 nerve root. Posterior cervical-thoracic segmental fixation was placed from C4-T1 using cervical lateral mass screws and thoracic pedicle screws (Figures 10, 11). Autologous bone harvested during the laminectomy was utilized for posterior cervical-thoracic fusion.

The patient did well after surgery. Post-operative MRI demonstrated excellent decompression of the spinal cord (Figure 12). The patient's motor exam improved to full strength, and he had resolved pain. At 10-months post-op, the patient had achieved solid bony fusion.

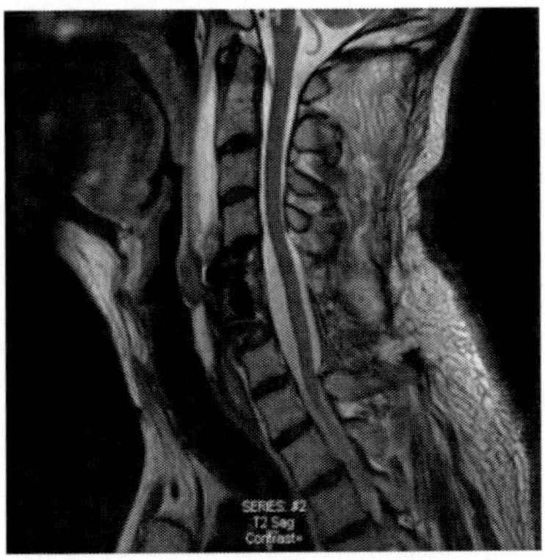

Figure 12. Post-Operative MRI.

REFERENCES

[1] Aita, I, K Hayashi, Y Wadano, and T Yabuki. 1998. "Posterior Movement and Enlargement of the Spinal Cord after Cervical Laminoplasty." *The Journal of Bone and Joint Surgery. British Volume* 80 (1): 33–37. doi:10.1302/0301-620X.80B1.7919.

[2] Ames, Christopher P, Benjamin Blondel, Justin K Scheer, Frank J Schwab, Jean-Charles Le Huec, Eric M Massicotte, Alpesh a Patel et al. 2013. "Cervical Radiographical Alignment: Comprehensive Assessment Techniques and Potential Importance in Cervical Myelopathy." *Spine* 38 (22 Suppl. 1): S149–60. doi:10.1097/ BRS.0b013e3182a7f449.

[3] Benzel, E C, J Lancon, L Kesterson, and T Hadden. 1991. "Cervical Laminectomy and Dentate Ligament Section for Cervical Spondylotic Myelopathy." *Journal of Spinal Disorders*. doi:10.1097/00002517-199109000-00005.

[4] Boden, Scott, D Davis, T Dina, A Mark, and S Wiesel. 1990. "Abnormal Magnetic-Resonance Scans of the Cervical Spine in Asymptomatic Subjects." *Journal of Bone and Joint Surgery* 72 (3): 403–8.

[5] Breig A, Turnbull I, Hassler O. 1966. "Effects of mechanical stresses on the spinal cord in cervical spondylosis. A study on fresh cadaver material." *Journal of neurosurgery* 25 (1): 45-56. Epub. 1966/07/01.

[6] Burkus, J Kenneth, Regis W Haid, Vincent C Traynelis, and Praveen V Mummaneni. 2010. "Long-Term Clinical and Radiographic Outcomes of Cervical Disc Replacement with the Prestige Disc: Results from a Prospective Randomized Controlled Clinical Trial." *Journal of Neurosurgery. Spine* 13 (3): 308–18. doi:10.3171/2010.3.SPINE095 13.

[7] Bydon, Mohamad, Dimitrios Mathios, and Mohamed Macki. 2014. "Long-Term Patient Outcomes after Posterior Cervical Foraminotomy: An Analysis of 151 Cases." *J. Neurosurgery Spine* 21 (November): 727–31. doi:10.3171/2014.7.SPINE131110.

[8] Chiles, Bennie W., Michael A. Leonard, Haroon F. Choudhri, and Paul R. Cooper. 1999. "Cervical Spondylotic Myelopathy: Patterns of Neurological Deficit and Recovery after Anterior Cervical Decompression." *Neurosurgery* 44 (4): 762–70.

[9] Clarke E, Robinson PK. 1956. "Cervical myelopathy: a complication of cervical spondylosis." *Brain: a journal of neurology* 79 (3): 483-510. Epub. 1956/09/01.

[10] Cooper PR. 2005. "Cervical spondylotic myelopathy." *Journal of neurosurgery Spine* 3 (3): 253-4; author reply 4. Epub. 2005/10/21.

[11] Eck JC, Humphreys SC, Lim TH, Jeong ST, Kim JG, Hodges SD et al. 2002. "Biomechanical study on the effect of cervical spine fusion on adjacent-level intradiscal pressure and segmental motion." *Spine* 27 (22): 2431-4. Epub. 2002/11/19.

[12] Edwards, W C, and H LaRocca. 1983. "The Developmental Segmental Sagittal Diameter of the Cervical Spinal Canal in Patients with Cervical Spondylosis." *Spine* 8 (1): 20–27. http://www.ncbi.nlm.nih.gov/pubmed/6867853.

[13] Epstein NE. 1998. "Circumferential surgery for the management of cervical ossification of the posterior longitudinal ligament." *Journal of spinal disorders* 11 (3): 200-7. Epub. 1998/07/10.

[14] Fehlings, Michael G, Sean Barry, Branko Kopjar, Sangwook Tim Yoon, Paul Arnold, Eric M Massicotte, Alexander Vaccaro et al. 2013. "Anterior Versus Posterior Surgical Approaches to Treat Cervical Spondylotic Myelopathy: Outcomes of the Prospective Multicenter AOSpine North America CSM Study in 264 Patients." *Spine* 38 (26): 2247–52. doi:10.1097/BRS.0000000000000047.

[15] Furlan, Julio C, Sukhvinder Kalsi-Ryan, Ahilan Kailaya-Vasan, Eric M Massicotte, and Michael G Fehlings. 2011. "Functional and Clinical Outcomes Following Surgical Treatment in Patients with Cervical Spondylotic Myelopathy: A Prospective Study of 81 Cases." *Journal of Neurosurgery. Spine* 14 (3): 348–55. doi:10.3171/2010.10.SPINE 0910 29.

[16] Garrido, Ben J, Tarek A Taha, and Rick C Sasso. 2010. "Clinical Outcomes of Bryan Cervical Disc Arthroplasty a Prospective, Randomized, Controlled, Single Site Trial with 48-Month Follow-Up." *Journal of Spinal Disorders and Techniques* 23 (6): 367–71. doi:10.1097/BSD.0b013e3181bb8568.

[17] Hamanishi, C, and S Tanaka. 1996. "Bilateral Multilevel Laminectomy with or without Posterolateral Fusion for Cervical Spondylotic Myelopathy: Relationship to Type of Onset and Time until Operation." *Journal of Neurosurgery* 85 (3): 447–51. doi:10. 3171/jns.1996. 85.3.0447.

[18] Hirabayashi, K, K Watanabe, K Wakano, N Suzuki, K Satomi, and Y Ishii. 1983. "Expansive Open-Door Laminoplasty for Cervical Spinal Stenotic Myelopathy." *Spine* 8 (7): 693–99. doi:10.1097/00007632-198310000-00003.

[19] Houten JK, Cooper PR. 2003. "Laminectomy and posterior cervical plating for multilevel cervical spondylotic myelopathy and ossification of the posterior longitudinal ligament: effects on cervical alignment, spinal cord compression, and neurological outcome." *Neurosurgery*. 52 (5): 1081-7; discussion 7-8. Epub. 2003/04/ 18.

[20] Huang, Russel C, Federico P Girardi, Ashley R Poynton, and Frank P Cammisa Jr. 2003. "Treatment of Multilevel Cervical Spondylotic Myeloradiculopathy with Posterior Decompression and Fusion with Lateral Mass Plate Fixation and Local Bone Graft." *Journal of Spinal Disorders and Techniques* 16 (2): 123–29. doi:10.1097/0002 4720-200304000-00002.

[21] Hukuda, S, T Mochizuki, M Ogata, K Shichikawa, and Y Shimomura. 1985. "Operations for Cervical Spondylotic Myelopathy. A Comparison

of the Results of Anterior and Posterior Procedures." *The Journal of Bone and Joint Surgery. British Volume* 67 (4): 609–15. http://www.ncbi.nlm.nih.gov/pubmed/4030860.

[22] Irvine, G B, and W E Strachan. 1987. "The Long-Term Results of Localised Anterior Cervical Decompression and Fusion in Spondylotic Myelopathy." *Paraplegia* 25 (1): 18–22. doi:10.1038/sc.1987.7.

[23] Kadanka, Z, J Bednarik, O Novotny, I Urbanek, and L Dusek. 2011. "Cervical Spondylotic Myelopathy: Conservative versus Surgical Treatment after 10 Years." *European Spine Journal* 20 (9): 1533–38.

[24] Kaptain, G J, N E Simmons, R E Replogle, and L Pobereskin. 2000. "Incidence and Outcome of Kyphotic Deformity Following Laminectomy for Cervical Spondylotic Myelopathy." *Journal of Neurosurgery* 93 (2 Suppl.): 199–204. doi:10.3171/spi.2000. 93.2.0199.

[25] Kato Y, Iwasaki M, Fuji T, Yonenobu K, Ochi T. 1998. "Long-term follow-up results of laminectomy for cervical myelopathy caused by ossification of the posterior longitudinal ligament." *Journal of neurosurgery*. 89 (2): 217-23. Epub. 1998/08/04.

[26] Kawaguchi, Y, M Kanamori, H Ishihara, H Nakamura, K Sugimori, H Tsuji, and T Kimura. 2001. "Progression of Ossification of the Posterior Longitudinal Ligament Following En Bloc Cervical Laminoplasty." *The Journal of Bone and Joint Surgery. American Volume* 83-A (12): 1798–1802. http://eutils.ncbi.nlm.nih.gov/entrez/eutils/elink.fcgi?dbfrom=pubmed&id=11741057&retmode=ref&cmd=prlinks.

[27] Kawakami, M, T Tamaki, H Iwasaki, M Yoshida, M Ando, and H Yamada. 2000. "A Comparative Study of Surgical Approaches for Cervical Compressive Myelopathy." *Clinical Orthopaedics and Related Research*, no. 381: 129–36. http://journals.lww.com/corr/Abstract/2000/12000/A{_}Comparative{_}Study{_}of{_}Surgical{_}Approaches{_}for.16.aspx\nhttp://www.ncbi.nlm.nih.gov/pubmed/11127649.

[28] Kumar, Vijay G R, Gary L. Rea, Lawrence J. Mervis, and John M. McGregor. 1999. "Cervical Spondylotic Myelopathy: Functional and Radiographic Long-Term Outcome after Laminectomy and Posterior Fusion." *Neurosurgery* 44 (4): 771–78.

[29] Law, M D, M Bernhardt, and a a White. 1993. "Cervical Spondylotic Myelopathy: A Review of Surgical Indications and Decision Making." *The Yale Journal of Biology and Medicine* 66 (3): 165–77. http://www.pubmedcentral.nih.gov/articlerender.fcgi?artid=2588867{&}tool=pmcentrez{&}rendertype=abstract.

[30] Lees F, Turner JW. 1963. "Natural History and Prognosis of Cervical Spondylosis." *British medical journal* 2 (5373): 1607-10. Epub. 1963/12/28.

[31] Leung, Clarence, Adrian Th. Casey, Jan Goffin, Pierre Kehr, Klaus Liebig, Bengt Lind, Carlo Logroscino, and Vincent Pointillart. 2005. "Clinical Significance of Heterotopic Ossification in Cervical Disc Replacement: A Prospective Multicenter Clinical Trial." *Neurosurgery* 57 (4): 759–63. doi:10.1227/01.NEU.0000175856.31210.58.

[32] Lubelski, Daniel, Andrew T. Healy, Michael P. Silverstein, Kalil G. Abdullah, Nicolas R. Thompson, K. Daniel Riew, Michael P. Steinmetz, Edward C. Benzel, and Thomas E. Mroz. 2015. "Reoperation Rates after Anterior Cervical Discectomy and Fusion versus Posterior Cervical Foraminotomy: A Propensity-Matched Analysis." *Spine Journal* 15 (6): 1277–83. doi:10.1016/j.spinee.2015.02.026.

[33] Maldonado, Carlos Valencia, R. D R Paz, and Claudia Balhen Martin. 2011. "Adjacent-Level Degeneration after Cervical Disc Arthroplasty versus Fusion." *European Spine Journal*. doi:10.1007/s00586-011-1916-1.

[34] Matsuda, Y, K Miyazaki, K Tada, A Yasuda, T Nakayama, H Murakami, and M Matsuo. 1991. "Increased MR Signal Intensity due to Cervical Myelopathy. Analysis of 29 Surgical Cases." *Journal of Neurosurgery* 74 (6): 887–92. doi:10.3171/jns.1991.74. 6.0887.

[35] Montgomery, D M, and R S Brower. 1992. "Cervical Spondylotic Myelopathy. Clinical Syndrome and Natural History." *The Orthopedic Clinics of North America* 23 (3): 487–93.

[36] Morio, Y, R Teshima, H Nagashima, K Nawata, D Yamasaki, and Y Nanjo. 2001. "Correlation between Operative Outcomes of Cervical Compression Myelopathy and Mri of the Spinal Cord." *Spine* 26 (11): 1238–45. doi:10.1097/00007632-200106010-00012.

[37] Muhle, C, D Weinert, A Falliner, J Wiskirchen, J Metzner, M Baumer, G Brinkmann, and M Heller. 1998. "Dynamic Changes of the Spinal Canal in Patients with Cervical Spondylosis at Flexion and Extension Using Magnetic Resonance Imaging." *Invest. Radiol.* 33 (8): 444–49. http://www.ncbi.nlm.nih.gov/entrez/query.fcgi?cmd=Retrieve&db=Pub Med&dopt=Citation&list_uids=9704283.

[38] Mummaneni, Praveen V, J Kenneth Burkus, Regis W Haid, Vincent C Traynelis, and Thomas A Zdeblick. 2007. "Clinical and Radiographic Analysis of Cervical Disc Arthroplasty Compared with Allograft Fusion:

A Randomized Controlled Clinical Trial." *Journal of Neurosurgery. Spine* 6 (3): 198–209. doi:10.3171/spi.2007.6.3.198.

[39] Nordqvist L. 1964. "The Sagittal Diameter of the Spinal Cord and Subarachnoid Space in Different Age Groups." A Roentgenographic Post-Mortem Study. *Acta radiologica: diagnosis* Suppl. 227:1-96. Epub. 1964/01/01.

[40] Nouri, Aria, Lindsay Tetreault, Anoushka Singh, Spyridon K Karadimas, and Michael G Fehlings. 2015. "Degenerative Cervical Myelopathy: Epidemiology, Genetics, and Pathogenesis." *Spine* 40 (12): E675–93. doi:10.1097/BRS.0000000000000913.

[41] Nurick S. 1972. "The pathogenesis of the spinal cord disorder associated with cervical spondylosis." *Brain: a journal of neurology*. 95(1): 87-100. Epub. 1972/01/01.

[42] Pickett, Gwynedd E, Demytra K Mitsis, Lali H Sekhon, William R Sears, and Neil Duggal. 2004. "Effects of a Cervical Disc Prosthesis on Segmental and Cervical Spine Alignment." *Neurosurgical Focus* 17 (3): E5. doi:170305 [pii].

[43] Ranawat, C S, P O'Leary, P Pellicci, P Tsairis, P Marchisello, and L Dorr. 1979. "Cervical Spine Fusion in Rheumatoid Arthritis." *The Journal of Bone and Joint Surgery*. American Volume 61: 1003–10.

[44] Raynor, R B, J Pugh, and I Shapiro. 1985. "Cervical Facetectomy and Its Effect on Spine Strength." *Journal of Neurosurgery* 63 (2): 278–82. doi: 10.3171/jns.1985.63.2. 0278.

[45] Sasai K, Saito T, Akagi S, Watanabe H. 1995. "[Clinical study of cervical radiculopathy after laminoplasty for cervical myelopathy]." *Nihon Seikeigeka Gakkai zasshi* 69 (12): 1237-47. Epub. 1995/12/01.

[46] Satomi, K, Y Nishu, T Kohno, and K Hirabayashi. 1994. "Long-Term Follow-up Studies of Open-Door Expansive Laminoplasty for Cervical Stenotic Myelopathy." *Spine*. http://www.ncbi.nlm.nih.gov/pubmed/8184342.

[47] Schwab, John S, Denis J Diangelo, and Kevin T Foley. 2006. "Motion Compensation Associated with Single-Level Cervical Fusion: Where Does the Lost Motion Go?" *Spine* 31 (21): 2439–48. doi:10.1097/01.brs.0000239125.54761.23.

[48] Sheikh Taha, Abdel Majid, Jennifer Shue, Darren Lebl, and Federico Girardi. 2015. "Considerations for Prophylactic Surgery in Asymptomatic Severe Cervical Stenosis: Review Article." *HSS Journal*. doi:10.1007/s11420-014-9426-4.

[49] Snow, Robert B, and Howard Weiner. 1993. "Cervical Laminectomy and Foraminotomy as Surgical Treatment of Cervical Spondylosis: A Follow-up Study with Analysis of Failures." *Journal of Spinal Disorders and Techniques* 6 (3): 245. http://journals.lww.com/jspinaldisorders/Fulltext/1993/06030/Cervical_Laminectomy_and_Foraminotomy_as_Surgical.11.aspx\npapers3://publication/uuid/011C79C1-CC00-473B-9142-0216CD93B961.

[50] Sodeyama, T, S Goto, M Mochizuki, J Takahashi, and H Moriya. 1999. "Effect of Decompression Enlargement Laminoplasty for Posterior Shifting of the Spinal Cord." *Spine* 24 (15): 1522–27. doi:10.1097/00007632-199908010-00005.

[51] Song, Kyung-Jin, and Byeong-Yeol Choi. 2014. "Current Concepts of Anterior Cervical Discectomy and Fusion: A Review of Literature." *Asian Spine Journal* 8 (4): 531. doi:10.4184/asj.2014.8.4.531.

[52] Suda, Kota, Kuniyoshi Abumi, Manabu Ito, Yasuhiro Shono, Kiyoshi Kaneda, and Masanori Fujiya. 2003. "Local Kyphosis Reduces Surgical Outcomes of Expansive Open-Door Laminoplasty for Cervical Spondylotic Myelopathy." *Spine* 28 (12): 1258–62. doi:10.1097/01.BRS.0000065487.82469.D9.

[53] T K, N T, H T. 1982. "Enlargement of spinal canal by the sagittal splitting of the spinous process." *Bessatsu Seikei Geka*. 2: 234-40.

[54] Teresi, L M, R B Lufkin, M a Reicher, B J Moffit, F V Vinuela, G M Wilson, J R Bentson, and W N Hanafee. 1987. "Asymptomatic Degenerative Disk Disease and Spondylosis of the Cervical Spine: MR Imaging." *Radiology* 164 (1): 83–88. doi:10.1148/radiology.164.1.3588931.

[55] Yang, K. Q., X. S. Lu, Q. L. Cai, L. X. Ye, and W. Q. Lu. 1985. "Anterior Multilevel Decompression and Fusion for Cervical Spondylotic Myelopathy. Report of 214 Cases." *Chinese Medical Journal* 98 (1): 1–6.

[56] Yonenobu, Kazuo, Takeshi Fuji, Keiro Ono, Kozo Okada, Tomio Yamamoto, and Norimasa Harada. 1985. "Choice of Surgical Treatment for Multisegmental Cervical Spondylotic Myelopathy." *Spine* 10 (8): 710–16. doi:10.1097/00007632-198510000-00004.

[57] Yoo, Do-Sung, Sang-Bok Lee, Pil-Woo Huh, Seok-Gu Kang, and Kyoung-Suok Cho. 2010. "Spinal Cord Injury in Cervical Spinal Stenosis by Minor Trauma." *World Neurosurgery* 73 (1): 50–52; discussion e4. doi:10.1016/j.surneu.2009.05.021.

[58] Zdeblick, T a, D Zou, K E Warden, R McCabe, D Kunz, and R Vanderby. 1992. "Cervical Stability after Foraminotomy. A Biomechanical *in Vitro* Analysis." *The Journal of Bone and Joint Surgery. American Volume* 74 (1): 22–27. http://www.ncbi.nlm.nih.gov/pubmed/1734010.

[59] Zhang ZH, Yin H, Yang K, Zhang T, Dong F, Dang G et al. 1983. "Anterior intervertebral disc excision and bone grafting in cervical spondylotic myelopathy." *Spine* 8 (1): 16-9. Epub. 1983/01/01.

In: Intervertebral Disc Degeneration
Editors: A. L. Ho and A. M. Desai

ISBN: 978-1-63485-829-8

Chapter 5

THORACIC DISC HERNIATIONS

***Nathan E. Simmons, MD*[1,*]**

Division of Neurosurgery, Dartmouth Hitchcock Medical Center,Lebanon, NH

[1]Department of Neurological Surgery, Stanford University School of Medicine, Stanford, California

ABSTRACT

Thoracic disc herniations occur less frequently than cervical or lumbar herniations, yet are common enough that surgeons should understand management strategies. Preoperative assessment of the size, location, presence of calcification, and spinal level are all important factors for deciding upon a surgical approach. While some disc herniations will require anterior approaches, these are typically associated with higher levels of morbidity and lengthier hospital stays, suggesting posterior approaches, when feasible, offer better outcomes. In most surgeries, the need for fusion is low but the final decision needs to be tailored for the individual patient.

Keywords: thoracic herniated disc, thoracotomy, lateral extracavitary, transpedicular, costotransversectomy

---

* Correspondence to: Nathan E. Simmons (Nathan.E.Simmons@hitchcock.org) Department of Neurosurgery, Dartmouth-Hitchcock Medical Center. One Medical Center Dr, Lebanon, NH 03753.

INTRODUCTION

Thoracic disc herniations comprise but a small portion of the total spectrum of degnerative spine conditions managed by surgeons. However, due to their location and variable presentation, they require as much, if not more, evaluation and strategic planning for successful operative intervention.

As opposed to the cervical and lumbar regions which experience a greater range of motion and force, the thoracic spine is relatively immobile due to its minimal anatomic curve and the presence of supporting skeletal elements such as theribcage and sternum. Consequently, the development of degenerative conditions such as herniated discs are much less frequent in the thoracic spine. Estimates suggest symptomatic thoracic herniated discs occur in one out of every 1,000,000 people [14, 18]. This translates to 0.15-4% of all surgical procedures for degnerative spinal conditions [22]. Therefore, while uncommon, spinal surgeons will undoubtedly encounter patients with symptomatic thoracic discs and need to understand the salient features of their management.

The thoracic region shares elements of both the cervical and lumbar area when considering surgical approaches. While the anatomy of the spinal column is similar to the lumbar region, the presence of the spinal cord complicates and limits posterior approaches. In the cervical region, this hindrance is managed by commonly addressing the degnerative disc via an anterior approach. However, unlike the cervical region, anterior approaches in the thoracic spine are much more involved and potentially morbid. Consequently, complication rates for thoracic disc surgery are higher than those for cervical or lumbar regions (*Figure 1*) [17].

A variety of anterior, posterior, and posterolateral vectors have been developed for the surgeon, each offering unique benefits and disadvantages. Likewise, the development of more minimally invasive has also been efficacious in the management of these conditions. This chapter will attempt to review these indications and surgical approaches.

Symptom Presentation

As in the cervical spine, patients can present with either or both of the following: radicular symptoms with more laterally located herniated discs compressing the exiting nerve roots and/or myelopathic findings associated with spinal cord compression in central disc hernations. Given that most thoracic herniated discs occur centrally or centrolaterally, it is not unsurprising that most patients will harbor some form of motor weakness (55 - 61%) and/or sensory deficit (61 - 64%) [15]. While bowel/bladder impairment is possible, these symptoms are seen in only a minority of patients [15].

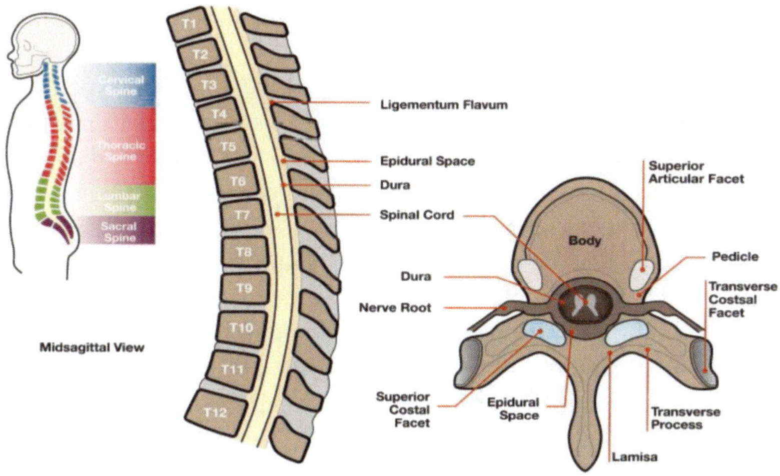

Figure 1. Anatomy of the Thoracic Spine.

It is noteworthy to consider axial pain and the presence of a herniated thoracic disc. Asymptomatic thoracic herniated discs can be discerned on imaging in 10-37% of random MRIs [12]. However, Stillerman has shown that a significant percentage of patients improve with respect to axial pain following treatment of thoracic herniated discs [15]. The correlation bewteen axial back pain and degenerative/herniated discs is problematic for patient and surgeon alike and will require individualized analysis.

Preoperative Management

One of the most important aspects of preoperative evaluation for these patients is the determination of the exact level of the pathology. For example, when a radiology report indicates the T9-T10 level, the surgeon will need to know how this level was labeled and whether that method can be simulated in the operating room. Generally, a lower level thoracic process can be counted from the sacrum. This will require assessment of whether or not transitional vertebrae exist in the lumbar spine. Likewise, if the body habitus is favorable, upper thoracic lesions can sometimes be counted caudally from the cranium and cervical spine. However, midthoracic lesions (and potentially any thoracic level depending on habitus) may require intraoperative anterior/posterior x-rays for localizationg and, thus, the surgeon needs to verify the presence or absence of cervical ribs and/or the vertebral count from whatever reference point which appears reproduceable.

In addition to the radiologic assessment of the level, the type of imaging also needs to be reviewed. Most surgeons will assess surgical patients based on MR images. However, given the surgical approach options, disc hernations laying with the anterolateral canal can be accessed through posterior, posterolateral, and anterior approaches. Often a key determinant is whether or not the disc herniation is calcified as calification increases the difficulty in removing disc herniations through posterior trajectories (*Figure 2*). Occasionally, the surgeon should consider obtaining preoperative CT to better assess for calcification. Softer discs can often be teased safely through posterior approaches while calcified discs often require more aggressive curettage and potentially drilling. If the disc is causing spinal cord compression, this may often be the deciding factor in addressing the lesion anteriorly.

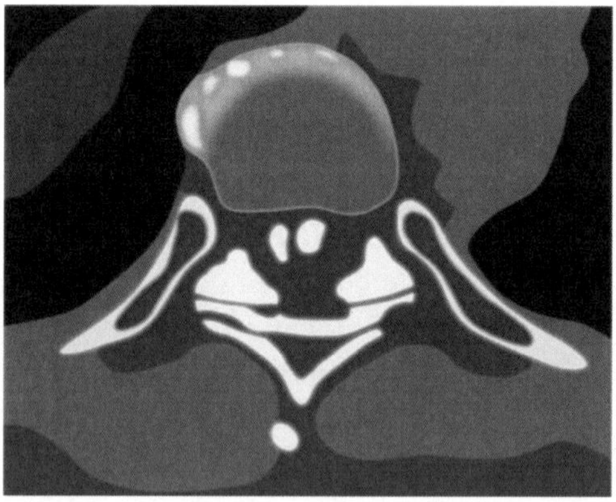

Figure 2. Calcified Thoracic Disc.

Neuromonitoring must also be considered in the preoperative planning. If the herniated disc lays within the foramen, monitoring may not be necessary as spinal cord manipulation will be minimal. However, if the disc is more centrally located and spinal cord manipulation may be necessary, it would be prudent to consider neuromonitoring. As such, preoperative testing of motor evoked potentials and somatosensory evoked potentials will give the operative team a baseline from which to compare any changes. While obviously not a guarantee of spinal cord injury avoidance, monitoring can serve as a useful tool to avoid unnecessary manipulation of the cord.

Surgery

In the operating room, a number of tenets will aid in the successful management of thoracic herniated discs. As mentioned earlier, localization is of prime importance in these cases. Various techniques have been reported for direct localization of levels including dye, PMMA vertebroplasty, Gugliemi coils, percutaneous wires [21]. However, these require the patient to undergo an additional procedure and probably are only needed in uncommon situations where traditional images might be difficult. Typically, thoughtful use of conventional xrays without markers will suffice.

Borrowing a rule from carpentry, the surgeon would be wise to "measure twice and cut once." As such, the patient will need to be positioned for ideal imaging. Lateral approaches lend themselves to anterior/posterior (A/P) radiographs, thus the surgeon should be ready and comfortable with counting ribs and have similar preoperative studies by which to compare. In the prone position, one may be able to count from cervical or lumbar references if the disc herniation is close to these junctions and the patient's body habitus allows. However, sometimes the surgeon will need to obtain A/P or P/A imaging. This would necessitate placing the patient on an operating table/frame suited for through-table imaging (*Figure 3*).

Neuromonitoring will need to be performed in many such cases. Anesthesia will need to rely primarily on total intravenous anesthesia (TIVA), propofol/narcotics and limit paralytics to only the period around induction. In addition, medications causing for decreases in cardiac output should be used cautiously for fear of compromising spinal cord perfusion during the operation. Neuro-anaesthesiologists will be familiar with these requests but surgeons should review goals of the anasthesia prior to induction.

Prior to incision, the patient is often bolused with intravenous steroid in order to prevent spinal cord injury. Blood pressure should be closely managed as the perfusion of the spinal cord can be limited from the herniation and subsequent surgical manipulation. Zuckerman, et al., reported on three patients in which a decline in mean arterial pressure was folllowed by worsened electrophysicalogical monitoring [23]. Recommendations vary, but mean arterial pressure should be maintained above at least 70-80 mmHg, though it also has been suggested above 90mmHg. Zuckerman, et al., uses a strategy of maintaining the mean arterial pressure at least 10% above baseline pre-induction levels [23].

Operative approaches (detailed descriptions of the approaches can be found at the respective references)

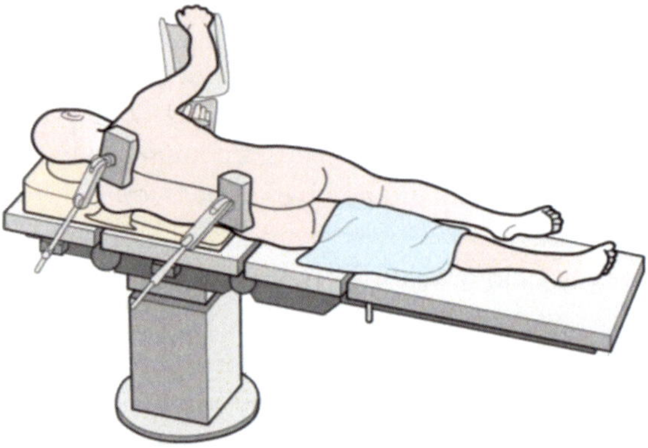

Figure 3. Lateral Positioning.

Posterior midline:

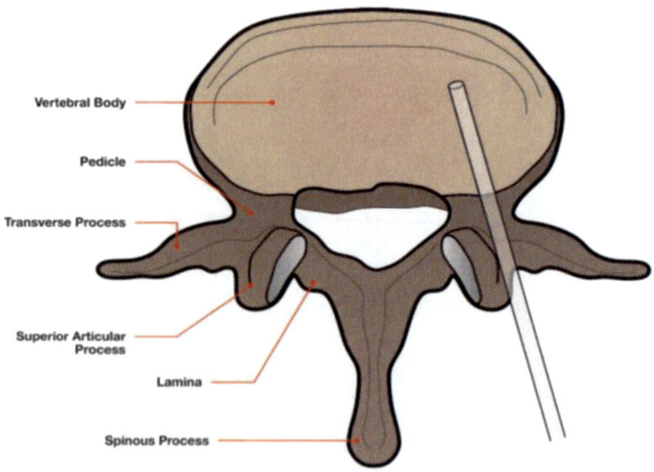

Figure 4. Transpedicular [16].

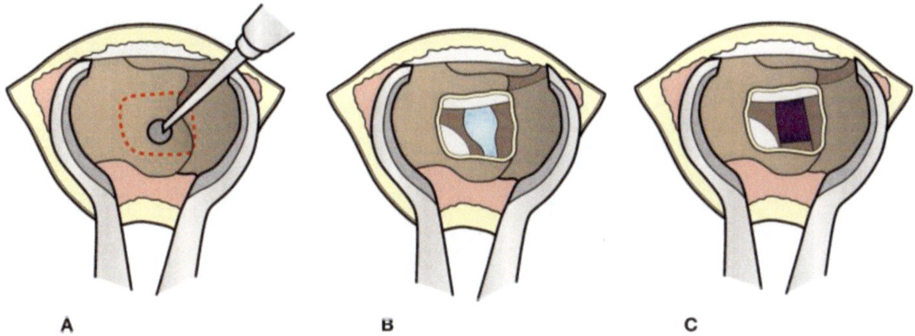

Figure 5. Transforaminal/Transfacet pedicle sparing [16].

These approaches are likely the most commonly used methods for thoracic disc surgery. Detailed descriptions of the techniques can be found elsewhere. Briefly, these procedures typically employ a midline incision on a prone patient. The ipsilateral musculature is elevated off the spinous processes, laminae, and facets. The transpedicular approach (*Figure 4*) starts with a lateral laminotomy, usually performed with a combination of a high speed drill and 1 and 2mm Kerrison rongeurs. As the lateral dura is identified, the medial facet joint is similarly removed and the exiting nerve root and pedicles are exposed. The high speed drill is used to drill into the medullary bone of the inferior pedicle, thinning the cortex medially and superiorly. This allows the surgeon to then fracture this portion of the pedicle laterally (away from the cord), thus developing a greater working space to the disc lying just above the pedicle. Disc herniations within the lateral canal can then be mobilized with down biting currettes and removed safely with rongeurs.

The transfacet/transforaminal technique (*Figure 5)* represents a slight refinement of the transpedicular route in which the pedicle is spared. As the facet joint overlies the foramen and disc, pedicle removal is not mandatory. This technique requires drilling through the facet, avoiding the pedicle, and working in the disc space adjancent to the exiting nerve root. Usually the nerve root exits throught the superior portion of the foramen, enabling a working corridor just inferior for disc retrieval.

Posterior lateral:

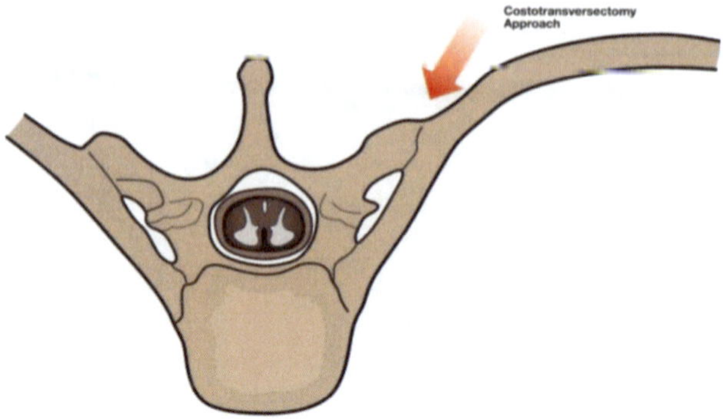

Figure 6. Costotransversectomy approach [8].

These approaches commonly employ a lateral incision (hockey stick, curivilinear, or straight) in order to allow for a shallower viewing angle toward the disc space (*Figures 6 and 7*). Each requires resection of the lamina, facet, transverse process, and rib/costovertebral joint. The major difference between these two proceudres is the amount of rib resected, with the lateral extracavitary approach resecting a larger amount of rib. Given the larger incisions and more extensive tissue dissection, these procedures typically create more postoperative pain and also bring forth the potential for inadvertent thoracic cavity entry as the pleura will require dissection from the rib before rib removal. Lubelski, et al., compared the two procedures in a restrospective review and noted a trend toward greater blood loss and length of stay in the lateral extracavitary group. However, complications proved similar in both groups, though the authors noted that both these procedures were inherently risky [8].

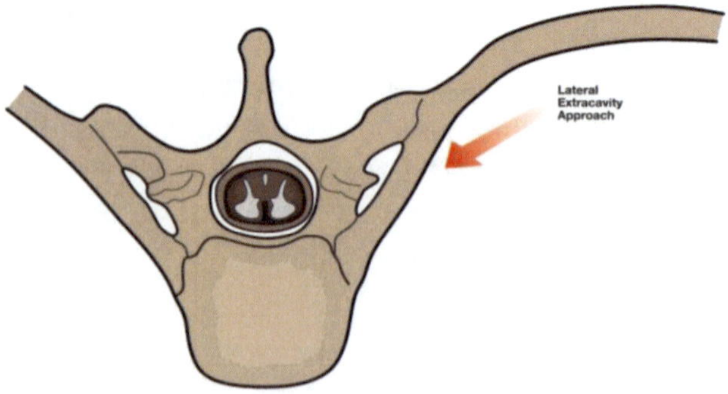

Figure 7. Lateral extracavitary approach [8].

Kshettry et al. recently published a cadaveric study quantifying the exposures obtained of the ventral spinal canal in various posterior approaches. [7] Their findings also drew attention to the fact that a given approach may have better exposure in certain regions of the spine than others, For instance, the lower thoracic spine typically has straighter pedicles which place the facet joints in a more medial location. Thus a transfacet approach in the lower spine may result in less ventral visualization than in the upper thoracic spine. The transpedicular approach provided superior visualization to the facetectomy only in the T1-2 and T11-12 regions. Similarly, the lateral extracavity approach gave a significant benefit over the costotransversectomy only in the T7-T10 location. While these measurements were only from cadaveric specimens, it emphasizes the variability of anatomy in the thoracic spine and the need for the surgeon to discerningly review the images in order to plan the best surgical approach.

Anterior/Anterior-lateral:

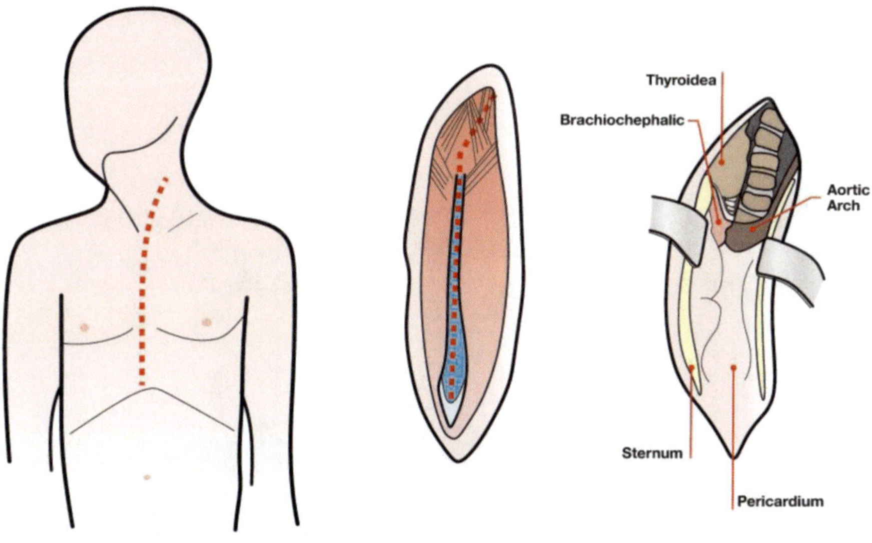

Figure 8. Transsternal or Modified Sternotomy approach [5].

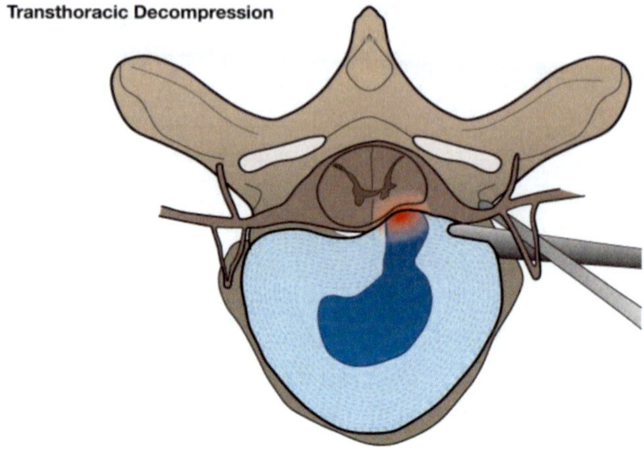

Figure 9. Transthoracic approach [20].

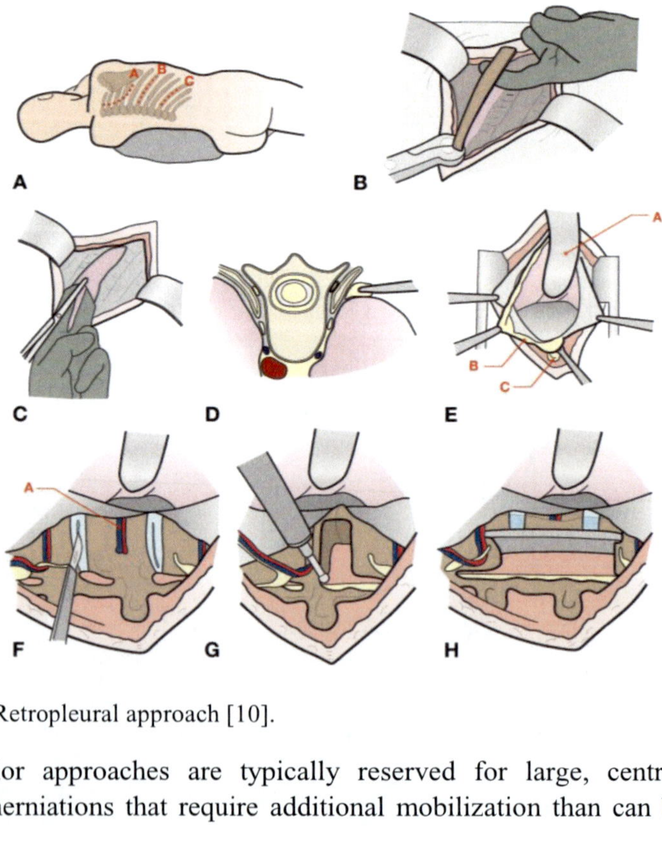

Figure 10. Retropleural approach [10].

Anterior approaches are typically reserved for large, central, and/or calcified herniations that require additional mobilization than can be offered through posterior access. The transsternal approach (*Figure 8)* is used exclusively in the upper thoracic region for rare herniations in the T1-T5 region. In the mid to lower thoracic region, anterior approaches are usually approached on the left side so as to avoid the vena cava, thoracic duct, and liver.

While the anterior approach offers the benefit of accessing the disc space directly and mobilizing the herniation away from the neural structures, the surgery is nevertheless a significant undertaking for patient and surgeon, alike. Yoshihara and Yoneoka reviewd data from the National Inpatient Sample and concluded a significant increase in morbidity associated with anterior approaches for thoracic disc herniations [22]. In their review, they demonstrated a significant increase in complications (particularly pulmonary), hospital length of stay, and hospital costs for anterior apporaches. Similarly, Arts and Bartels reviewed 100 consecutive patients undergoing either a mini-transthoracic discectomy or transpedicular discectomy and concluded the former was associated with a longer surgical time, lengthier hospital stay, increased blood loss, and higher complication rate [3]. While both studies are limited by selection bias, they suggest that while necessary in some situations, herniated discs not mandating an anterior approach are probably best addressed from posterior corridors.

Minimally Invasive:

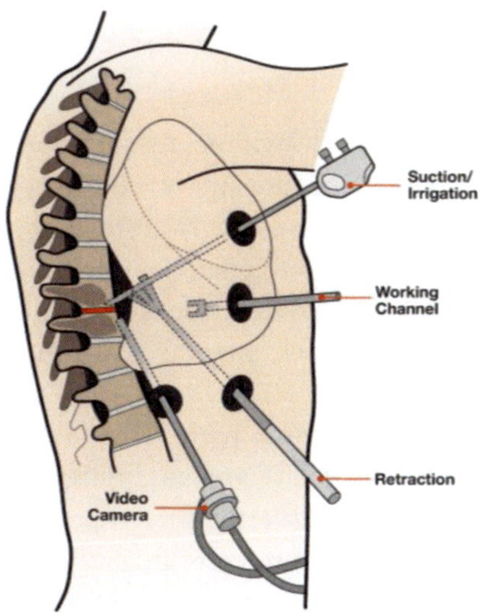

Figure 11. Video assisted thoracoscopic procedure [1].

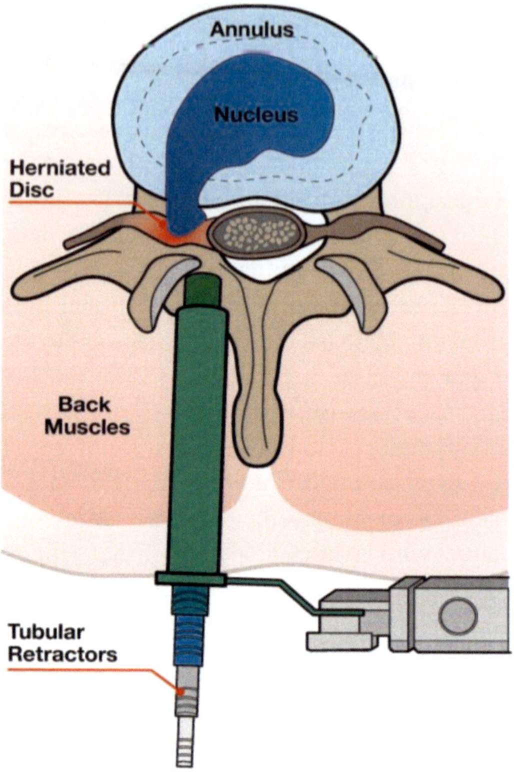

Figure 12. Tubular retractor [4, 11, 13].

As with many surgical procedures, an increasing emphasis on "minimal invasive" procedures is growing within the treatment of thoracic disc herniations. The first of these procedures involved modifying the techniques of thoracic surgeons in using video-assited thoracoscopic surgery (VATS) (*Figure 11*). As with thoracoscopic or general endoscopic surgeries, the patient will require multiple small incisions for camera and working port access sites. As the thoracic cavity is entered, these patients will require postoperative chest tubes in most cases.

Though a number of surgeons have shown excellent results with thoracoscopic surgery, most surgeons are unfamiliar with these instruments and techniques [2]. The learning curve for such a procedure is very steep and likely can only be maintained by surgeons in facilities with relatively high volumes of such pathology. Not surprisingly, thoracoscopic techniques are practiced by a relatively small number of surgeons.

Surgeons have since adopted tubular retractors from the lumbar spine to the thoracic spine. (*Figure 12)* The tubular retractor systems offer the benefit of minimal incision length, familiarity with approach and instrumentation, and avoidance of thoracic cavity complications. A number of successful techniques have been reported using tubular retractors including the use of primary microscopic views, endoscopic views through the retractor, transfacet approaches, and even lateral extracavitary tubular approaches [4, 11, 13]. Uribe and colleagues have modified the McCormick's retropleural approach with the introduction of a "mini-open" approach utiliziing a smaller incision and retractor blades from lumbar approaches [19]. These approaches will need to be further evaluated for their efficacy in treating thoracic herniated discs and for incorporation into mainstream surgical techniques.

To Fuse or Not to Fuse?

The thoracic spine is unique in that it has a greater inherent stability owing to the presence of the ribs/sternum and a minimal curvature. As a result, the majority of thoracic discectomies, both posterior and anterior, do not require fusion. While some surgeons advocate for the routine use of fusion so as to eliminate the risk of postoperative instability, the fusion can bring with it the risk of hardware failure/pseudoarthorsis, misplaced hardware, and longer operative times for the patient. Therefore, the surgeon can most likely defer on a fusion following thoracic discectomies unless there exists significant abnormal alignment (scoliosis, exaggerrated kyphosis), osteoporosis, or an overly aggressive bone removal during the surgery. Krauss, et al., reviewed 18 patients having undergone transthoracic discectomies and demonstrated that none developed a kyphosis nor scoliosis at the operative site with a follow-up of 22 months [6]. While not randomized, the suggestions through case series and clinical observations are that most discectomies, anterior or posterior, can be safely performed without fusions.

Complications

Durotomy

Cerebrospinal fluid (CSF) leaks during posterior/posterolateral surgeries are managed similarly to lumbar and cervical procedures. When possible, the dural violation is directly sutured and tissue, synthetic pathches, and/or glue can be used to augment a closure. In cases where the dural injury is not well visualized, an indirect repair may need to suffice with an onlay patch of tissue/synthetic material, carefully administered glue along the gutters, and a meticulous fascial closure. Lumbar drainage can also be considered for the early postoperative period.

Dural leaks during anterior procedures pose a much greater challenge. The risk of a leak during an anterior procedure may be greater due to the selection bias for larger and more calcified disc hernations. Direct dural closures are the ideal solution but are more often technically challenging due to the depth of anatomy and the method of surgery (thoracoscopic, tubular retractor). Again, indirect closure is often employed yet in these cases and a thoracic fistula can complicate the postoperative course. In cases of CSF leak, a postoperative chest tube can be placed to water seal to prevent fistula formation and the use of a lumbar drain can additionally promote adequate closure.

Intercostal Neuralgia

A thoracic radiculopathy is not uncommonly encountered after anterior approaches. Most of these will resolve, however, in some cases, the patient will complain on ongoing pain that can be debilatating. Strategies to avoid intercostal nerualgia have included care in the dissection of the neuro-vascular bundle off the rib, watching for of excessive retraction against the underside of the rib, and avoiding resection of the rib head at the entry site for mini-open procedures [17]. In the event of intercostal neuralgia, pain specialists can often perform percutaneous blocks and/or radiofrequency ablations to lessen the pain.

Conclusion

Given their infrequent presentation, thoracic disc herniations offer a range of challenges and surgical approaches for the surgeon to consider. Most spine surgeons need not be experts in all these methods but need to know of the options and maintain a variety of mastered techniques by which to address these lesions.

CHECKLIST FOR THORACIC DISC SURGERY

Preoperative

- o Confirming level and verifying intraoperative counting strategy
- o Assessment of calcification
- o Estimating access via posterior/anterior approaches
- o Baseline MEP/SSEP
- o OR table selection (AP vs lateral imaging)
- o Consideration of preoperative marking for incision
- o Need for fusion

Perioperative

- o Arterial line for maintenance of MAP > 80mmHG
- o Steroid administration
- o Imaging modality
- o Neuromonitoring

REFERENCES

[1] Ammerman, Joshua M, and Anthony J. Caputy. 2012. Video assisted thoracoscopic discectomy: indications and techniques. In *Schmidek and Sweet Operative Neurosurgical Techniques: Indications, Methods, and Results*, edited by Alfredo Quiones-Hinojosa, 1843-1851. Philadelphia, PA: Elsevier Saunders.

[2] Anand, Neal, and John J. Regan. 2002. Video-assisted thoracoscopic surgery for thoracic disc disease. *Spine*. 27: 871-879.

[3] Arts, Mark P. and Ronald H.M.A. Bartels. 2013. Anterior or posterior approach
of thoracic disc herniation? A comparative cohort of mini-transthoracic versus transpedicular discectomies. *The Spine Journal*. 14: 1654-1662.

[4] Khoo, Larry T., Zachary A. Smith, Farbod Asgarzadie, Yorgios Barlas, Sean S. Armin, Vartan Tashjian, and Baron Zarate. 2011. Minimally invasive extracavitary approach for thoracic discectomy and interbody fusion: 1-year clinical and radiographic outcomes in 13 patients compared with a cohort of traditional anterior transthoracic approaches. *Journal of Neurosurgery: Spine*. 14: 250-260.

[5] Knoller, S.M., and L. Brethner. 2002. Surgical treatment of the spine at the cervicothoracic junction: an illustrated review of a modified sternotomy approach with the description of tricks and pitfalls. *Archives of Orthopedic and Trauma Surgery.* 122: 365-368.

[6] Krauss, William E., Diane A. Edwards, and Aaron A. Cohen-Gadol. 2004. Transthoracic discectomy without interbody fusion. *Surgical Neurology*. 63: 403-409.

[7] Kshettry, Varun R., Andrew T. Healy, Noble G. Jones, Thomas E. Mroz, and Edward C. Benzel. 2015. A quantitative analysis of posterolateral approaches to the ventral thoracic spinal canal. *The Spine Journal*. 15: 2228-2238.

[8] Lubelski, Daniel, Kalil G. Abdullah, Thomas E. Mroz, John H. Shin, Matthew D. Alvin, Edward C. Benzel, and Michael P. Steinmetz. 2012. Lateral Extracavitary vs costotransversectomy approaches to the thoracic spine : reflections on lessons learned. *Neurosurgery*. 71: 1096-1102.

[9] Lubelski, Daniel, Kalil G. Abdullah, Michael P. Steinmetz, Frank Masters, Edward C. Benzel, Thomas E. Mroz, and John H. Shin. 2013. Lateral extracavitary, costotransversectomy, and transthoracic thoracotomy approaches to the thoracic spine : review of techniques and complications. *Journal of Spinal Disorders and Techniques*. 26: 222-232.

[10] McCormick, Paul C. 1995. Retropleural approaches to the thoracic and thoracolumbar spine. *Neurosurgery*. 37: 908-914.

[11] Regev, Gilad J., Khalil Salame, Eyal Behrbalk, Ory Keynan, and Zvi Lidar. 2012. Minimally invasive transforaminal, thoracic microscopic discectomy: technical report and preliminary results and complications. *The Spine Journal.* 12: 570-576.

[12] Simmons, Nathan E. 2012. Surgical techniques in the management of thoracic disc herniations. In *Schmidek and Sweet Operative Neurosurgical Techniques: Indications, Methods, and Results*, edited by Alfredo Quiones-Hinojosa, 1833-1842. Philadelphia, PA: Elsevier Saunders.

[13] Smith, Justin S., Kurt M. Eichholz, Stephen Shafizadeh, Alfred T. Ogden, John E. O'Toole, and Richard Fessler. 2013. Minimally invasive thoracic microendoscopic diskectomy: surgical technique and case series. *World Neurosurgery*. 80: 421-427.

[14] Snyder, Laura A., Zachary A. Smith, Nader S. Dahdaleh, and Richard G. Fessler. 2014. Minimally invasive treatment of thoracic disc herniations. *Neurosurgery Clinics of North America*. 25: 271-277.

[15] Stillerman, Charles B, Thomas C. Chen, William T. Couldwell, Wei Zheng, and Martin H. Weiss. 1998. Experience in the surgical management of 82 symptomatic herniated thoracic discs and review of the literature. *Journal of Neurosurgery*. 88: 623-633.

[16] Stillerman, Charles B., Paul C. McCormick, and Edward C. Benzel. 1999. Thoracic Discectomy. *Spine Surgery: Techniques, complication avoidance, and management*, edited by Edward C. Benzel, 369-388. New York : Churchill Livingstone.

[17] Strom, Russell G., Vin Marthur, Heather Givans, Douglas S. Kondziolka, and Noel I. Perin. 2015. Technical modifications and decision-making to reduce morbidity in thoracic disc surgery: An institutional experience and treatment algorithm. *Clinical Neurology and Neurosurgery*. 133: 75-82.

[18] Tan, Lee A., Demetrius K. Lopes, and Ricardo B.V. Fontes. 2014. Ultrasound-guided posterolateral apporach for midline calcified thoracic disc herniation. *The Journal of the Korean Neurosurgical Society*. 55 : 383-386.

[19] Uribe, Juan S., William D. Smith, Luiz Pimenta, Roger Härtl, Elias Dakwar, Urvij M. Modhia, Glen A. Pollock, Vamsi Nagineni, Ryan Smith, Ginger Christian, Leonardo Oliveira, Luis Marchi, and Vedat Devieren. 2012. Minimally invasive lateral approach for symptomatic thoracic disc herniation: initial multicenter clinical experience. *Journal of Neurosurgery: Spine*. 16: 264-279.

[20] Vollmer, Dennis G. and Nathan E. Simmons. 2000. Transthoracic approaches to thoracic disc herniations. *Neurosurgical Focus*. 9: 1-6.

[21] Yoshihara, Hiroyuki. 2014. Surgical treatment for thoracic disc herniation. *Spine*. 39: E406-E412.

[22] Yoshihara, Hiroyuki, and Daisuke Yoneoka. 2014. Comparison of in-hospital morbidity and mortality rates between anterior and nonanterior approach procedures for thoracic disc hernation. *Spine*. 39: E728-E733.

[23] Zuckerman Scott L., Jonathan A. Forbes, Akshitkumar M. Mistry, Harish Krishnamoorthi, Sheena Weaver, Letha Mathews, Joseph S. Cheng, and Matthew J. McGirt. 2014. Electrophysiological deterioration in surgery for thoracic disc herniation: impact of mean arterial pressures on surgical outcome. *European Spine Journal*. 23: 2279-2290.

In: Intervertebral Disc Degeneration
Editors: A. L. Ho and A. M. Desai
ISBN: 978-1-63485-829-8

Chapter 6

SURGICAL MANAGEMENT OF CERVICAL DISC HERNIATION

Vinod K. Ravikuzmar[1,2], BS, Jennifer L. Quon[2], MD, Allen L. Ho[2], MD and Ali K. Ozturk[3*], MD

[1]Department of Neurosurgery, New York Medical College, Valhalla, New York, US

[2]Department of Neurological Surgery, Stanford University School of Medicine. Stanford, California, US

[3]Department of Neurosurgery, University of Pennsylvania Perelman School of Medicine. Philadelphia, Pennsylvania, US

ABSTRACT

Cervical disc herniation (CDH) occurs with regular frequency and is the most common indication for cervical spine surgery. While conservative treatment is the first line of defense when managing CDH, severe cases may be treated with anterior, posterior, or combined approaches. Choice of an approach is dependent on careful synthesis of symptoms, exam findings, and imaging results by the surgeon. Studies offer conflicting views regarding which approach results in superior outcomes. The eventual decision on surgical approach, if determined to be necessary, must be individually tailored for each patient.

* Corresponding Author address. Email: Ali.Ozturk@uphs.upenn.edu. Washington Square West Building, 235 South 8th Street, Philadelphia, PA.

Keywords: cervical herniated disc, ACDF, arthroplasty, decompression, foraminotomy, disc replacement

INTRODUCTION

Cervical disc herniation (CDH) is a source of neck and arm pain whose incidence peaks in the sixth decade of life [30]. The etiology of CDH is multifactorial, and known risk factors include lifting heavy objects, cigarette smoke, select occupations, and the male gender. Certain studies report that CDHs occur in 19 out of every 100,000 people, making it a relatively prevalent source of spinal cord and nerve root compression [39]. Most patients experience either neck or arm pain, accompanied by motor weakness in the upper extremity as well as sensory symptoms (e.g., tingling) presenting in a dermatomal distribution [4].

The pathophysiology of cervical disc disease is related to continual mechanical stress and the wide range of motion of the cervical spine that leads to overstretching of the annulus fibrosis leading the annular tears and intradiscal tissue displacement. The horizontal fissures are the primary sites of these changes, which lead to disc protrusions in the direction of the neural foramen. Large disc protrusions occur predominantly in younger patients given that elderly individuals tend to have desiccated disc tissue that were less likely to protrude.

Conservative therapy of CDH should be attempted for six to twelve weeks before surgery is considered [4]. However, if the patient presents with a loss of significant motor function or signs of myelopathy, surgery may need to be performed more urgently.

Despite its prevalence and potential for progression of severe symptoms over time, the clinical course of CDH is largely not understood [30]. Since it is difficult to characterize, CDH treatments and prognosis of these interventions are difficult to predict. Successful identification of risk factors and addressing problems before severe symptoms manifest is thus the preferred solution. This chapter will attempt to review all aspects of CDH care, beginning with diagnosis and conservative treatment options, and terminating with an analysis of various possible surgical approaches to treat the condition.

DIAGNOSIS

Symptoms

CDH results from protrusion of the intervertebral disc centrally into the spinal canal causing cervical myelopathy or laterally into the foramen causing radiculopathy. The three main clinical symptoms associated with CDH are pain, radiculopathy, and myelopathy. Pain associated with cervical syndrome is typically sudden onset, positional, and worse at night. Axial pain can originate from the sinuvertebral nerve innervating the disc, PLL, and meninges, or from the dorsal primary ramus innervating the facets [1, 2]. Radicular pain and symptoms result from nerve root irritation from foraminal disc herniation and can include upper extremity pain, diffuse weakness/numbness of the hands, sometimes in a dermatomal distribution, problems with gait and balance, fine motor impairment, as well as noticeable clumsiness. When CDH causes narrowing of the spinal canal or cervical stenosis, myelopathy symptoms typically develop insidiously manifesting as weakness and spasticity of all extremities, gait imbalance, loss of dexterity, or autonomic dysfunction of the bowel and bladder [9].

Exam

The signs can vary widely in CDH patients: motor weakness, hyper or hypo-reflexia, Hoffmann's or Babinski reflex, inversion of the brachioradialis reflexes, crossed radial reflexes, or clonus. The onset of problems is often sudden for radiculopathy but can be more insidious with myelopathyand caused by direct impingement of nerve roots and the associated inflammation [43].

Imaging

CDH can be seen on plain radiographs, myelography, computerized tomography (CT) or magnetic resonance imaging (MRI). Myelograms can directly demonstrate compression of the nerve or its root. Radiographs may indirectly demonstrate pathology via osteophytes, a decrease in disc height between vertebra, or protrusions/extrusions of calcified disc. MRI is useful for its high soft tissue resolution and multi-planar images and is currently the most frequently used modality in the diagnosis of CDH [44]. It can be utilized to identify herniated disk fragments as well as compressed nerve roots. It can also determine the amount of degeneration and the level of fibrosis of the disc [5].

While MRI is superior for soft tissue anatomy, CT imaging is the preferred modality for demonstrating the bony anatomy, calcification/ ossification, gas within the herniated disc space, or dural indentation. Thus, CT and MRI have complimentary roles and the clinician should have a low threshold to order both if necessary.

Kuijper et al. estimate that 89.7% of patients with radiculopathy present with parasthesias, whereas 24%, 15.3%, and 64.2% of patients present with sensory loss, weakness, and hypoactive tendon reflexes, respectively. Even when a patient does not present with one of the classic symptoms physical exam findings alone cannot rule out CDH [19].

Conservative Treatment

Conservative treatment is recommended for patients in the absence of neurologic deficit and/or intolerable pain and discomfort. Non-medical therapies such as heat packs, soft collars for comfort, and positional and activity changes to limit mechanical stress on the neck can be powerful adjuncts. Patients should avoid heavy lifting, spinal vibration-inducing activities such as running and prolonged neck extension. Medications such as NSAIDs, ibuprofen, COX-2 inhibitors, or oral steroids may reduce inflammation in the area of disc herniation, and are widely considered a first line treatment for pain management of CDH. Physical therapy can complement medical therapy and help reduce pain and increase mobility. Epidural steroid injections (ESI) can also be considered if the prior first line treatments are ineffective, and the patients' symptoms relatively mild.

For patients with more severe CDH with significant neurologic deficit or myelopathy, surgical treatment is recommended. Surgical options can be categorized into the anterior, posterior, and combined approaches.

Anterior Approaches

Anterior approaches for treating CDH include anterior cervical discectomy and fusion (ACDF) and cervical disc replacement (CDR). The standard anterior approach involves dissection, discectomy, and grafting. This approach is utilized primarily when there is stenosis at three or fewer cervical levels or when the patient presents with a kyphotic deformity. It is overall considered to be a safe procedure with successful symptomatic relief.

Anterior Cervical Discectomy and Fusion (ACDF)

Smith and Robinson were the first to apply the anterior approach to the cervical spine, using an iliac crest bone graft to replace the removed disc. In essence, the ACDF involves removing the offending intervertebral disc via discectomy and inserting a spacer to allow for spinal fusion. Driven by the poor prognosis of posterior approaches in treating posterior osteophyte nerve root compression, they were pleased to find that the ACDF was associated with less mortality, less disruption of the spinal canal, and better fusion at the pathological intervertebral region. Since then, modifications of Smith and Robinson's basic principles have enhanced the efficacy of the ACDF. For example, the Cloward technique is very similar to Smith-Robinson's, but modifies the decompression to focus on direct anterior decompression of central or lateralized pathology and he was the first to advocate for allograft fusion [14, 36] (Figure 1).

Anterior cervical plates provide sufficient anterior stability and mobility without the need for posterior stabilization, optimize conditions for arthrodesis, and are highly efficacious in the setting of multi-level fusions [7]. Plates have been associated with the development of dysphagia, esophageal injury, as well as adjacent level ossification, including osteophyte formation and ligament ossification. These adverse effects may be largely minimized with proper plate placement, as well as continued advancements in plate technology [7]. The lower profile of newer anterior plating systems minimizes esophageal trauma and post-operative swallow difficulties. Internal fixation with plates and screws may also be a source of hardware failure if arthrodesis is not achieved. Hardware breakage can occur as a result of differences in tensile strength and elasticity between the bone and hardware. Depending on the extent of hardware failure, it may be necessary to re-operate and remove the broken construct, particularly if the patient has recurrent neck pain and a non-union is present. Smaller locking screws prevent the plate from causing spinal cord damage by obviating the need for bicortical fixation and have decreased screw backouts and subsequent esophageal damage. Dynamic plates allow for the appropriate distribution of stress onto bone as well as a reduction in screw loosening and breakage. This leads to earlier bony fusion by providing stress shielding onto the bone graft [3]. Finally, resorbable plates have demonstrated improved hardware longevity and stress distribution compared to metal plates, and are a promising therapy for the future.

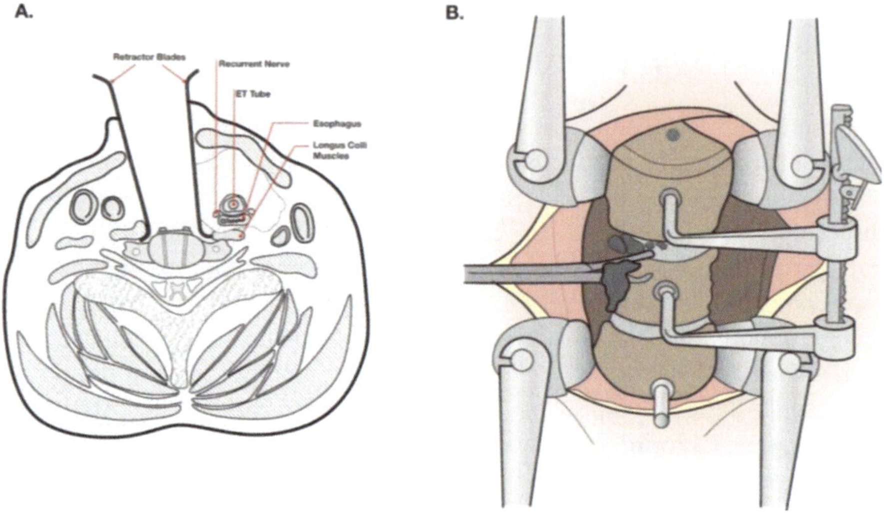

Figure 1. Anterior Cervical Discectomy and Fusion (ACDF) via Cloward technique. A) Axial view of ACDF anatomic exposure. B) Operative view of ACDF Cloward technique exposure and disectomy.

An ideal graft should exhibit osteogenesis, osteoconduction, and osteoinduction. Currently only a few types of grafts demonstrate all three of these characteristics [37]. Grafts should be at least 7mm in height and 2 mm greater than the original disc height to allow of restoration of prior normal disc height. Autografts have been traditionally considered the gold standard graft due to high fusion rates. However, they are associated with donor site morbidity, additional OR time and issues with variable patient bone quality. Donor site complications have lead to a morbidity rate of 20% of higher [33]. and can include, myalgias, paresthesias, hematomas, hip fractures, and infections [28, 33]. Allografts avoids issues of donor site morbidity, is more readily available, and lead to decreased blood loss and operative times. Demineralized Bone Matrix (DBM) is another type of allograft that requires a synthetic cage or mineralized allograft to support the disc space. Xenografts such as bovine bone exhibits biocompatibility problems, creating complications that can sometimes lead to repeated operations. Besides a lower rate of fusion compared to autografts, other significant risks of allograft include immunologic reaction, necrosis of graft, fracture, or delayed union/non-union [24]. Pseudarthrosis or an irreparable bone fracture, can occur in approximately 2-20% of procedures, thus requiring revision typically from a posterior approach [11, 32]. However, when utilized in conjunction with cervical plate fixation, fusion rates are comparable to autograft [31]. Finally, ceramics can also be utilized as graft material and are advantageous in that they avoid donor site morbidity, have sufficient biocompatibility, and have no inherent risks of infection or disease transmission. Hydroxyapatite and tricalcium phosphate are the most widely used and demonstrated favorable fusion rates and outcomes [8, 46].

Cages also can preserve and augment disc height and improve cervical lordosis without the risk of donor site morbidity and complications [32]. They are typically made with stainless tell, titanium, tantalum, or synthetics, and are especially useful in multi-level fusions that involve corpectomies. They can, however, cause a delay in fusion, which may subsequently lead to nonunion and kyphosis due to cage migration, subsidence, and loss of lordosis [16]. Cages also have some potential magnetic artifact, which may decrease imaging visualization [12]. In addition, ceramic materials including tricalcium phosphate or calcium hydroxyapatite can be used that are cost effective, biocompatible, and present almost no infection risk. Though initially problematic because of fracture risk and slippage, modern ceramics have minimized these risks. Bone morphogenic protein (BMP) is no longer approved in the anterior cervical spine due to concerns with ectopic bone formation, dysphagia, and severe edema. However, utilization of autologous cancellous bone packed into cages can obviate the risk of donor site complications and have demonstrated comparable fusion rates to autografts [16, 38]. Advances in technique have chiefly involved the development of novel grafts and spacers to improve fusion.

There are also synthetic materials that can be used in place of autografts and allografts. For example, interbody spacers, such as those made from porous tantalum, polyether-ether-ketone (PEEK), and the zero-Profile (Zero-P) anchored spacer, are becoming increasingly popular. These cages are typically box shaped within which cancellous autobone, DBM or ceramics can be packed. In a recent study, Vanichkachorn et al. demonstrate that the use of PEEK interbody spacers in single-level ACDF produces a high rate of fusion without the associated complications of allografts [37]. Further, Cho et al. demonstrate the potential of Zero-P for lowering the failure rate of ACDFs [6].

More recently, microdiscectomy and endoscopic techniques have been pioneered as minimally invasive strategies to improve patient outcomes [42].

Full endoscopic cervical discectomy (FECD) can involve either an anterior or posterior approach tailored to the offending pathology. FECD is thought to have less soft tissue damage, faster rehabilitation, as well as fewer and easier surgical revisions when compared with more invasive decompressive techniques. Therefore, FECD is not only a good stand-alone treatment, but may also be beneficial as a supplement to conventional procedures [42]. Other noninvasive techniques include the cervical microendoscopic foraminotomy/discectomy (CMEF/D) and the cervical microendoscopic decompression of stenosis (CMEDS) [15]. When the canal diameter is decreased at the level of the midvertebral body or the compression extends beyond the disc space, corpectomy should be implemented following discectomy in order to remove the offending vertebral body. Cages are often helpful in these scenarios in order to help maintain and restore cervical kyphosis lost with corpectomies.

Surgical Approach and Considerations

Positioning for the anterior cervical approach should take into account the angle of the disc space to be fused. The head and neck should be supported and hyperextended if possible (if there is no concern about posterior instability) by raising the height of the shoulders with supports. Depending on the level, mobilizing the shoulders as far inferior as possible may help optimize visualization of the lower cervical levels. There is considerable debate regarding optimal side of approach for the anterior approach [21-23, 25, 26]. The anatomically variant course of the recurrent laryngeal nerve is on the right, thus a left side should be protective against nerve injury. However, many surgeons are right handed and prefer approaching from the right. The thoracic duct is also located on the left side, thus, a right-sided approach can avoid a chylothorax complication [14]. Still others suggest allowing pathology to dictate side of approach, that is, approaching from the side opposite the compressive pathology for ease of access.

With respect to avoiding nerve and esophageal injury and devastating vocal cord paralysis, many of these injuries occur as a result of retraction and recognition of the structures held in retraction for exposure is critical. Releasing intubation cuff pressure periodically and use of blunt versus sharp dissection during exposure is prudent to avoid complications. After localization of desired level with XR fluoroscopy, an incision made along a convenient skin crease is preferred for a better cosmetic result. A horizontal incision along the skin crease is adequate for exposure of multiple cervical levels, if necessary. After dividing the skin and subcutaneous fat layer, the platysma is encountered and divided horizontally. Deep cervical fascia enveloping the sternocleidomastoid muscle (SCM) laterally and the omohyoid muscle deep to the SCM. This deep cervical fascia must be released in order to mobilize the trachea and esophagus medially. Often times, the omohyoid muscle may need to be divided with impunity for adequate exposure. The carotid pulse is palpated with a finger laterally and blunt dissection of the deep cervical fascia is completed medial to the carotid and lateral to the trachea and esophagus until the anterior vertebral bodies are felt. The alar fascia attaching the trachea and esophagus is divided and the longus colli muscles are visualized.

The mid-point between the longus colli approximate the mid-line and the longus colli are dissected off the vertebral bodies via cautery. The target disc space is then identified and confirmed with fluoroscopy and soft tissue dissected off the anterior portion of the target vertebral bodies for fusion. Self-retaining cervical retractors are utilized to maintain retraction soft tissue structures and are typically anchored under the longus colli muscles. These retractors optimize the operative window for the discectomy and ensure adequate protection of soft tissue structures from injury. The annulus of the disc is incised and the discectomy completed in standard fashion with a curette or high-speed drill if necessary for hard disk with exposure, incision, and resection of the PLL if possible to ensure optimal posterior decompression. Direct visualization of the dura after removal of the PLL ensures complete removal of soft disc herniation. Resection of disc material within the uncal-vertebral joints with Kerrison rongeurs is also essential to relieve radicular compression and a small blunt probe should the utilized to inspect the neural foramen to ensure adequate nerve root decompression.

At this point, several different options exist for interbody grafting or placement of a cage (especially following a corpectomy) as discussed above. The plating options are also various, but generally both interbody graft or cage and anterior plates are implanted to maintain or restore disc height, avoid foraminal stenosis, cervical kyphosis, maintain anterior cervical stability, and promote bony fusion across levels.

Disc Replacement – Arthroplasty

Cervical disc arthroplasty (CDA) is a form of total disc replacement that arose as a motion-preserving alternative treatment to ACDF [20, 22]. With standard anterior fusion there is decreased motion of the fused segments, which increases the stress on the adjacent levels, with leads to adjacent segment disease overtime. Disc replacement via CDA allows for preservation of motion at the disease level to decrease stress at adjacent levels and avoidance of adjacent segment disease. First described by Fernstrom with a steel ball design, [13]. the designs have evolved significantly to include ball-and-trough, semi-constrained metal endplate-on-polyethylene insert, or cross-linked polyethylene annulus design. These differing designs allow for rotational and translational movements while at the same time mimicking the 'cushion' of a IVD with prosthetic annulus and nucleus. Indications for CDA include single or two-level disc herniations and spondylosis with radiculopathy and/or myelopathy. Contraindications include pre-operative instability, facet join arthritis, osteoporosis, previous local infection or ankylosis. Hu et al. demonstrate in their long-term meta-analysis that CDA resulted in superior outcomes compared to ACDF with regards to neurological outcomes, improvement in pain symptoms, number of follow-up procedures, and the rate of adverse events [20]. Conflicting studies, however, make it difficult to determine differences in cost-effectiveness and quality of life between these two treatments [21, 27]. Improvements or maintenance of sagittal balance with CDA was similar to ACDF [29]. Disc replacement can be complicated by migration of the prosthesis, ossification, kyphosis, and failure of the device. In fact, severe heterotopic ossification in a subset of cases may restrict range of motion (ROM) and cause pain [20, 47]. Prostheses are currently being tested and implemented alongside arthroplasty in order to improve clinical and radiological outcomes [22, 25].

Posterior Approaches

Posterior approaches to CDH treatment involve decompression, disc removal, and cervical fusion. The earliest cervical spine operations were performed posteriorly, prior to the development of anterior techniques. Posterior approaches may lead to more post-operative pain due to dissection of the paraspinal muscles and therefore longer hospital stays. Complications from posterior approaches are often related to positioning and can include ocular injury, postlaminectomy kyphosis or instability, air embolism, pseudomeningoceles, vertebral artery injury, or brachial plexopathies. Cervical laminectomy can also lead to a C5 or C6 nerve radiculopathy due to traction of the extradural components of the roots following shift and expansion of the cord after decompression. Nonetheless, posterior approaches are particularly relevant for treating patients with extensive cervical lordosis, pathology located dorsal or lateral. Many suggest that lordosis should be a prerequisite for a posterior approach in order to facilitate spinal cord movement away from anterior structures. Posterior approaches are relatively straightforward and avoid many of the critical structures encountered in an anterior approach. Patients are positioned prone and three-pin Mayfield fixation is used to position the head in a tucked fashion. A neutral or lordotic position should be assumed and over flexion avoided if a fusion is being performed. Fluoroscopy can help identify the relevant level. Palpation of the spinous processes can identify midline and dissection follows the ligamentum nuchae. This allows minimal blood loss and minimizes dissection of the paraspinal muscles. A bovie and Cob can be used for muscle dissection. Aggressive devascularization or thermal damage can prevent fusion and wound healing. It is also important to stay within the borders of the lateral masses because beyond these borders are the venous plexi surrounding the vertebral arteries. For closure the fascia should be reapproximated with absorbable sutures.

Decompression

Decompression-based approaches remain part of the standard for treating cervical disk disease. They can be divided into three subtypes: laminoplasty, laminectomy, and foraminotomy.

Laminoplasty and Laminectomy

The goals of surgery are to decompress the spinal cord at the level of pathology. Preservation of cervical lordosis lends itself to a cervical laminoplasty or laminectomy. These approaches allow the surgeon to decompress at multiple levels with preservation of motion. Fusion can be performed if there are concerns about stability. Some studies have suggested that posterior fusions, with lateral mass screw fixation, may be prudent in all cervical laminectomies in order to prevent such complications and post laminectomy kyphosis.

In a laminoplasty, the vertebral lamina is cut unilaterally, creating a hinge that widens the spinal canal and relieves pressure on the spinal cord. If necessary, the spinous process can be extracted, and wedges can be used to maintain the patency of the opening. Bilateral gutters are created using a high-speed burr and kerrison rongeurs, followed by a green stick osteotomy, bone graft insertion, and finally plate insertion for stabilization. Endoscopic techniques can also allow for a minimally invasive technique. Patients who have undergone a laminoplasty experience fewer complications and have preserved cervical mobility compared to those who have undergone a laminectomy [45]. Laminoplasty is contraindicated in patients with an ossified ligamentum flavum, epidural scars, or pre-operative kyphosis [23].

Laminectomy, on the other hand, involves complete excision of the posterior spinal ligament and spinous processing order to relieve pressure on the spinal cord. As described above, the paraspinal muscles are dissected off of the spinous process. The lateral dissection should expose the entirety lateral masses unless instrumentation is also planned. Careful dissection of the subperiosteal plane should be performed prior to using the drill in order to ensure that there is no soft tissue damage. A Leksell rongeur and high-speed bur can be used to thin the laminae and subsequently remove it en-bloc. A small cutting bur allows the outer cortical and cancellous bone to be removed, leaving only a thin layer of cortical bone. Notably, at the cervical levels the dura is not protected by the ligamentum flavum at the superior extent of the lamina. The laminae at these levels are also shingled and often the inferior lamina of the level above must also be removed in the laminectomy. Importantly, surgeons should be wary of placing instruments underneath bone at the stenotic level. Intersegmental motion should be avoided in areas of cord compression. Finally, the facets must be spared in the laminectomy so that the spine is not destabilized, and the patient doesn't subsequently develop a kyphotic deformity (Figure 2).

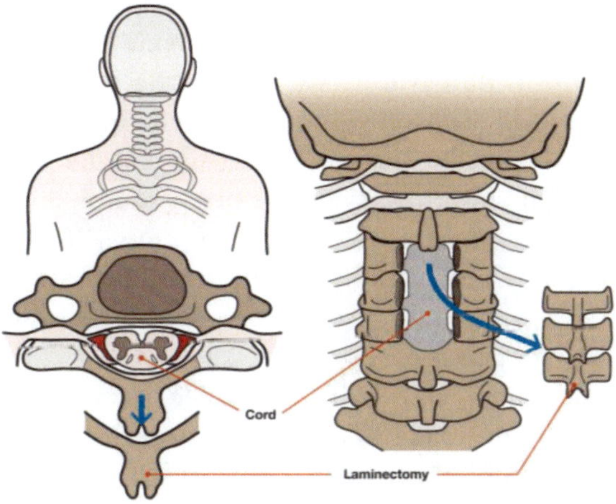

Figure 2. Posterior cervical laminectomy.

Posterior Cervical Foraminotomy

Posterior cervical foraminotomy (PCF) was first described in 1944 by Spurling and Scoville and is a motion-preserving alternative to ACDF [34]. This technique is reserved for cases of nerve root compression, rather than myelopathy, favoring lateral disc herniations. Clinical symptoms must correlate with radiographic findings. It is appropriate to use this approach after conservative management has failed. Advantages to this approach are that it does not destabilize the disk space and therefore require a fusion, and it avoids many of the critical structures involved in anterior approaches. Contraindications to PCF include cervical instability, posterior longitudinal ligament ossification, cervical spine kyphosis, and axial neck pain [34].

In a posterior cervical formaninotomy, the patient is positioned either prone or sitting, though the later is more difficult. The prone position requires the torso to be supported with a Wilson frame, and the head is typically stabilized with three-pin Mayfield fixation. The head should be slightly tucked in a “military” position, and the surgeon should be cautious not to hyperextend the neck. Intraoperative x-ray or fluoroscopy can identify the pathologic level optimize the placement of the incision. Generally, a 1-2 inch incision allows adequate dissection of muscle and fascia off the spinous processes as well as minimizes the amount of muscle retraction. The medial 50% of the facet should be exposed. A high-speed drill is used to decorticate the lamina of the vertebral levels on the pathologic side. A kerrison or drill can be used to remove bone, starting just medial to the junction of the lamina and the facet, in order to expose the lateral most portion of the lamina. Removal of the superior portion of the inferior lamina will expose the inferior pedicle. The ligamentum flavum can be dissected with off with a nerve hook or small dissector. The nerve root is then visualized exiting the thecal sac and the foramen is palpated with a nerve hook. The bone overlying the nerve root is thinned with a drill. The shell of bone can be removed with sharp curette then kerrison. These instruments are then used to carefully decompress the nerve root by removing the offending tissue, which often presents as bony overgrowth, ligament, or disk overlying the dorsal surface of the nerve root. Small osteophytes anteriorly can be carefully curetted. The bony decompression can be extended accordingly. Typically only 30-50% of the foramen needs to be unroofed to ensure adequate decompression. The nerve root should be palpated out laterally and the color observed for signs of longstanding compression. Careful hemostasis should be obtained, but care should be taken not to leave too much hemostatic material at the site. The facia is reapproximated and the incision closed (Figure 3).

Since its inception, PCF has developed into a minimally invasive surgery, which has resulted in reduced blood loss, shorter hospital durations, and decreased post-operative narcotic requirements. Minimally invasive techniques, first implemented in 2000 have since dramatically reduced the postoperative morbidity of posterior approaches.

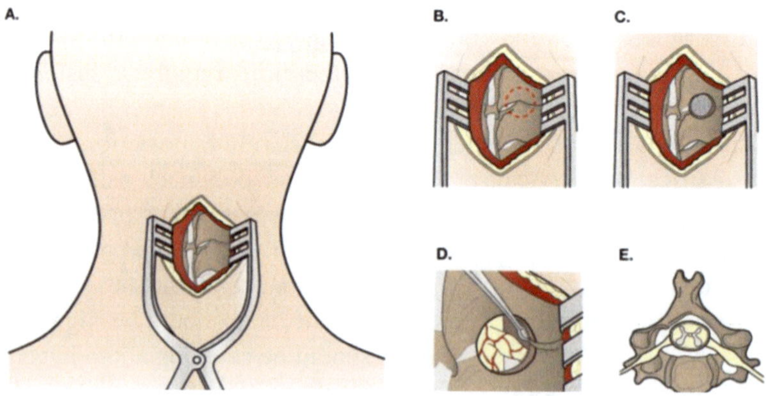

Figure 3. Posterior cervical foraminotomy. A) Paramedian incision and unilateral exposure of the lamina. B) Identification of lamina and target facet joint. C) Facetectomy is performed. D) Removal of overlying ligamentum flavum to visualize nerve root and ensure adequate decompression. E) Axial view of ideal foraminal decompression of target nerve root.

Disc Replacement

Posterior disc replacement strategies arose as an alternative to the ACDF, given the concerns for adjacent segment disease and post-operative dysphagia [18, 26]. Disc replacement was originally devised in the late 1980s and featured a metal ball-and-socket device, secured in place with screws. Over time, a titanium alloy with a porous coating was used to facilitate bone ingrowth. Current variants include polyethylene coats and calcium phosphate layers.

Advantages of a posterior cervical discectomy include less destabilization of the disc space and therefore no need for a fusion, less risk of damaging surrounding structures, and the ability to simultaneously address foraminal stenosis. Nevertheless, the need to dissect spinal muscle in this approach leads to greater post-operative pain and longer recovery times.

Anterior vs. Posterior Approaches

A purely anterior or posterior approach for CDH can lead to varying complications either in the immediate post-operative period or in the long-term. Herkowitz et al. compared anterior and posterior approaches and characterized disc herniations as one of two types. Type 1 represented single level anterolateral herniations and includes patients who presented with radiculopathies. In contrast, type 2 represented central soft disc herniations and included patients who presented with myelopathy as well as potential upper extremity paresthesias. Patients who were treated with anterior approaches had better long-term outcomes than those treated with either laminectomy or foraminotomy [17]. In contrast, Dohrmann et al. suggest that posterior approaches had a 94% success rate at long-term follow-up compared with 80% for anterior approaches [10].

Combined Approaches

A combination of anterior and posterior approaches has demonstrated efficacy in treating certain pathologies. Yang et al. describe retrospective study of patients undergoing either an ACDF or combined anterior-posterior approaches for the treatment of CDH with concurrent ossification of the posterior longitudinal ligament. They include 5 who underwent combined

ACDF and either single- or multi-stage posterior laminectomies and fusions. Outcomes for the combined approach did not differ significantly from the standard ACDF [41].

Microsurgical discectomy with laminoplasty (MDTL) is another combined technique that was pioneered to address some of the disadvantages of a purely anterior approach. Introduced by Fujimoto et al. in 2002, the technique utilizes simultaneous discectomy and laminoplasty to preserve motion in the operated spinal segments. A surgical microscope is used to reduce the risk damaging surrounding neurological structures [35].

Another combined approach involves discectomy and nucleoplasty. Discectomy is first performed to remove the herniated disc. The disc is subsequently coagulated using the nucleoplasty technique [40]. Potential complications are similar to nucleoplasty alone, and include hematoma, disc infection, nerve damage, and equipment breakage inside the wound.

Conclusion

Due to their variable presentation, CDH treatment selection is highly individualized, requiring many factors and challenges to be considered. Though it is not necessary for all spine surgeons to be experts in these detailed surgical methods, it is imperative to understand the fundamental differences and advantages of each procedure.

References

[1] Aprill, Charles, Anthony Dwyer, and Nikolai Bogduk. "Cervical zygohypophyseal joint patterns, II: a clinical evaluation." 1990. *Spine* 15 (6): 458-61.

[2] Bogduk, Nikolai, and Anthony Marshland. "The cervical zygohypophyseal joints as a source of neck pain." 1988. *Spine* 13 (6): 610-7.

[3] Brodke, Darrel S., Sohrab Gollogly, R. Alexander Mohr, Bao-Khang Nguyen, Andrew T. Dailey, and Kent N. Bachus. "Dynamic cervical plates: biomechanical evaluation of load sharing and stiffness." *Spine (Phila Pa 1976)* 26 (12): 1324-9.

[4] Carette, Simon, and Michael G Fehlings. 2005. "Clinical Practice. Cervical Radiculopathy." *The New England Journal of Medicine* 353 (4): 392–99. doi:10.1056/NEJMcp043887.

[5] Chen, Yue-Yao, Xiao-Feng Lin, Fang Zhang, Xiang Zhang, Hui-Jun Hu, Dong-Ye Wang, Lie-Jing Lu, and Jun Shen. 2013. "Diffusion Tensor Imaging of Symptomatic Nerve Roots in Patients with Cervical Disc Herniation." *Academic Radiology* 21 (3): 338–44. doi:10.1016/j.acra.2013.11.005.

[6] Cho, Hyun Jun, Junseok W. Hur, Jang Bo Lee, Jin Sol Han, Tai Hyoung Cho, and Jung Yul Park. 2015. "Cervical Stand-Alone Polyetheretherketone Cage versus Zero-Profile Anchored Spacer in Single-Level Anterior Cervical Discectomy and Fusion: Minimum 2-Year Assessment of Radiographic and Clinical Outcome." *Journal of Korean Neurosurgical Society* 58 (2): 119–24. doi:10.3340/jkns.2015.58.2.119.

[7] Chung, Jae Yoon, Sung Kyu Kim, Sung Taek Jung, and Keun Bae Lee. 2014. "Clinical Adjacent-Segment Pathology after Anterior Cervical Discectomy and Fusion: Results after a Minimum of 10-Year Follow-Up." *Spine Journal* 14 (10): 2290–98. doi:10.1016/j.spinee.2014.01.027.

[8] Cook, Stephen D., Jeanette E. Dalton, Edward H. Tan, William V. Tejeiro, Michael J. Young, and Thomas S. Whitecloud III. 1994. "3rd In vivo evaluation of anterior cervical fusions with hydroxylapatite graft material." *Spine (Phila Pa 1976)* 19 (16): 1856-66.

[9] Crandall, Paul H., and Ulrich Batzdorf. 1966. "Cervical spondylotic myelopathy." *Journal of Neurosurgery* 25 (1): 57-66.

[10] Dohrmann GJ, JC Hsieh. 2014. "Long-term results of anterior versus posterior operations for herniated cervical discs: analysis of 6,000 patients." *Med Princ. Pract.* 23 (1): 70-3. doi:10.1159/000351887.

[11] Elder, Benjamin D., Eric W. Sankey, Debebe Theodros, Mohamad Bydon, C. Rory Goodwin, Sheng-Fu Lo, Thomas A. Kosztowski, Allen J. Belzberg, Jean-Paul Wolinsky, Daniel M. Sciubba, Ziya L. Gokaslan, c, Ali Bydon, Timothy F. Witham. 2016. "Successful anterior fusion following posterior cervical fusion for revision of anterior cervical discectomy and fusion pseudarthrosis." *J Clin Neurosci* 24: 57-62. doi:10.1016/j.jocn.2015.07.019.

[12] Elliott, C A, R Fox, R Ashforth, S Gourishankar, and A Nataraj. 2015. "Magnetic Resonance Imaging Artifact Following Anterior Cervical

Discectomy and Fusion with a Trabecular Metal Cage." *Journal of Neurosurgery. Spine*, 1–6.

[13] Fernstrom, U. 1996. "Arthroplasty with intercorporal endoprothesis in herniated disc and in painful disc." *Acta Chir Scand Suppl* 357: 154-9.

[14] Fessler, Richard Glenn, and Laligam Sekhar. 2006. *Atlas of Neurosurgical Techniques: Spine and Peripheral Nerves*. New York: Thieme Medical Publishers, Inc.

[15] Gala, Vishal C., John E. O'Toole, Jean Marc Voyadzis, and Richard G. Fessler. 2007. "Posterior Minimally Invasive Approaches for the Cervical Spine." *Orthopedic Clinics of North America*. doi:10.1016/j.ocl.2007.02.009.

[16] Gercek E, Arlet V, Delisle J, Marchesi D. Subsidence of stand-alone cervical cages in anterior interbody fusion: warning. Eur Spine J. 2003;12:513–516.

[17] Herkowitz, H N, L T Kurz, and D P Overholt. 1990. "Surgical Management of Cervical Soft Disc Herniation. A Comparison between the Anterior and Posterior Approach." *Spine* 15 (10): 1026–30. http://www.ncbi.nlm.nih.gov/pubmed/2263967.

[18] Jackson, Robert J., Reginald J. Davis, Gregory A. Hoffman, Hyun W. Bae, Michael S. Hisey, Kee D. Kim, Steven E. Gaede, Pierce Dalton Nunley. 2016. "Subsequent surgery rates after cervical total disc replacement using a Mobi-C Cervical Disc Prosthesis versus anterior cervical discectomy and fusion: a prospective randomized clinical trial with 5-year follow-up." *J Neurosurg Spine* 24 (5): 734-45. doi:10.3171/2015.8.SPINE15219.

[19] Kujper, B., J. Th. J. Tans, R.J. Schimsheimer, B.F.W. van der Kallen, A. Beelen, F. Nollet, M. de Visser. 2009. "Degenerative Cervical Radiculopathy: Diagnosis and Conservative Treatment. A Review." *European Journal of Neurology.* 16 (1): 15-20. doi:10.1111/j.1468-1331.2008.02365.x.

[20] Lei, Tao, Yaming Liu, Hui Wang, Jiaxin Xu, Qinghua Ma, Linfeng Wang, Yong Shen. 2016. "Clinical and radiological analysis of Bryan cervical disc arthroplasty: eight-year follow-up results compared with anterior cervical discectomy and fusion." *Int Orthop.* doi:10.1007/s00264-015-3098-7.

[21] Lewis, Daniel J, Mark a Attiah, Neil R Malhotra, Mark G Burnett, and Sherman C Stein. 2014. "Anterior Surgical Management of Single-Level Cervical Disc Disease: A Cost-Effectiveness Analysis." *Spine* 39 (25): 2084–92. doi:10.1097/BRS.0000000000000612.

[22] Loumeau, Thomas P., Bruce V. Darden, Thomas J. Kesman, Susan M. Odum, Bryce A. Van Doren, Eric B. Laxer, Daniel B. Murrey. 2016. "A RCT comparing 7-year clinical outcomes of one level symptomatic cervical disc disease (SCDD) following ProDisc-C total disc arthroplasty (TDA) versus anterior cervical discectomy and fusion (ACDF)." *Eur Spine J.* doi:10.1007/s00586-016-4431-6.

[23] Luk, Keith D., Vijay Kamath, Ashwin Avadhani, S. Rajasekaran. 2010. "Cervical laminoplasty." *Eur Spine J.* 19 (2): 347-8. doi:10.1007/s00586-010-1314-0.

[24] Norman-Taylor, FH, and RN Villar. 1997. "Bone allograft: a cause for concern?" *J Bone Joint Surg Br* 79 (2): 178-80.

[25] Obernauer, J, J. Landscheidt, S. Hartmann, G. A. Schubert, C. Thomé, C. Lumenta. 2016. "Cervical arthroplasty with ROTAIO® cervical disc prosthesis: first clinical and radiographic outcome analysis in a multicenter prospective trial." *BMC Musculoskelet. Disord.* 17:11. doi: 10.1186/s12891-016-0880-7.

[26] Ozdol, Cagatay, Cezmi Cagri Turk, Ali Erdem Yildirim, Ali Dalgic. 2015. "Anterior Herniation of Partially Calcified and Degenerated Cervical Disc Causing Dysphagia." *Asian Spine J.* 9 (4): 612-6. doi:10.4184/asj.2015.9.4.612.

[27] Qureshi, Sheeraz A, Steven McAnany, Vadim Goz, Steven M Koehler, and Andrew C Hecht. 2013. "Cost-Effectiveness Analysis: Comparing Single-Level Cervical Disc Replacement and Single-Level Anterior Cervical Discectomy and Fusion: Clinical Article." *Journal of Neurosurgery. Spine* 19 (5): 546–54. doi:10.3171/2013.8.SPINE12623.

[28] Samartzis Dinos, Francis H. Shen, Edward J. Goldberg, and Howard S. An. 2005. "Is autograft the gold standard in achieving radiographic fusion in one-level anterior cervical discectomy and fusion with rigid anterior plate fixation?" *Spine (Phila Pa 1976)* 30 (15): 1756-61.

[29] Sasso, Rick C., Newton H. Metcalf, John A. Hipp, Nicholas D. Wharton, Paul A. Anderson. 2011. "Sagittal alignment after Bryan cervical arthroplasty." *Spine (Phila Pa 1976)* 36 (13): 991-6. doi: 10.1097/BRS.0b013e3182076d70.

[30] Schoenfeld, Andrew J, Alan a George, Julia O Bader, and Pedro M Caram. 2012. "Incidence and Epidemiology of Cervical Radiculopathy in the United States Military: 2000 to 2009." *Journal of Spinal Disorders and Techniques*. doi:10.1097/BSD.0b013e31820d77ea.

[31] Shapiro, Scott. 1996. "Banked fibular and the locking anterior cervical plate in anterior cervical fusions following cervical discectomy." *Journal of Neurosurgery* 84 (2): 161-5.

[32] Shiban, Ehab, Karina Gapon, Maria Wostrack, Bernhard Meyer, Jens Lehmberg. 2015. "Clinical and radiological outcome after anterior cervical discectomy and fusion with stand-alone empty polyetheretherketone (PEEK) cages." *Acta Neurochir (Wien)* 158 (2): 349-55. doi:10.1007/s00701-015-2630-2.

[33] Silber, Jeff S., D. Greg Anderson, Scott D. Daffner, Brian T. Brislin, J. Martin Leland, Alan S. Hilibrand, Alexander R. Vaccaro, Todd J. Albert. 2003. "Donor site morbidity after anterior iliac crest bone harvest for single-level anterior cervical discectomy and fusion." *Spine* 28 (2): 134-9.

[34] Skovrlj, Branko, Yakov Gologorsky, Raqeeb Haque, Richard G. Fessler, and Sheeraz A. Qureshi. 2014. "Complications, Outcomes, and Need for Fusion after Minimally Invasive Posterior Cervical Foraminotomy and Microdiscectomy." *Spine Journal* 14 (10): 2405–11. doi:10.1016/j.spinee.2014.01.048.

[35] Tanaka, Nobuhiro, Yoshinori Fujimoto, Tadayoshi Sumida, Hideki Manabe, Kazuyoshi Nakanishi, Yasushi Fujiwara, Naosuke Kamei, Toshio Nakamae, Bunichiro Izumi, and Mitsuo Ochi. 2013. "Long-term clinical results of microsurgical transdural discectomy with laminoplasty: follow-up results over 10 years." *J Neurosurg Spine* 18 (6): 653-60. doi:10.3171/2013.3.SPINE12673.

[36] Vaccaro, Alexander R., and Jason C. Eck. 2010. *Controversies in Spine Surgery: Best Evidence Reccomendations.* New York: Thieme Publishers, Inc.

[37] Vanichkachorn, Jed, Timothy Peppers, Dennis Bullard, Scott K. Stanley, Raymond J. Linovitz, James T. Ryaby. 2016. "A prospective clinical and radiographic 12-month outcome study of patients undergoing single-level anterior cervical discectomy and fusion for symptomatic cervical degenerative disc disease utilizing a novel viable allogeneic, cancellous, bone matrix (trinity evolution™) with a comparison to historical controls." *Eur Spine J.* doi:10.1007/s00586-016-4414-7.

[38] Wang, Jeffrey C., Paul W. McDonough, Kevin K. Endow, Rick B. Delamarter. 2000. "Increased fusion rates with cervical plating for two-level anterior cervical discectomy and fusion." *Spine (Phila Pa 1976)* 25 (1): 41-5.

[39] Wong, Jessica J., Pierre Côté, Jairus J. Quesnele, Paula J. Stern, and Silvano A. Mior. 2014. "The Course and Prognostic Factors of Symptomatic Cervical Disc Herniation with Radiculopathy: A Systematic Review of the Literature." *Spine Journal.* doi:10.1016/j.spinee.2014.02.032.

[40] Yang, Bo, Jingkai Xie, Biao Yin, Le Wang, Shibing Fang, and Shengyu Wan. 2013. "Treatment of Cervical Disc Herniation through Percutaneous Minimally Invasive Techniques." *European Spine Journal: Official Publication of the European Spine Society, the European Spinal Deformity Society, and the European Section of the Cervical Spine Research Society*, 382–88. doi:10.1007/s00586-013-3063-3.

[41] Yang, Hai-song, De-yu Chen, Xu-hua Lu, Li–li Yang, Wang-jun Yan, Wen Yuan, Yu Chen. 2010. "Choice of surgical approach for ossification of the posterior longitudinal ligament in combination with cervical disc hernia." *Eur Spine J.* 19 (3): 494–501. doi:10.1007/s00586-009-1239-7.

[42] Yang, Jun-Song, Lei Chu, Liang Chen, Fu Chen, Zhen-Yong Ke, Zhong-Liang Deng. 2014. "Anterior or posterior approach of full-endoscopic cervical discectomy for cervical intervertebral disc herniation? A comparative cohort study." *Spine (Phila Pa 1976)* 39 (21): 1743-50. doi:10.1097/BRS.0000000000000508.

[43] Yeung, Jacky T, John I Johnson, and Aftab S Karim. 2012. "Cervical Disc Herniation Presenting with Neck Pain and Contralateral Symptoms: A Case Report." *Journal of Medical Case Reports* 6 (1): 166. doi:10.1186/1752-1947-6-166.

[44] Yi, Sook Ji, Jang Gyu Cha, Jong Kyu Han, Hyun-Joo Kim. 2015. "Imaging of Herniated Discs of the Cervical Spine: Inter-Modality Differences between 64-Slice Multidetector CT and 1.5-T MRI." *Korean Journal of Radiology* 16 (4): 881-8. doi: 10.3348/kjr.2015.16.4.881.

[45] Yue, B, Bohua Chen, Xue-Xiao Ma, Yong-Ming Xi, Hong-Fei Xiang, You-Gu Hu, Guoqing Zhang. 2015. "One stage laminoplasty and posterior herniotomy for the treatment of myelopathy caused by cervical stenosis with cervical disc herniation." *Int J Clin Exp Med.* 8 (6): 9565-9.

[46] Zdeblick, Thomas A., Mary E. Cooke, David N. Kunz, David Wilson, Ronald P. McCabe. 1994. "Anterior cervical discectomy and fusion

using a porous hydroxyapatite bone graft substitute. " *Spine (Phila Pa 1976)* 19 (20): 2348-57.

[47] Zhao, Yan Bin, Yu Sun, Zhong Qiang Chen, and Zhong Jun Liu. 2010. "Application of Cervical Arthroplasty with Bryan Cervical Disc: Long-Term X-Ray and Magnetic Resonance Imaging Follow-up Results." *Chinese Medical Journal* 123 (21): 2999–3002. doi:10.3760/cma.j.issn.0366-6999.2010.21.009.

In: Intervertebral Disc Degeneration
Editors: A. L. Ho and A. M. Desai
ISBN: 978-1-63485-829-8

Chapter 7

LUMBAR STENOSIS: PREVALENCE, RISK FACTORS, AND TREATMENT

Daniel Shepherd[1,2], MD, Panagiotis Kerezoudis[1,2], MD, Michelle J. Clarke[1], MD and Mohamad Bydon[1,2,*], MD

[1]Department of Neurologic Surgery, Mayo Clinic, Rochester, MN, US
[2]Mayo Clinic Neuro-Informatics Laboratory, Rochester, MN, US

ABSTRACT

Lumbar spinal stenosis (LSS) is a clinical syndrome characterized by buttock and/or lower extremity pain with or without back pain secondary to degenerative spinal canal narrowing and compression of the neurovascular elements. LSS is the most common reason for spinal surgery in patients over 65 years of age. It results in significant pain and disability, compromising the quality of life and everyday activities of the affected patients. Pain is aggravated by certain postures, including walking, standing or lumbar extension and characteristically alleviated by recumbency, sitting and forward flexion. Initial treatment options include conservative management such as lifestyle modification, physiotherapy, epidural injections and medications. Very few randomized controlled clinical trials have assessed the role and the efficacy of non-surgical

* Correspondence to: Mohamad Bydon (bydon.mohamad@mayo.edu), Department of Neurosurgery, Mayo Clinic, 200 First Street SW, Rochester, MN, US.

modalities for the management of patients with LSS and therefore there is a lack of sufficient evidence to suggest a specific method is superior. Surgical intervention is performed when there is failure of conservative management or neurologic emergency. Current techniques include open or minimally invasive approaches that aim at restoring spinal canal diameter and relieving neurovascular compromise.

Keywords: lumbar stenosis, spinal canal narrowing, aging, intervertebral disc

1. Introduction

Lumbar spinal stenosis (LSS) or lumbar stenosis is a degenerative condition secondary to the normal aging process that affects the intervertebral discs, the ligamentum flavum and the facet joints causing narrowing of the spaces that surround the spinal neurovascular structures.

LSS was described back in the 1880s [1] but it was Verbiest in 1954 who first tried to define central lumbar spinal stenosis. He reported a "particular form of narrowing of the lumbar vertebral canal" that was not associated with any other anomaly of the spine. He also noted that with walking and standing these patients presented with signs of disturbance of the cauda equina: bilateral radicular pains, disturbances of sensation and impairment of motor power in the legs, However, when the patient was in recumbent position the symptoms immediately disappeared. The neurological examination during testing revealed nothing abnormal [2].

North American Spine Society defines lumbar stenosis as "a clinical syndrome of buttock or lower extremity pain, which may occur with or without back pain, associated with diminished space available for the neural and vascular elements in the lumbar spine" [3].

2. Prevalence – Epidemiology

LSS is the most common indication for surgical intervention in the spine in people older than 65 years of age [4], translating to more than 37,000 laminectomies in Medicare alone and an aggregated hospital cost of nearly $1.65 billion [5]. It has been found that LSS affects more than 200,000 people in the US [5].

According to the Framingham population study, the incidence of anatomic spinal stenosis in people older than 60 based on cross-sectional imaging studies, ranges between 19 to 47%. [6] Moreover, data from the National Spine Network and the National Ambulatory Medical Care Survey, have shown that LSS is diagnosed in 13-14% of patients with chronic low back pain who seek a specialist's opinion and 3-4% who see a general physician [7, 8].

3. Signs and Symptoms

Patients with acquired lumbar stenosis typically present in the sixth and seventh decade of life, whereas patients with congenital lumbar stenosis typically present in the third to fifth decade. Low back pain is one of the most common symptoms and main reasons patients seek medical care [9–11]. Other common sites of pain include the buttocks, the thighs and the legs. Patients usually describe the pain as burning or cramping in nature, with symptom varying from gradual, dull aching pain in the sacroiliac area and posterior thighs to sharp, shooting radicular pain along the lower extremity. When central canal stenosis is present, pain is often bilateral, but not always symmetrical. In contrast, with pure lateral recess and foraminal stenosis, the symptoms typically resemble unilateral radiculopathy.

Patients report symptom relief with positions that decrease lumbar lordosis and increases central canal diameter such as sitting, squatting and recumbency as these tend to reduce the inward buckling of the ligamentum flavum and distract the facet joints thus enlarging the neural foramina and relieving pressure on neurovascular structures.

The most cardinal manifestation of spinal stenosis is neurogenic claudication. It is moderately sensitive (~60%), but highly specific for LSS. [12] It consists of progressive onset of pain, weakness, numbness and tingling in unilateral or bilateral buttocks, hips, thighs or legs, that is provoked by standing and lumbar extension, aggravated by prolonged walking and characteristically relieved by a change in posture. [13] Patients may occasionally exhibit the "shopping cart sign," where the patient is walking in a flexed or a stooped position in order to relieve the symptoms. Intermittent claudication secondary to peripheral vascular disease poses an important diagnostic challenge, as it also presents with leg pain during walking (Table 1). The key difference lies on whether the symptoms exacerbate with posture versus exertion. Patients with neurogenic claudication improve with sitting down and leaning over, whereas those with intermittent (vascular) claudication report pain alleviation with rest. Nadeau et al. found that the positive "shopping cart sign," which is a constellation of symptoms, including pain located above the knee, triggered by walking and relieved with sitting, is highly suggestive of neurogenic claudication. (Positive Likelihood Ratio of 13) [14]. Conversely, pain located below the knees that is alleviated with standing alone provides strong evidence of intermittent claudication (Positive Likelihood Ratio of 20) [14].

Interestingly, the neurologic exam can be normal in up to 18% of cases, including normal lower extremity muscle strength, normal reflexes and negative straight leg raising test. Pain is typically reproduced by lumbar extension and diminished knee reflexes and reduced or absent ankle reflexes are also common finding.

Table 1. Neurogenic vs vascular claudication

Clinical Feature	Neurogenic Claudication	Intermittent Claudication
Pain distribution	dermatomal (nerve distribution)	Sclerotomal (muscle groups with common vascular supply)
Quality of pain	Shooting, electric shock-like	Cramping
Pain onset	can be immediate, inconsistent	Gradual, consistent
Aggravating factors	standing, waking, coughing variable amount of exercise	fixed amount of exercise
Alleviating factors	posture-dependent sitting, bending over	posture-independent standing still
Sensory loss	dermatomal distribution	stocking distribution
Distance to claudication	Variable day-to-day	Constant day-to-day
Legs affected	usually both	usually one
Foot pallor on elevation	none	mild to marked
Peripheral pulses	normal	decreased or absent
Feet skin temperature	normal	decreased

Neurological findings include motor, sensory, reflex and autonomic signs that correspond to the level(s) of involvement [15]. The most common affected root is the L5, followed by the L4, the L3 and the S1 [15, 16]. Bladder dysfunction can also be seen and is most frequently encountered in the geriatric population. Deen et al. performed two- to four- level laminectomies in patients averaging 71 years of age for severe LSS and a variable degree of bladder compromise. Although only 45% of patients exhibited improved urinary function (post-void residual urinary volume, cystoscopy and urodynamic studies) and 60% reported subjective recovery of bladder function, the authors concluded that laminectomy can have a beneficial effect on bladder function in patients with severe LSS [17].

In summary, LSS is a significant cause of chronic pain and disability. Its symptoms can have significant impact on patient mobility and physical activity. Most patients with LSS have limited walking capacity and the use of walking aids is often necessitated. Compromised functional autonomy forces most patients to follow a sedentary lifestyle behavior with serious repercussions for overall health and physical performance.

4. Causes and Associated Conditions

LSS can be classified into congenital and acquired (or both).

- *Congenital LSS* is a condition in which abnormalities during postnatal development cause narrowing of the spinal canal [18]. According to the Framingham study, the prevalence of congenital LSS in the population ranges between 2.6 and 4.7% [6]. It has also been associated with congenital spondylolisthesis and achondroplasia [19].
- *Acquired LSS* is the result of degenerative changes to the spine secondary to aging. These changes include loss of intervertebral disc height, disc bulging, facet joint hypertrophy and osteophyte formation and hypertrophy of the ligamentum flavum. (Figure 1 and 2) Other less common causes include trauma, excessive scar tissue after back surgery, ankylosing spondylitis and infection [18].

It is important to mention that LSS is a process with dynamic component: the association of symptoms with patient's posture, such as standing, walking and recumbency correlate with the dynamic changes in the spine. These changes occur in a normal spines as well but in a degenerative spine with baseline narrowing, lumbar spine extension and axial loading reduce lumbar spinal canal diameter critically compressing neurovascular structures [20, 21].

4.1. Degenerative Spondylolisthesis

Spondylolisthesis is a degenerative spine pathology that is caused by one vertebral body slipping forward or backward relative to the level below. Patients are typically women (female-to-male ratio 2:1) aged 50 to 60 years whose symptoms evolved over decades and exacerbated over months and years. Neurological deficits late in the course and are correlated with the onset of neurogenic claudication or radiculopathy associated with proximal weakness or footdrop. The most commonly involved level is the L4-5, followed by L3-4, L2-3 and L5-S1 (Figure 1a).

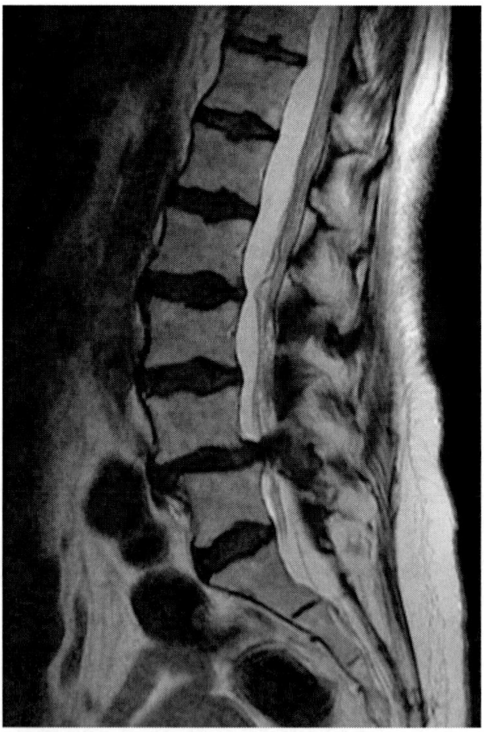

Figure 1a. Sagittal lumbar spine MRI without IV contrast of a 74 year old female with a 1 year history of L5 radiculopathy. Imaging shows a marked central spinal stenosis at L4-5. There is concurrent grade I spondylolisthesis at L4-5.

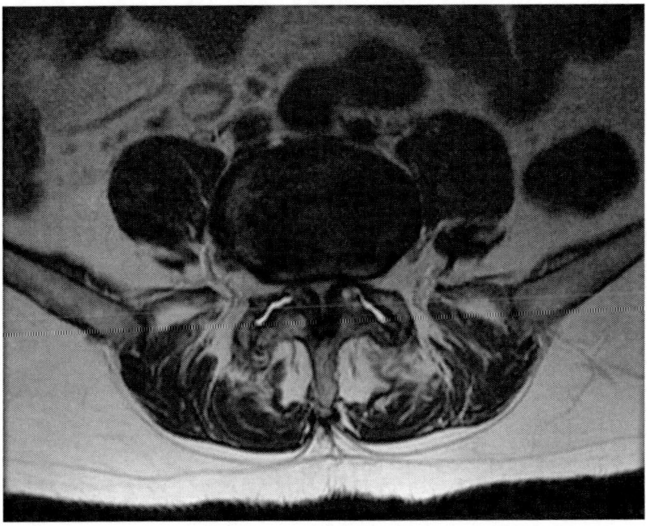

Figure 1b. Axial lumbar spine MRI scan without IV contrast showing severe spinal canal stenosis at the L4-L5 level with advanced degenerative facet changes and bilateral L4-L5 neural foraminal stenosis.

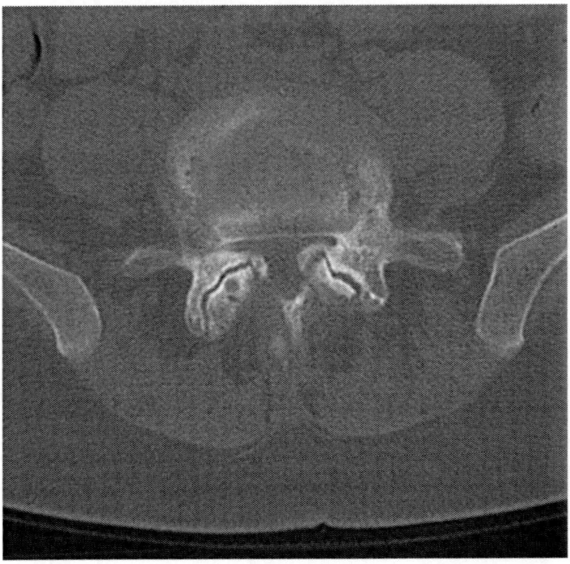

Figure 1c. Axial lumbar spine CT scan without IV contrast showing severe spinal canal stenosis at the L4-L5 level with advanced degenerative facet changes and moderate bilateral L4-L5 neural foraminal narrowing.

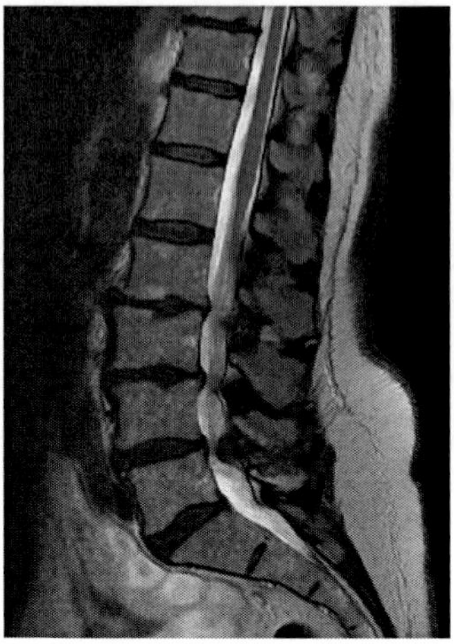

Figure 2a. Sagittal lumbar spine MRI without IV contrast of an 84 year old female with a 1 year history of neurogenic claudication. Imaging shows multilevel congenital and degenerative changes within the lumbar spine that is contributing to severe central spinal stenosis at L4-L5 with compression of the cauda equina. There is also moderate spinal stenosis L2-L3 and L3-L4.

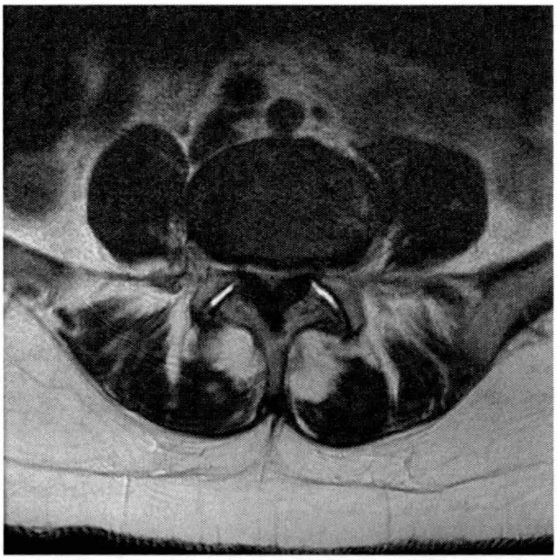

Figure 2b. Axial lumbar spine MRI without IV contrast showing bilateral facet joint, periarticular and interspinous inflammation at the L4-L5 level. There is also moderate foraminal narrowing.

Guidelines for the management of patients with LSS and associated degenerative spondylolisthesis are lacking, but general recommendations include patient education, analgesic medication as well as flexion strengthening and stabilizing exercises [22]. The SPORT trial is the highest quality study to date that has evaluated the outcomes of surgical versus nonsurgical treatment for patients with LSS and degenerative spondylolisthesis. The study found no difference between the two groups in the intention-to-treat analysis, although the as-treated analysis after the crossover showed significant improvement in pain and function in favor of the surgical group during a 2-year follow-up period [23, 24].

4.2. Disc Herniation

A herniated disc is a condition in which the annulus fibrosis of the vertebral disc is ruptured, enabling the inner nucleus pulposus to herniate outwards. The extruded disc materials may compress the surrounding nerves and create pain or other neurological symptoms. Up to 45% of patients undergoing surgery for LSS with or without spondylolisthesis will have some form of disc herniation. [15] In a study of 100 patients that underwent multilevel laminectomy (mean = 3.6 levels) with one-level (78 patients) and two-level (22 patients) instrumented fusion, 57 herniated discs were identified in 50 patients: 21 central, 7 foraminal, 24 far lateral and 5 recurrent disc herniations.

4.3. Ossification of Ligamentum Flavum (OLF)

Ossification of the ligamentum flavum is a phenomenon in which there is calcification of the ligamentum flavum which may result in central or lateral recess stenosis. It can be a significant contributor to LSS. It presents as an initial ingrowth of fibrocartilage and formation of ossific-calcific components in the ligamentum flavum attributed to type II collagen proliferation. It is more common in East Asians and sometimes coexists with ossification of the posterior longitudinal ligament (OPLL) [25]. Hypertrophy or OLF usually begins laterally and extend medially [26]. It is an important risk factor for incidental durotomy: in a study of 110 predominantly geriatric patients, all of the 10 cases that developed intraoperative dural tears exhibited severe OLF, which extended to or through the dura in 3. For the remaining 100 patients without dural tears, 57 exhibited moderate/hypertrophied yellow ligament and 22 showed marked OLF.

4.4. Ossification of the Posterior Longitudinal Ligament (OPLL)

OPLL is a condition that results in hypertrophy and calcification of the posterior longitudinal ligament, which just lies anterior to the spinal dura. Although the majority of OPLL is found in the cervical spinal canal (80%), the frequency in the proximal lumbar spinal canal is around 10%, with the remaining 10% being found in the proximal thoracic spine [27]. OPLL and OLF can both contribute to lumbar stenosis [27]. In a study of 1100 patients that underwent decompressive surgery for spinal stenosis, 23 patients (2.3%) had OPLL and/or OYL (only OPLL-11, only OLF-12, OPLL and OLF-3) [27].

4.5. Limbus Vertebral Fractures

A limbus vertebral fracture, also called a posterior apophyseal ring fracture, is an uncommon fracture pattern that may result in LSS. The pathogenesis of this fracture still remains controversial. Mechanisms of injury that have been reported to be important for this type of injury are acute trauma and strenuous sports activity [28, 29]. They are classified into four types and are best visualized by CT [30]. Type I lesions consist of avulsions of the posterior cortical vertebral rim, Type II fractures are composed of central cortical and cancellous bone fractures, Type III lesions are more lateralized chip fractures and Type IV fractures span the entire length and breadth of the posterior vertebral margin between the end plates [30]. The fragments are typically large and warrant an extensive exposure and resection to afford adequate decompression. Unilateral facetectomy is usually necessitated in the setting of foraminal and far lateral lesions. Furthermore, piecemeal removal is the safest method for resection, by first creating a depression or a defect at the level of the disk space and then morcellating the fracture segment using a curette, tamp and mallet technique [15]. Intraoperative somatosensory evoked potentials (SEPs) and electromyography (EMG) can prove to be useful in order to minimize excess manipulation and retraction of neural elements and consequent neurological injury.

4.6. Synovial Cysts

Synovial cysts are small, benign, fluid filled sacs that can form around facet joints as a result of degenerative joint changes. Similar to disc herniations, they may compress the surrounding neural elements and contribute to the pathology of LSS [31]. Epstein et al. compared patients with a diagnosis of synovial cysts and LSS without (45 patients) versus with coexisting spondylolisthesis (35 patients) based on the SF-36 questionnaire [32]. Laminectomy was performed in both groups at an average of 3.8 vs 3.5 levels, respectively. Post-operatively, five patients from the first group developed instability and 11 patients with Grade 1 preoperative spondylolisthesis progressed to Grade 2. Two years following surgical intervention, good/excellent results in SF-36 Function scale (+44 and +38 points) were documented in only 58% and 63% of patients, respectively. As synovial cysts reflect intrinsic disruption and pathology of the facet joint and therefore instability, spinal fusion should be considered in order to achieve optimal operative results.

4.7. Scoliosis

Degenerative lumbar scoliosis (DLS) is mainly a disease of the elderly population with an estimated prevalence ranging from 6% to 68% [34–36]. It can be the sequelae of childhood scoliosis or be developed de novo with age, as a result of degenerative disc and joint disease. Spine malalignment can lead to gait instability as well as difficulty standing upright and walking with severe repercussions on patient's quality of life [33].

There are no current evidence-based guidelines for the treatment of adult patients with DLS and therefore decision making and surgical candidacy largely depends on the provider's expertise and the patient's preferences. The benefits of correcting the spinal deformity and addressing the symptoms should outweigh the associated risks, such as nerve injury, infection, pseudarthrosis and further spinal instability [37]. The complication rates can be as high as 60% for long fusion procedures [38]. An alternative to spinal fusion, decompression with nonfusion dynamic stabilization is a safe and effective procedure for patients with LSS and mild to moderate DLS (<30°) with satisfactory outcomes, including correction of the scoliotic angle, visual analog scale and Oswestry Disability Index [39]. There is an ongoing trial comparing surgical vs non-operative management for adult patients with DLS (clinicaltrials.gov; NCT00854828) and hopefully it will provide further insight into the management of this complex disorder.

5. Differential Diagnosis

Differential diagnosis includes, but it is not limited to

1. Intermittent (vascular) claudication
2. Disc herniation
3. Degenerative disc disease: trochanteric bursitis
4. Facet joint arthropathy
5. Juxtafacet cyst
6. Arachnoiditis
7. Intraspinal tumor
8. Diabetic nephropathy
9. Spinal dural arteriovenous malformation

6. Natural History of LSS

Given the fact that most patients with LSS seek medical care, particularly those with incapacitating symptoms that limit everyday life activities, the natural history of this condition is still largely unknown. The North American Spine Society (NASS) has recently released guidelines concluding that the natural course is favorable in approximately one third to a half of patients with clinically mild to moderately symptomatic LSS. [3] Moreover, several older studies have shown that the condition can improve in up to one third of patients and most patients remain unchanged for up to eight years of follow-up [40, 41]. A more recent study by Minamide et al. [42] followed up 34 patients with a diagnosis of LSS and leg or low back pain with serial magnetic resonance imaging and found that symptoms remained the same or improved in 60% of patient, despite progressive anatomic changes. Interestingly, Haig et al. [43] suggest that spinal stenosis is a fluctuating disease process with potentially improving continuum, where anatomic and neurologic deficits do not necessarily predict future function.

7. Imaging Studies

According to current guidelines, the imaging studies provide the most definitive diagnostic information for patients with suspicion of LSS [44]. In clinical practice, imaging is not a routine part of initial patient evaluation but it is rather reserved for diagnostic confirmation and procedural planning of surgical candidates.

7.1. X-Rays (XR)

Plain anteroposterior (AP) lumbosacral radiographs demonstrate the number of lumbar vertebrae and may disclose concurrent bony anomaly, such as spondylolisthesis. Lateral films reveal the lumbar spine curvature and the presence of static or dynamic instability and olisthesis. This is defined as translation greater than 4 mm and degrees of angulation at the level of olisthy greater than 10-12 [45]. Lastly, oblique views demonstrate the pars interarticularis and any associated defects.

7.2.Computed Tomography (CT)

Reconstructed CT scan images in axial, sagittal and coronal planes can confirm the diagnosis of LSS. In addition to demonstrating AP spinal canal diameter, computed tomography can contribute to revealing disk disease (degenerative disk, bulging annulus, herniated disk), hypertrophied ligaments, facet arthropathy, ossification of the posterior longitudinal ligament (OPLL) and ossification of the ligamentum flavum. (Figure 1c) CT myelograms are rarely performed for LSS, as the combination of CT and MRI evaluation can noninvasively establish the diagnosis in the majority of the cases. [44] On the other hand, a CT myelogram may provide useful information in instances when MRI evaluation is not available.

7.3.Magnetic Resonance Imaging (MRI)

MRI is considered the gold-standard noninvasive imaging modality for soft-tissue structures assessment but not for bony pathology. It allows the examination of the shape, the size and the anatomic association between spinal, neural and vascular elements [44]. Nevertheless, a systematic review found no difference in the accuracy between CT and MRI for the diagnosis of LSS [46]. MRI is best utilized to demonstrate degenerative disk disease and associated compressive changes of the nerve roots and the thecal sac, hypertrophy or ossification of the posterior longitudinal ligament and ligamentum flavum, olisthesis and other neural pathology [47] (Figure 2a).

In addition, increased fluid within the facet joints can be visualized on routine axial MRI views [48] and it is positively correlated with sagittal spinal instability documented by MRI and dynamic radiographs obtained at the L4-5 level. Three-dimensional enhanced MRI offer "myelographic" views that may capture surgical findings in 82.6% of the time [49]. MRI has a sensitivity of 87-96% and specificity of 68-75% for the diagnosis of LSS [50]. Moreover it has variability for assessment of the different spinal characteristics, with central canal stenosis showing the highest reliability and foraminal stenosis and subarticular zone stenosis the lowest reliability [51] (Figure 1b and 2b).

Regarding parameters that are used to quantify LSS, anteroposterior diameter less than 10 mm and cross sectional area less than 70 mm^2 of the spinal canal are most commonly reported. [52] Moreover, developmental spinal stenosis is defined as anteroposterior canal diameter of <20 mm at L1, <19 mm at L2, <19 mm at L3, L4 <17 mm at L4, and <16 mm at L5 and S1 [53]. Lastly, according to a Delphi study, perineural intraforaminal fat and disc protrusion are the most important diagnostic indicators of LSS [54].

Contrast-enhanced MRI is not a part of routine evaluation of a patient with possible LSS but it can help differentiate between among tumors, scar, arachnoiditis, demyelinating syndromes and infection [55].

Although spinal canal narrowing and neurovascular compression visualization on imaging is needed for LSS diagnosis, it is not sufficient; many asymptomatic lesions might be identified on MRI in the elderly population. An old case series conducted in patients older than 60 years, showed that herniated discs (36%) and lumbar stenosis (21%) were symptomatic in only about one third of the subjects [47]. Therefore, abnormalities on MRI images must always be correlated with age and any clinical signs and symptoms before surgical intervention is contemplated.

8. Management

8.1. Non-Surgical

Non-surgical management is generally considered the first-line treatment option for LSS. It includes lifestyle modification, physiotherapy, medication, spinal injections and multidisciplinary rehabilitation. Corroborating conservative treatment, a study in 1996 [56] compared Oswestry Disability

Index (ODI) and surgeons' clinical assessment for 54 matched pairs of patients with lumbar stenosis treated surgically (laminectomy) vs non-surgically and found no statistically significant differences in the outcomes between the two groups. There are very few high quality randomized clinical trials that have investigated non-surgical management strategies for LSS. There is an ongoing trial that has assigned patients with radiographically confirmed LSS into 3 groups, comparing usual medical care with individualized manual therapy and rehabilitation exercise versus community based group exercise [57]. Another study is assessing the effect of a pedometer-based physical activity promotion and nutrition lifestyle intervention on overall health and quality of life of patients with symptomatic LSS [58, 59].

Although there is a lack of consensus regarding treatment recommendations, most patients who seek medical care are initially managed conservatively and surgical management is recommended after failure of conservative treatment [60].

8.1.1. Physiotherapy

Physiotherapy is a well-established and accepted treatment for LSS. Physiotherapy-related options include [61]:

1. Aerobic exercise
2. Balance training
3. Flexion-based exercises
4. Spinal manipulation
5. Postural instruction
6. Body weighted supported treadmill ambulation
7. Muscle coordination training
8. Manual stretching of the back and hip musculature

Tomkins et al. carried out a telephone survey on patients diagnosed with lumbar stenosis and found that the most common physical therapy treatments used are massage (27%), strengthening exercises (23%), flexibility exercises (18%) and heat/ice (14%) [62]. Unfortunately, there is paucity of studies regarding the efficacy of physiotherapy for LSS. A recently published systematic review of nonoperative treatments for patients with LSS and neurogenic claudication found only low quality evidence from single small trials, concluding that exercise might provide short-term benefit for leg pain and function compared to no treatment [60]. Another systematic review by Macedo et al. failed to reach conclusions regarding which physical therapy treatment is superior for LSS [63]. The authors found that physiotherapy modalities offer no additional benefit to exercise alone. Moreover, when physiotherapy was compared to surgical intervention, surgery lead to better long-term (2-year) outcomes for pain and disability but not for walking distance. Lastly, a secondary data analysis of the Spine Patient Outcomes Research Trial (SPORT) showed that physiotherapy was not associated with improvement in pain and physical function after 1 year, although patients were less likely to receive surgery within one year [64]. The most recent randomized controlled trial was published in 2015 and compared standard physiotherapy regimen of lumbar flexion, conditioning exercises and patient education with lumbar decompression [65]. Interestingly, intention-to-treat analysis revealed no difference between the two groups at one and two years. Nevertheless, the results of the study are difficult to interpret as a high proportion of the participants assigned to physiotherapy crossed over to surgery.

In summary, physiotherapy for patients with LSS has not yet been established as a successful alternative to surgical intervention. This can be attributed to the fact that physiotherapy's main role is to address the patient's symptoms and functionality, rather than the pathology itself. For example, flexion exercises and other postural dynamic changes during physiotherapy alter spinal canal diameter, thus relieving spinal compression. The mechanisms underlying these effects remain to be determined and further investigation is therefore warranted.

8.1.2. Medications

Various over-the-counter and prescription drugs can be used to treat LSS symptoms. Despite their anti-inflammatory and analgesic properties, non-steroidal anti-inflammatory drugs (NSAIDS) are no more effective than acetaminophen in the treatment of LSS. The same holds true for opioids and muscle relaxants as well; according to well controlled studies, they are not more effective than acetaminophen and NSAIDS for pain control [66, 67]. The role of long term opioids is still unclear [66]. Corticosteroids and antidepressants are often prescribed for patients with LSS, but their efficacy is not yet fully elucidated [69, 70].

Prostaglandins, gabapentin and vitamin B6 are some drugs that have been in used small clinical trials and were found to improve pain and walking distance [56, 65]. Prostaglandin (PG) E1 has been suggested to improve symptoms in patients with LSS by vasodilation and improving blood flow to cauda equina and nerve roots. In short term follow-up studies, PGE1 led to improvement in pain, Japanese Orthopedic Association Score and walking distance [68]. Calcitonin is no better than placebo and acetaminophen (paracetamol) [59, 66].

8.1.3. Epidural Injections

Epidural injections are often used to help alleviate LSS symptomatology, but the evidence surrounding the effectiveness of epidural injections is controversial. Some studies have reported that epidural injections improve pain, function and quality of life when compared to home exercise and inpatient physical therapy alone [60]. However, other trials have failed to show any benefit. A recent meta-analysis showed that epidural steroid injections provide limited short-term and long-term pain relief and walking distance improvement in LSS patients [68].

Local anesthetics may also be injected to assist with pain control in patients with LSS. A systematic review of the literature of injections for central LSS found that local anesthetics either alone or with steroids offer low back and lower extremity pain relief [69]. There is lack of evidence to suggest that epidural steroid injections are better than local lidocaine injections alone, regardless of the mode of the epidural injection. One large, double-blind controlled trial found no benefit of epidural injections with glucocorticoids and lidocaine over lidocaine alone after 6 weeks of follow-up [70].

Steroid injections are not without risks. They are associated with hyperglycemia, anxiety, sleeplessness, transient immunity suppression, and they have even been associated with an increased rate of fungal meningitis [71]. Steroid injections are contraindicated in the setting of an infection. Despite these risks, in select patients with LSS, epidural injections may be a good alternative for patients who do not have adequate symptom relief from physiotherapy or oral medications.

8.2. Surgery

8.2.1. When to Operate?

Surgical intervention can be an appropriate treatment modality for patients who have failed conservative medical management and who lack severe comorbidities prohibiting intervention. In selected circumstances, surgery can improve pain control and can potentially reverse existing neurological deficits. Some studies have shown superiority of surgical intervention versus medical management alone [23, 72, 73]. A randomized controlled trial of 94 patients comparing nonsurgical (44 patients) and surgical (50 patients) interventions for treatment of LSS, the surgical group reported a greater degree of back and leg pain relief, and they demonstrated less overall disability compared to the nonsurgical cohort [72]. This is consistent with multiple other studies that have also reported improved pain relief and functional outcomes with surgical patients [23, 73, 74]. Surgery for LSS consists of either decompression alone or decompression with spinal fusion.

8.2.2. Laminotomy

Lumbar laminotomy is a procedure that involves removal of the inferior portion of the rostral hemilamina and mesial one third of the ipsilateral facet while simultaneously preserving the spinous process, interspinous ligament, and lateral two thirds of the ipsilateral facet joint. Laminotomies may be performed in a unilateral or bilateral fashion. One study followed 102 patients who had underwent a unilateral laminotomy for an average of 5.6 years, and 92.2% noted sustained improvement post operatively [75]. Another study of bilateral laminotomies showed a 76% incidence of good or excellent results based on patient outcome questionnaires and a 71% of good or excellent outcomes based on surgeon outcome measures [76]. Given the preservation of the spinous process and interspinous ligaments, laminotomies may help preserve spinal stability. One study compared clinical results and postoperative stability of 41 patients treated by laminectomy with those of 26 patients who underwent bilateral laminotomy after a mean follow-up period of 3.7 years. The clinical outcomes were comparable (78 versus 81% good outcome), but spinal instability was more frequent in the laminectomy group [77].

8.2.3. Laminectomy without Fusion

Lumbar laminectomy is an effective and safe treatment for severe LSS. It involves surgical removal of the entire dorsal spinous process, bilateral lamina, and underlying ligamentum flavum. With this technique, compression of the neural foramina can be palpated, and foraminotomies can easily be performed if there is evidence of concurrent foraminal stenosis. There is class III evidence to suggest that a decompression without fusion is acceptable in patients without evidence of spinal instability [78]. One study of 500 patients showed statistically significant differences in back pain, radiculopathy, neurogenic claudication, motor deficits, and sensory deficits in patients who underwent laminectomy for LSS [74]. The surgeon should carefully evaluate the radiographic images in order to determine the level of diseased segments and provide an adequate decompression.

Success rates associated with a decompressive lumbar laminectomy for LSS range from 78 to 91% [79–82]. A prospective study found a success rate of 78-88% at six weeks and 6 months, but this dropped to 70% at 1 year and 5 year follow up post operatively [82]. A second study of 50 patients with LSS and degenerative spondylolisthesis demonstrated that a lumbar laminectomy had 91% frequency of good to excellent results at three years and an 87% success rate at six years [79]. Other studies have also found comparable success rates (80% to 84%) following decompression alone for LSS [80, 81].

8.2.4. Laminectomy with Instrumented Fusion

In some series, the addition of instrumented fusion techniques following decompressive laminectomy has been associated with improved outcomes. For instance, one study of 50 patients with LSS and olisthesis compared decompression alone (25 patients) to decompression with instrumented fusion (25 patients) and found that the fusion cohort had improved outcomes at 3 years. [83] Common indications for a fusion include presence of spondylolisthesis, radiographic evidence of facet joint laxity at the site of stenosis, scoliotic deformity, excessive kyphosis, and excessive surgical removal of facet joint or ligaments that may result in iatrogenic spinal instability.

Careful patient selection and extensive preoperative discussions are essential as fusion procedures place patients at a greater risk for perioperative morbidity and mortality compared to decompressive procedures alone [84, 85]. Deyo et al. report that fusion procedures in the elderly can have a twofold increased mortality rate, a 20% increased perioperative morbidity rate, and that patients were 5.6 times more likely to require a blood transfusion [84, 85].

8.2.5. Minimally Invasive Surgery

Minimally invasive spine surgery (MIS) techniques are becoming increasingly popular in spinal surgery. Studies suggest that MIS decompression techniques may be comparable to open decompression procedures. One prospective study of 885 patients comparing the effectiveness of MIS decompression versus traditional open laminectomy concluded that the Oswestry Disability Index (ODI) in patient undergoing MIS decompression was equivocal to that of the laminectomy cohort [86]. Multiple other studies have also ascertained that MIS decompression procedures are associated with significantly less blood loss, reduced hospital stays, and often have decreased need for ancillary support upon dismissal [87, 88].

Certain patient populations, such as the geriatric patients or patients with medical comorbidities that limit more invasive procedures, may have increased benefit from MIS techniques. Multiple studies have shown MIS decompression to be a safe and effective treatment strategy for LSS in elderly patients and improve their quality of life [89–91].

Overall, MIS procedures have a similar complication profile when compared to open approaches [87]. However, due to decreased maneuverability, certain complications such as dural tears may be more difficult to repair intraoperatively. Careful patient selection and adequate surgical experience with MIS techniques is crucial to perform a safe and effective minimally invasive lumbar decompression.

8.3. Surgical Failures and Operative Complications

Surgical failures in patients with LSS can usually be classified into two broad groups: patients who did not get any pain relief following surgery (early treatment failures), and those who initially experienced pain relief but later developed recurrent symptoms (late treatment failures). One study showed that most early treatment failures were secondary to either poor patient selection (the absence of actual neurogenic claudication coupled with the absence of severe stenosis on preoperative radiographic studies) or inadequate surgical decompression [92]. Late treatment failures often occur due to recurrent stenosis. Recurrent stenosis can occur either at or adjacent to the previously operated level. In one series of 100 patients, 16 demonstrated recurrent stenosis [93]. Most patients with recurrent stenosis respond to further surgery.

Similarly, lumbar decompression surgery both with or without fusion techniques are associated with certain surgical risks. One of the more common complications associated with spinal decompression surgery is durotomy. The incidental durotomy rate with laminectomy procedures may be as high as 5 to 11% [74, 94–96]. A dural tear does predispose patient to subsequent complications such as low pressure headaches, meningeal pseudocyst formation, and dural-cutaneous cerebrospinal fluid (CSF) fistulas [97, 98]. Some studies suggest that an incidental durotomies during a first time lumbar decompression did not adversely affect the long-term outcomes in affected patients [99]. Other common surgical complications for surgery include superficial and deep wound infections (0.9 - 5%) [100], and temporary increased motor deficit (1-8%). Less common surgical complications include direct neural injury, deep vein thrombosis, pulmonary embolism, and post-operative visual loss secondary to posterior ischemic optic neuropathy [101, 102].

9. CONCLUSION

LSS is a common disease primarily affecting the elderly that is characterized by degenerative changes causing progressive compression of neurovascular structures, leading to debilitating symptoms of neurogenic claudication and radiculopathy. Patients should be informed of the generally favorable natural course of the disease and the expected benefits and risks of each treatment option. Management strategies should be applied in a stepwise fashion leading with initial conservative treatment options, including physiotherapy, medications and epidural injections. Surgical intervention should be considered in patients that fail conservative measures or develop significant neurologic compromise, such as cauda equina syndrome. Individualized decision making should consider the patient's expectations and goals. Minimally invasive spinal surgery represents a promising surgical technique that offers optimal surgical outcomes while minimizing complications. Future research should focus on defining the different phenotypes within the broad spectrum of LSS pathophysiology with the goal of enhancing personalized health care delivery.

REFERENCES

[1] Szpalski M, Gunzburg R. Lumbar spinal stenosis in the elderly: an overview. *Eur Spine J* 2003;12 Suppl 2:S170–5.

[2] Verbiest H. A radicular syndrome from developmental narrowing of the lumbar vertebral canal. *J Bone Joint Surg Br* 1954;36-B:230–7.

[3] Watters WC 3rd, Baisden J, Gilbert TJ, Kreiner S, Resnick DK, Bono CM, et al. Degenerative lumbar spinal stenosis: an evidence-based clinical guideline for the diagnosis and treatment of degenerative lumbar spinal stenosis. *Spine J* 2008;8:305–10.

[4] Deyo RA. Treatment of lumbar spinal stenosis: a balancing act. *Spine J* 2010;10:625–7.

[5] Deyo RA, Mirza SK, Martin BI, Kreuter W, Goodman DC, Jarvik JG. Trends, major medical complications, and charges associated with surgery for lumbar spinal stenosis in older adults. *JAMA* 2010;303:1259–65.

[6] Kalichman L, Cole R, Kim DH, Li L, Suri P, Guermazi A, et al. Spinal stenosis prevalence and association with symptoms: the Framingham Study. *Spine J* 2009;9:545–50.

[7] ECRI Health Technology Assessment Group. Treatment of degenerative lumbar spinal stenosis. *Evid Rep Technol Assess* 2001:1–5.

[8] Lurie J, Tomkins-Lane C. Management of lumbar spinal stenosis. *BMJ* 2016;352:h6234.

[9] Amundsen T, Weber H, Nordal HJ, Magnaes B, Abdelnoor M, Lilleâs F. Lumbar spinal stenosis: conservative or surgical management?: A prospective 10-year study. *Spine* 2000;25:1424–35; discussion 1435–6.

[10] Iversen MD, Katz JN. Examination findings and self-reported walking capacity in patients with lumbar spinal stenosis. *Phys Ther* 2001;81:1296–306.

[11] Lin S-I, Lin R-M. Disability and walking capacity in patients with lumbar spinal stenosis: association with sensorimotor function, balance, and functional performance. *J Orthop Sports Phys Ther* 2005;35:220–6.

[12] Turner JA, Ersek M, Herron L, Deyo R. Surgery for lumbar spinal stenosis. Attempted meta-analysis of the literature. *Spine* 1992;17:1–8.

[13] Porter RW. Spinal stenosis and neurogenic claudication. *Spine* 1996;21:2046–52.

[14] Nadeau M, Rosas-Arellano MP, Gurr KR, Bailey SI, Taylor DC, Grewal R, et al. The reliability of differentiating neurogenic claudication from vascular claudication based on symptomatic presentation. *Can J Surg* 2013;56:372–7.

[15] Epstein NE. Lumbar Spine Stenosis. Youmans Neurological Surgery, Elsevier; 2011, p. 2923–34.

[16] Epstein JA, Epstein BS, Lavine L. Nerve rot compression associated with narrowing of the lumbar spinal canal. *J Neurol Neurosurg Psychiatry* 1962;25:165–76.

[17] Deen HG Jr, Zimmerman RS, Swanson SK, Larson TR. Assessment of bladder function after lumbar decompressive laminectomy for spinal stenosis: a prospective study. *J Neurosurg* 1994;80:971–4.

[18] Ciricillo SF, Weinstein PR. Lumbar spinal stenosis. *West J Med* 1993;158:171–7.

[19] Soldatos T, Chalian M, Thawait S, Belzberg AJ, Eng J, Carrino JA, et al. Spectrum of magnetic resonance imaging findings in congenital lumbar spinal stenosis. *World J Clin Cases* 2014;2:883–7.

[20] Chad DA. Lumbar spinal stenosis. *Neurol Clin* 2007;25:407–18.

[21] Penning L. Functional pathology of lumbar spinal stenosis. *Clin Biomech* 1992;7:3–17.

[22] Kalichman L, Hunter DJ. Diagnosis and conservative management of degenerative lumbar spondylolisthesis. *Eur Spine J* 2008;17:327–35.

[23] Weinstein JN, Lurie JD, Tosteson TD, Hanscom B, Tosteson ANA, Blood EA, et al. Surgical versus nonsurgical treatment for lumbar degenerative spondylolisthesis. *N Engl J Med* 2007;356:2257–70.

[24] Weinstein JN, Tosteson TD, Lurie JD, Tosteson ANA, Blood E, Hanscom B, et al. Surgical versus nonsurgical therapy for lumbar spinal stenosis. *N Engl J Med* 2008;358:794–810.

[25] Miyazawa N, Akiyama I. Ossification of the ligamentum flavum of the cervical spine. *J Neurosurg Sci* 2007;51:139–44.

[26] Baba H, Maezawa Y, Furusawa N, Imura S, Tomita K. The role of calcium deposition in the ligamentum flavum causing a cauda equina syndrome and lumbar radiculopathy. *Paraplegia* 1995;33:219–23.

[27] Epstein NE. Ossification of the yellow ligament and spondylosis and/or ossification of the posterior longitudinal ligament of the thoracic and lumbar spine. *J Spinal Disord* 1999;12:250–6.

[28] Clark JE. Apophyseal fracture of the lumbar spine in adolescence. *Orthop Rev* 1991;20:512–6.

[29] Takata K, Inoue S, Takahashi K, Ohtsuka Y. Fracture of the posterior margin of a lumbar vertebral body. *J Bone Joint Surg Am* 1988; 70:589–94.

[30] Epstein NE, Epstein JA. Limbus lumbar vertebral fractures in 27 adolescents and adults. *Spine* 1991;16:962–6.

[31] Epstein NE. Lumbar synovial cysts: a review of diagnosis, surgical management, and outcome assessment. *J Spinal Disord Tech* 2004;17:321–5.

[32] Epstein NE. Lumbar laminectomy for the resection of synovial cysts and coexisting lumbar spinal stenosis or degenerative spondylolisthesis: an outcome study. *Spine* 2004;29:1049–55; discussion 1056.

[33] Pellisé F, Vila-Casademunt A, Ferrer M, Domingo-Sàbat M, Bagó J, Pérez-Grueso FJS, et al. Impact on health related quality of life of adult spinal deformity (ASD) compared with other chronic conditions. *Eur Spine J* 2015;24:3–11.

[34] Kobayashi T, Atsuta Y, Takemitsu M, Matsuno T, Takeda N. A prospective study of de novo scoliosis in a community based cohort. *Spine* 2006;31:178–82.
[35] Schwab F, Dubey A, Gamez L, El Fegoun AB, Hwang K, Pagala M, et al. Adult scoliosis: prevalence, SF-36, and nutritional parameters in an elderly volunteer population. *Spine* 2005;30:1082–5.
[36] Hong JY, Suh SW, Modi HN, Hur CY, Song HR, Park JH. The prevalence and radiological findings in 1347 elderly patients with scoliosis. *J Bone Joint Surg Br* 2010;92:980–3.
[37] Daubs MD, Lenke LG, Cheh G, Stobbs G, Bridwell KH. Adult spinal deformity surgery: complications and outcomes in patients over age 60. *Spine* 2007;32:2238–44.
[38] Wang G, Hu J, Liu X, Cao Y. Surgical treatments for degenerative lumbar scoliosis: a meta analysis. *Eur Spine J* 2015;24:1792–9.
[39] Lee SE, Jahng T-A, Kim H-J. Decompression and nonfusion dynamic stabilization for spinal stenosis with degenerative lumbar scoliosis: Clinical article. *J Neurosurg Spine* 2014;21:585–94.
[40] Johnson K-E, ROS??AN I, UD??AN A. The Natural Course of Lumbar Spinal Stenosis. *Clin Orthop Relat Res* 1992;&NA;82???86.
[41] Hurri H, Slätis P, Soini J, Tallroth K, Alaranta H, Laine T, et al. Lumbar spinal stenosis: assessment of long-term outcome 12 years after operative and conservative treatment. *J Spinal Disord* 1998;11:110–5.
[42] Minamide A, Yoshida M, Maio K. The natural clinical course of lumbar spinal stenosis: a longitudinal cohort study over a minimum of 10 years. *J Orthop Sci* 2013;18:693–8.
[43] Haig AJ, Tong HC, Yamakawa KSJ, Parres C, Quint DJ, Chiodo A, et al. Predictors of pain and function in persons with spinal stenosis, low back pain, and no back pain. *Spine* 2006;31:2950–7.
[44] de Schepper EIT, Overdevest GM, Suri P, Peul WC, Oei EHG, Koes BW, et al. Diagnosis of lumbar spinal stenosis: an updated systematic review of the accuracy of diagnostic tests. *Spine* 2013;38:E469–81.
[45] Dvorák J, Panjabi MM, Novotny JE, Chang DG, Grob D. Clinical validation of functional flexion-extension roentgenograms of the lumbar spine. *Spine* 1991;16:943–50.
[46] de Graaf I, Prak A, Bierma-Zeinstra S, Thomas S, Peul W, Koes B. Diagnosis of lumbar spinal stenosis: a systematic review of the accuracy of diagnostic tests. *Spine* 2006;31:1168–76.

[47] Boden SD, Davis DO, Dina TS, Patronas NJ, Wiesel SW. Abnormal magnetic-resonance scans of the lumbar spine in asymptomatic subjects. A prospective investigation. *J Bone Joint Surg Am* 1990;72:403–8.

[48] Rihn JA, Lee JY, Khan M, Ulibarri JA, Tannoury C, Donaldson WF 3rd, et al. Does lumbar facet fluid detected on magnetic resonance imaging correlate with radiographic instability in patients with degenerative lumbar disease? *Spine* 2007;32:1555–60.

[49] Ross JS, Modic MT. Current assessment of spinal degenerative disease with magnetic resonance imaging. *Clin Orthop Relat Res* 1992:68–81.

[50] Wassenaar M, van Rijn RM, van Tulder MW, Verhagen AP, van der Windt DAWM, Koes BW, et al. Magnetic resonance imaging for diagnosing lumbar spinal pathology in adult patients with low back pain or sciatica: a diagnostic systematic review. *Eur Spine J* 2012;21:220–7.

[51] Lurie JD, Tosteson AN, Tosteson TD, Carragee E, Carrino JA, Carrino J, et al. Reliability of readings of magnetic resonance imaging features of lumbar spinal stenosis. *Spine* 2008;33:1605–10.

[52] Steurer J, Roner S, Gnannt R, Hodler J, LumbSten Research Collaboration. Quantitative radiologic criteria for the diagnosis of lumbar spinal stenosis: a systematic literature review. *BMC Musculoskelet Disord* 2011;12:175.

[53] Cheung JP-Y, Samartzis D, Shigematsu H, Cheung KM-C. Defining clinically relevant values for developmental spinal stenosis: a large-scale magnetic resonance imaging study. *Spine* 2014;39:1067–76.

[54] Mamisch N, Brumann M, Hodler J, Held U, Brunner F, Steurer J, et al. Radiologic criteria for the diagnosis of spinal stenosis: results of a Delphi survey. *Radiology* 2012;264:174–9.

[55] Djukic S, Lang P, Morris J, Hoaglund F, Genant HK. The postoperative spine. Magnetic resonance imaging. *Orthop Clin North Am* 1990;21:603–24.

[56] Herno A, Airaksinen O, Saari T, Luukkonen M. Lumbar spinal stenosis: a matched-pair study of operated and non-operated patients. *Br J Neurosurg* 1996;10:461–5.

[57] Schneider M, Ammendolia C, Murphy D, Glick R, Piva S, Hile E, et al. Comparison of non-surgical treatment methods for patients with lumbar spinal stenosis: protocol for a randomized controlled trial. *Chiropr Man Therap* 2014;22:19.

[58] Tomkins-Lane CC, Lafave LMZ, Parnell JA, Rempel J, Moriartey S, Andreas Y, et al. The spinal stenosis pedometer and nutrition lifestyle intervention (SSPANLI): development and pilot. *Spine J* 2015;15:577–86.

[59] Tomkins-Lane CC, Lafave LMZ, Parnell JA, Krishnamurthy A, Rempel J, Macedo LG, et al. The spinal stenosis pedometer and nutrition lifestyle intervention (SSPANLI) randomized controlled trial protocol. *BMC Musculoskelet Disord* 2013;14:322.

[60] Ammendolia C, Stuber K, de Bruin LK, Furlan AD, Kennedy CA, Rampersaud YR, et al. Nonoperative treatment of lumbar spinal stenosis with neurogenic claudication: a systematic review. *Spine* 2012;37:E609–16.

[61] Whitman JM, Flynn TW, Childs JD, Wainner RS, Gill HE, Ryder MG, et al. A comparison between two physical therapy treatment programs for patients with lumbar spinal stenosis: a randomized clinical trial. *Spine* 2006;31:2541–9.

[62] Tomkins CC, Dimoff KH, Forman HS, Gordon ES, McPhail J, Wong JR, et al. Physical therapy treatment options for lumbar spinal stenosis. *J Back Musculoskelet Rehabil* 2010;23:31–7.

[63] Macedo LG, Hum A, Kuleba L, Mo J, Truong L, Yeung M, et al. Physical therapy interventions for degenerative lumbar spinal stenosis: a systematic review. *Phys Ther* 2013;93:1646–60.

[64] Fritz JM, Lurie JD, Zhao W, Whitman JM, Delitto A, Brennan GP, et al. Associations between physical therapy and long-term outcomes for individuals with lumbar spinal stenosis in the SPORT study. *Spine J* 2014;14:1611–21.

[65] Delitto A, Piva SR, Moore CG, Fritz JM, Wisniewski SR, Josbeno DA, et al. Surgery versus nonsurgical treatment of lumbar spinal stenosis: a randomized trial. *Ann Intern Med* 2015;162:465–73.

[66] Atlas SJ, Delitto A. Spinal stenosis: surgical versus nonsurgical treatment. *Clin Orthop Relat Res* 2006;443:198–207.

[67] van Tulder MW, Scholten RJ, Koes BW, Deyo RA. Nonsteroidal anti-inflammatory drugs for low back pain: a systematic review within the framework of the Cochrane Collaboration Back Review Group. *Spine* 2000;25:2501–13.

[68] Liu K, Liu P, Liu R, Wu X, Cai M. Steroid for epidural injection in spinal stenosis: a systematic review and meta-analysis. *Drug Des Devel Ther* 2015;9:707–16.

[69] Manchikanti L, Singh V, Pampati V, Falco FJ, Hirsch JA. Comparison of the efficacy of caudal, interlaminar, and transforaminal epidural injections in managing lumbar disc herniation: is one method superior to the other? *Korean J Pain* 2015;28:11–21.

[70] Friedly JL, Comstock BA, Turner JA, Heagerty PJ, Deyo RA, Sullivan SD, et al. A randomized trial of epidural glucocorticoid injections for spinal stenosis. *N Engl J Med* 2014;371:11–21.

[71] Disease Control C, Others. Multistate fungal meningitis outbreak investigation. *Internet Document* 2012;29.

[72] Malmivaara A, Slätis P, Heliövaara M, Sainio P, Kinnunen H, Kankare J, et al. Surgical or nonoperative treatment for lumbar spinal stenosis? A randomized controlled trial. *Spine* 2007;32:1–8.

[73] Athiviraham A, Yen D. Is spinal stenosis better treated surgically or nonsurgically? *Clin Orthop Relat Res* 2007;458:90–3.

[74] Bydon M, Macki M, Abt NB, Sciubba DM, Wolinsky J-P, Witham TF, et al. Clinical and surgical outcomes after lumbar laminectomy: An analysis of 500 patients. *Surg Neurol Int* 2015;6:S190–3.

[75] Oertel MF, Ryang Y-M, Korinth MC, Gilsbach JM, Rohde V. Long-term results of microsurgical treatment of lumbar spinal stenosis by unilateral laminotomy for bilateral decompression. *Neurosurgery* 2006;59:1264.

[76] Caspar W, Papavero L, Sayler MK, Harkey HL. Precise and limited decompression for lumbar spinal stenosis. *Acta Neurochir* 1994; 131:130–6.

[77] Postacchini F, Cinotti G, Perugia D, Gumina S. The surgical treatment of central lumbar stenosis. Multiple laminotomy compared with total laminectomy. *J Bone Joint Surg Br* 1993;75:386–92.

[78] Resnick DK, Choudhri TF, Dailey AT, Groff MW, Khoo L, Matz PG, et al. Guidelines for the performance of fusion procedures for degenerative disease of the lumbar spine. Part 9: fusion in patients with stenosis and spondylolisthesis. *J Neurosurg Spine* 2005;2:679–85.

[79] Alexander E Jr, Kelly DL Jr, Davis CH Jr, McWhorter JM, Brown W. Intact arch spondylolisthesis: a review of 50 cases and description of surgical treatment. *J Neurosurg* 1985;63:840–4.

[80] Hall S, Bartleson JD, Onofrio BM, Baker HL, Okazaki H, DESMOND O'DUFFY J. Lumbar Spinal Stenosis: Clinical Features, Diagnostic Procedures, and Results of Surgical Treatment in 68 Patients. *Ann Intern Med* 1985;103:271–5.

[81] Mauersberger W, Nietgen T. Surgical treatment of lumbar stenosis: long-term results. *Neurosurg Rev* 1989;12:291–5.

[82] Javid MJ, Hadar EJ. Long-term follow-up review of patients who underwent laminectomy for lumbar stenosis: a prospective study. *J Neurosurg* 1998;89:1–7.

[83] Herkowitz HN, Kurz LT. Degenerative lumbar spondylolisthesis with spinal stenosis. A prospective study comparing decompression with decompression and intertransverse process arthrodesis. *J Bone Joint Surg Am* 1991;73:802–8.

[84] Deyo RA, Cherkin DC, Loeser JD, Bigos SJ, Ciol MA. Morbidity and mortality in association with operations on the lumbar spine. The influence of age, diagnosis, and procedure. *J Bone Joint Surg Am* 1992;74:536–43.

[85] Deyo RA, Ciol MA, Cherkin DC, Loeser JD, Bigos SJ. Lumbar spinal fusion. A cohort study of complications, reoperations, and resource use in the Medicare population. *Spine* 1993;18:1463–70.

[86] Nerland US, Jakola AS, Solheim O, Weber C, Rao V, Lønne G, et al. Minimally invasive decompression versus open laminectomy for central stenosis of the lumbar spine: pragmatic comparative effectiveness study. *BMJ* 2015;350:h1603.

[87] Phan K, Mobbs RJ. Minimally Invasive Versus Open Laminectomy for Lumbar Stenosis: A Systematic Review and Meta-Analysis. *Spine* 2016;41:E91–100.

[88] Shih P, Wong AP, Smith TR, Lee AI, Fessler RG. Complications of open compared to minimally invasive lumbar spine decompression. *J Clin Neurosci* 2011;18:1360–4.

[89] Dagistan Y, Dagistan E, Gezici AR, Cancan SE, Bilgi M, Cakir U. Effects of minimally invasive decompression surgery on quality of life in older patients with spinal stenosis. *Clin Neurol Neurosurg* 2015; 139:86–90.

[90] Aleem IS, Rampersaud YR. Elderly patients have similar outcomes compared to younger patients after minimally invasive surgery for spinal stenosis. *Clin Orthop Relat Res* 2014;472:1824–30.

[91] Khashan M, Lidar Z, Salame K, Mangel L, Lador R, Drexler M, et al. Minimally invasive spinal decompression in patients older than 75 years of age: Perioperative risks, complications and clinical outcomes compared with patients younger than 45 years of age. *World Neurosurg* 2016. doi:10.1016/j.wneu.2016.02.018.

[92] Deen HG Jr, Zimmerman RS, Lyons MK, Wharen RE Jr, Reimer R. Analysis of early failures after lumbar decompressive laminectomy for spinal stenosis. *Mayo Clin Proc* 1995;70:33–6.

[93] Caputy AJ, Luessenhop AJ. Long-term evaluation of decompressive surgery for degenerative lumbar stenosis. *J Neurosurg* 1992;77:669–76.

[94] Epstein NE. The frequency and etiology of intraoperative dural tears in 110 predominantly geriatric patients undergoing multilevel laminectomy with noninstrumented fusions. *J Spinal Disord Tech* 2007;20:380–6.

[95] Bawany FI, Emaduddin M, Shahid M, Hussain M, Yousuful Islam M, Khan MS. Incidence of Pinhole Type Durotomy and Subsequent Cerebrospinal Fluid Leakage Following Simple Laminectomy. *Asian Spine J* 2015;9:529–34.

[96] Jankowitz BT, Atteberry DS, Gerszten PC, Karausky P, Cheng BC, Faught R, et al. Effect of fibrin glue on the prevention of persistent cerebral spinal fluid leakage after incidental durotomy during lumbar spinal surgery. *Eur Spine J* 2009;18:1169–74.

[97] Saxler G, Krämer J, Barden B, Kurt A, Pförtner J, Bernsmann K. The long-term clinical sequelae of incidental durotomy in lumbar disc surgery. *Spine* 2005;30:2298–302.

[98] Cammisa FP Jr, Girardi FP, Sangani PK, Parvataneni HK, Cadag S, Sandhu HS. Incidental durotomy in spine surgery. *Spine* 2000;25: 2663–7.

[99] Desai A, Ball PA, Bekelis K, Lurie J, Mirza SK, Tosteson TD, et al. SPORT: Does incidental durotomy affect longterm outcomes in cases of spinal stenosis? *Neurosurgery* 2015;76 Suppl 1:S57–63; discussion S63.

[100] Shektman A, Granick MS, Solomon MP, Black P, Nair S. Management of infected laminectomy wounds. *Neurosurgery* 1994;35:307–9; discussion 309.

[101] Lee LA, Roth S, Posner KL, Cheney FW, Caplan RA, Newman NJ, et al. The American Society of Anesthesiologists Postoperative Visual Loss RegistryAnalysis of 93 Spine Surgery Cases with Postoperative Visual Loss. *The Journal of the American Society of Anesthesiologists* 2006;105:652–9.

[102] Soheilian M, Yazdani S. Ischemic optic neuropathy. *Ophthalmology* 2007;114:2102–3; author reply 2103–4.

In: Intervertebral Disc Degeneration
Editors: A. L. Ho and A. M. Desai
ISBN: 978-1-63485-829-8

Chapter 8

LUMBAR DISC HERNIATIONS

Ajit Jada, MD, Roger Härtl, MD and Ali Baaj, MD*
New York-Presbyterian Hospital/Weill Cornell Medical Center, NY, US

ABSTRACT

Lumbar disc herniations occur with relatively high frequency such that surgeons should be aware of prevention, management, and treatment strategies. Clinical presentation including assessment of location, morphology, symptoms, and imaging are crucial sources of information in the determination of the necessity for surgery. Conservative management may include one or a combination of medication, physical therapy, and epidural steroid injections. If needed and depending on the surgeon's preference, minimally invasive microdiscectomies or endoscopic procedures may be utilized to treat patients. Ultimately, the ongoing debate between non-interventional and interventional approaches to treatment requires surgeons to make final decisions tailored to each patient.

Keywords: lumbar disc herniation, degenerative disc disease, adjacent level disease, management of disc herniations

* Corresponding Author address: New York-Presbyterian Hospital/Weill Cornell Medical Center 525 East 68 Street, Box 99, New York NY 10065. Email: alb9140@med.cornell.edu.

INTRODUCTION

Degenerative disc disease and its sequelae, disc herniations, comprise the most common cause for low back pain related physician office visits [1, 3]. In addition, lumbar disc herniations (LDH) are a significant source of morbidity and both operative and non-operative management of LDHs are associated with rising health care costs.

This chapter discusses the epidemiology, anatomy, risk factors, clinical features, and management and outcomes of lumbar disc herniations. The emphasis of the chapter will be on management and outcomes. The biomechanics and pathophysiology of disc disease are discussed in earlier chapters.

EPIDEMIOLOGY

Low back pain is the most commonly reported type of pain and affects approximately 29% of the adult population in the United States [1]. Total medical costs for both the non-operaive and operative management of low back pain in the U.S. ranges from $84 to $624.8 billion, with more recent estimates of spending exceeding $100 billion annually [2, 24]. Furthermore, degenerative disc disease and disc herniations comprise the most common cause for low back pain related physician office visits [3]. Degenerative disc disease comprises most of the back pain seen at visits, while disc herniations result in more radicular pain at presentation.

From 1992 to 2003 there has been a 500% increase in lumbar spine fusion surgery from $75 million to $482 million, respectively [23], with fusion surgery from recurrent lumbar disc herniations contributing to this total. With regard to lumbar disc herniation surgery alone, approximately 200,000 to 300,000 lumbar discectomies are performed annually in the U.S. [25-28].

Demographics

The highest prevalence of disc herniations are found in patients with an age range of 30-50 years, with a male to female ratio of 2:1 [39, 42]. In Western countries, the annual incidence of sciatica from lumbar disc herniations is 5 cases per 1000 adults [41]. The lifetime prevalence of lumbar disc herniation varies depending on the study but is commonly reported at 40% [43]. Furthermore, studies have reported a risk of approximately 3.6% in patients younger than 35 and 22% in those aged 45 to 54 [40]. In patients between 25 and 55 years 95% of herniated discs occur at the L4-5 and L5-1 levels, with younger patients having a predilection for herniations at L5-S1 (average age 39) whereas older patients (average age 42) had herniations at L4-5 [46]. In patients over 55 disc herniations are more common above the L4-5 level [44-46].

Sparse data exist on the frequency of lumbar disc herniations in patients < 21 years of age, with the most recent review citing only 1963 surgically treated LDH patients below the age of 21 in the literature [49] with pediatric patients constituting only 0.5-6.8% of all patients hospitalized for LDH [50, 51, 52]. Zitting et al. [53] performed an epidemiologic study following 12,058 Finnish babies from birth up to 28 years of age. The authors found that none of the subjects were hospitalized for LDH until the age of 15. The prevalence of hospitalization from LDH increased to 0.1-0.2% by age 20, and by age 28, 9.5% of males and 4.2% of females were admitted to the hospital with a diagnosis of LDH.

Anatomy

In order to appreciate how lumbar disc herniations occur, the anatomy of the lumbar spine needs to be briefly reviewed:

The lumbar spine has 2 basic functions, to house the spinal canal and to provide mechanical support to the axial skeleton [12]. The lumbar spine consists of 5 vertebral bodies, each containing 5 motion segments. The motion segments consist of the intervertebral disc (IVD), vertebral body, pedicles, apophyseal joints, lamina, and spinous process (Figure 1). The normal physiologic movement of the spine is maintained by ligaments and joint capsules. The major ligaments include the anterior longitudinal ligament (ALL) which runs along the anterior border of the vertebral body and limits extension, the posterior longitudinal ligament (PLL) which runs along the posterior border of the vertebral body and limits flexion, the interspinous and supraspinous ligaments, and the ligamentum flavum. The IVD has 3 structural components which include the nucleus pulposis (NP), annulus fibrosus (AF), and the vertebral endplate [12].

Intervertebral discs (IVD) are avascular fibro-cartilaginous pads that lie between the vertebral bodies. During development, blood vessels enter the AF and NP and remain patent until approximately 8 years of age, regressing over the next two decades of life, leaving the IVD as the largest avascular structure in the body [18-22].

The intervertebral discs serve to distribute loading forces evenly to the vertebral bodies during loading [4]. The IVD consists of a soft nucleus pulposus (NP) that is contained within a tough annulus fibrosus (AF). The NP consists of cells derived from embryonic notochord [5-8] and as the NP matures, chondrocyte-like cells remain in a highly hydrated gelatinous tissues matrix which resists and redistributed spinal compressive loads [9].

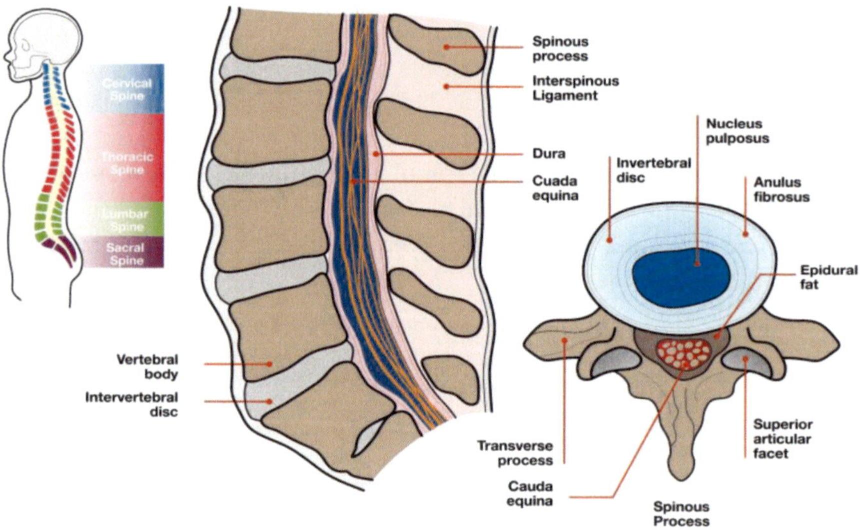

Figure 1. Lumbar Disc Anatomy.

The extracellular matrix (ECM) of the NP consists of primarily water, proteoglycans, namely aggrecan, and randomly oriented type II collagen, with minor ECM contribution from minor collagens Types III, VI, IX, and small proteoglycans [9]. The AF consists of both type I and type II collagen fiber bundles arranged circumferentially into distinct laminate layers. Fibers in the outer annulus form Sharpey's fibers which are entrenched within the vertebral bodies above and below the disc [9]. The inner annulus lacks the organized lamellar structure that the outer annulus contains, and in the inner annulus, Sharpey fibers combine with the cartilaginous endplate of the vertebral body [17].

As we discuss disc herniations further in this chapter it is important to correlate the anatomy of the lumbar spine with the pathology of disc herniations. Of note, there is a transitional area in the posterolateral junction of the disc which is the intersection of maximum and minimum concentrations of the laminate layers which comprise the external layer of the AF. In the posterolateral quadrant of the disc, there is also a change in the inclination of the fiber bundles from 0 degrees parallel to as much as 90 degrees inclination [10]. These structural phenomena may explain the high frequency of disc herniations from the posterolateral quadrant where tensile strain is highest in flexion and extension modalities [11].

The endplate consists of a cartilaginous bony components. The cartilaginous endplate is usually less than 1 mm in thickness and overlies the bony endplate. The bony endplate is thin sheet of bone which comprises the cortical rim of the vertebral body [16]. Cranial endplates are thinner and weaker than the caudal endplates, both of which are weakest in their central regions [14, 15]. The avascular IVD receives nutrients from diffusion through the capillary beds in the vertebral endplates.

The intervertebral disc is avascular and immunoprivileged, as a result the IVD has no exposure to the immune system [18-22]. Thus when a disc herniation occurs, it can elicit an inflammatory, auto-immune response [13].

Neuronal Innervation

The PLL, vertebrae, apophyseal joints, dura mater, and outer 1/3 of the annulus are innervated by the dorsal ramus and sinuvertebral nerves branching from the spinal nerve of the corresponding lumbar level [29-37]. Whereas, the lateral and anterior annular areas are innervated by branches of the gray rami communicans [37], the inner annulus and NP are not innervated [54]. The somatic afferent information is collected in the dorsal root ganglia (DRG), transmitted to the dorsal horn of the spinal cord and travels via the spinothalamic tract to the thalamus and somatosensory and pain cortical areas. Information from the grey rami communicans and autonomic afferents below the level of L2 is collected at the level of the L2 DRG and transmitted to the dorsal horn of the spinal cord and then relayed to the CNS.

Disc Herniations

Disc herniation occurs when a tear develops in the AF and the NP extrudes through the tear. When the NP herniates, nerve injury may occur from the NP pressing on adjacent nerve roots. Disc biomechanics are also altered, with higher compression forces exerted on the annulus [38]. Furthermore, sclerotic changes in the endplates and osteophytes are sequelae of long standing altered biomechanics secondary to disc herniations [38.]

Classifications of Disc Herniations

There are various classifications for disc herniations. They can be described by either location (Figure 2) or morphology (Figure 3). With regard to location, herniations are characterized as:

- Central
- Lateral Recess
- Foraminal
- Extra-foraminal
- Far Lateral (discussed later in the chapter)

From a morphology perspective, Spengler et al. [47] divided disc herniations into:

- Protruded Disc (Disc bulge with an intact annulus fibrosus)
- Extruded Disc (Disc material that passes the annulus fibrosus but is contiguous with the nucleus pulposus)
- Sequestered Disc (Disc material not contiguous with the nucleus pulposus, otherwise characterized as a “floating fragment.”)

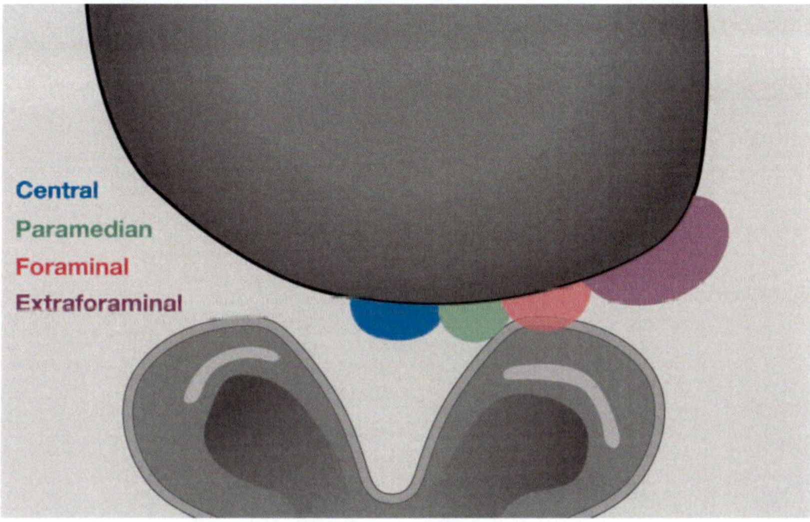

Figure 2. Disc Herniation Location.

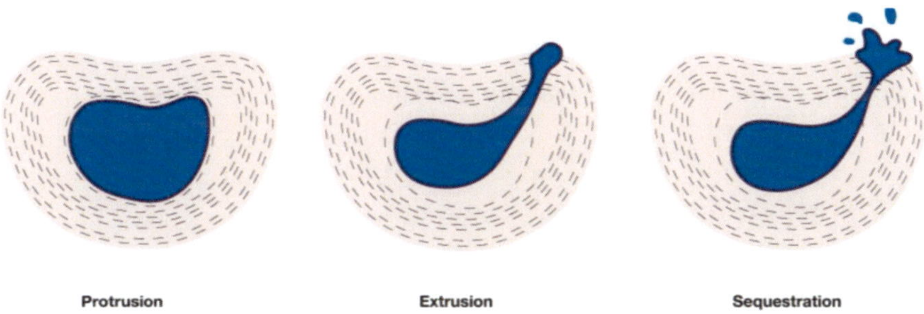

Figure 3. Disc Herniation Morphology.

Other literature have described disc herniations as Contained or Uncontained (Figure 4) [48]:

- Contained: The disc material has not passed beyond the PLL and is subligamentous.
- Uncontained: The disc material has herniated beyond the PLL.

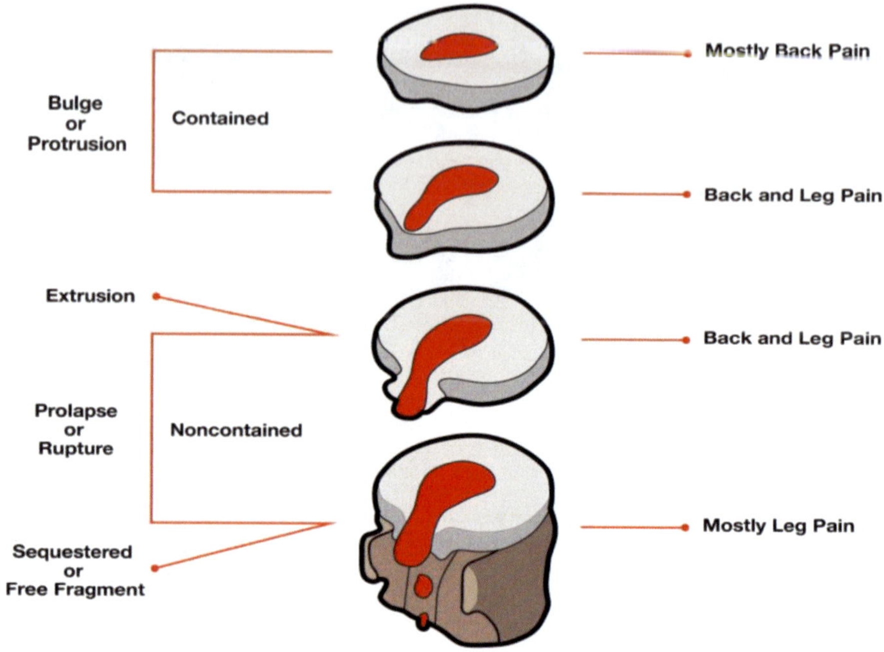

Figure 4. Contained and Uncontained Disc Herniations.

Onset of Herniation

Timing of onset of herniation is arbitrarily divided into acute or chronic. Most authors refer to herniations as acute for up to 3 months and chronic thereafter. From a surgical perspective, timing of herniation will factor into outcomes, so this classification is of importance.

Symptomatology and Pain

After LDH, inflammatory factors, in addition to direct compression on the nerve root; are suspected to play a role in the symptomatology of the patient [59]. As previously discussed, the NP is contained within an immunoprivileged environment, and when herniated out of the annulus, the disc material causes an inflammatory cascade by the body. These findings have been validated in animal and human studies from specimens obtained intra-operatively [60-62]. This immunologic cascade involves inflammatory cytokines including tumor necrosis factor-alpha, and IL-1 [63].

Risk Factors

Certain risk factors have been studied in the literature and there are activities associated with an increased risk of LDH. A review of activities are described below and the correlation with LDH is explained.

Sports

A retrospective study performed by Mundt et al. [65] analyzed 355 patients with disc herniations; both cervical and lumbar, that were between the ages of 20 and 64 for 2 years. Subjects were questioned regarding their participation in sports and control group of individuals free of disc herniations was used to determine whether the frequency of exposures in the case group was different from what would be expected in the subjects' age group and sex. The data showed that participation in recreational sports did not increase the risk for low back pain and herniated discs, either cervical or lumbar, and even offered a slight protective benefit against disc herniation.

There was an association with free weight lifting and increased risk of cervical disc herniation, not lumbar disc herniation. This was the case for the use of light weights, 3 sets of 10 repetitions, and heavy weights with 2 or more repetitions. No increased risk of disc herniations were apparent for use of weight lifting equipment, e.g., Nautilus, Universal Gym Equipment, etc. The authors hypothesized the difference was related to lack of stability of free weights and unequal distribution of weight to the cervical spine.

In another retrospective review of weight lifting as an independent risk factor for LDH [66], the authors found that lifting with the knees straight and back bent was consistently associated with LDH. This included lifting: weights > 25lbs, children 10-24lbs, and children > 25lbs. These results are correlated with biomechanical studies demonstrating increased intra-discal pressures and intra-abdominal pressures associated with lifting with the knees straight and back bent [67-70]

Driving

In older studies analyzing risk of disc herniation and driving, the data showed that individuals who spent at least half of their day driving had a three-fold increased risk of LDH as compared to non-drivers [71]. The risk was found to be five-fold in truck drivers and two-fold in car drivers, and correlated with the time spent driving [71]. Furthermore, the risk of LDH appeared to be correlated with the amount of vibration transmitted to the spine, road surface, speed of the vehicle, low seat position [71-75]. In addition, animal studies have shown that vibration of the spine at 5 Hz can adversely affect the intervertebral discs and facilitate degeneration [71, 76, 77].

However, the most recent literature published in the Lancet in 2002 [78] was a retrospective cohort studying 45 male monozygotic twins and lumbar disc disease associated with driving. The study group had 5.4 times more driving exposure than their twin, control counterpart. With all other variables controlled, driving exposure was not associated with accelerated lumbar degeneration and structural abnormalities. This was measured through MRI imaging of the lumbar spine and there were no significant differences in disc signal, annual tears, disc bulges, herniations, disc height, or endplate irregularities.

Smoking

Smoking has often been considered an independent risk factor for LDH. There is some conflict in the literature whether smoking has a direct causal effect on LDH, but there is a preponderance of evidence that demonstrates smoking is a risk factor for LDH as well as recurrent disc herniations (RDH).

A study by Kelsey et al. demonstrated cigarette smoke is associated with an increased risk of LDH by 20%, when 10 cigarettes are smoked per day for 1 year [79]. The Twin Spine Study [88] demonstrated a more modest effect on lumbar degeneration. When comparing smokers to non-smokers, they found an 18% increase in their lumbar disc degeneration score among twins, but less than a 2% difference among all subjects when comparing smokers to non-smokers, in their cohort.

A meta-analysis by Shiri et al. [80] demonstrated smoking was independent risk factor for lumbar radicular pain and experimental studies have shown smoking reduces perfusion around the intervertebral discs [80-82] possibly exacerbating disc degeneration [83-86]. Furthermore, smoking increases the production and release of inflammatory cytokines in intervertebral discs [86, 87] also contributing to degeneration and pain.

Gill et al. compared the ligament healing process in passively smoking mice with non-smoking mice and found decreased cellular density in the healing ligaments of smoking mice. Furthermore, the smoke exposed mice exhibited lower type I collagen expression in the injured ligament than their non-smoking counterparts [159]. A study by Nemoto et al., exposed 4-week old rats to passive smoking for 8 weeks. The authors found that the intervertebral discs exhibited tears, cracks, and misalignment of the annulus [160].

Diabetes

Diabetes has also been studied as an independent risk factor for LDH and RDH. The studies have unequivocally shown that diabetic patients are at an increased risk for both LDH and RDH [155, 161]. Robinson et al., compared intervertebral disc tissue removed during surgery for LDH between diabetics and non-diabetics [162]. The authors found that the proteoglycans of diabetic patients are banded at a lower buoyant density, indicating a lowered glycosylation rate and a lower number of sugar side chains per core protein. Furthermore, in discs of diabetic patients, there was a slight increase in the chain length of chondroitin sulfate. Further analysis of the glycosaminoglycan chains showed a decreased amount of keratan sulfate, compared with that in nondiabetic subjects. Thus, the authors concluded that discs in diabetic patients have lower buoyant density and undersulfated glycosaminoglycans which may lead to an increased susceptibility to lumbar disc herniation [162].

Clinical Presentations of Lumbar Disc Herniation

Patients may describe an incident attributable to a disc herniation such as a fall, lifting a heavy object, or rotational forces e.g., golf swing. Patients with LDH present with radicular pain more than axial low back pain, and axial back pain alone is poor indication for microdiscectomy. Axial and mechanical low back pain may indicate a more structural etiology for the pain, which would require a fusion surgery. Further investigations with flexion extension studies and even CT scans may be indicated.

The pattern of the radicular pain with LDH can correlate with the dermatomal distribution of the nerve affected by the disc herniation. The pain can be characterized as sharp, dull, or burning, and may be associated with paresthesias and weakness. These symptoms can be exacerbated with coughing, bending, or lifting [55].

The most common location of disc herniations, as previously described, is the posterolateral quadrant of the disc. When a disc herniation occurs, it commonly affects the traversing nerve root at that level. The traversing root exits under the pedicle of the vertebral body below the level of the herniation. For example, an L4-5 central disc herniation would usually compress the traversing L5 nerve root, resulting in an L5 radiculopathy.

Physical Examination

The patient's gait should be observed initially. In some cases, patients may lean away from the side of the leg pain, which is indicative of a paracentral herniation lateral to the nerve root. Whereas, with axillary herniations patients may lean toward the side of the herniation. It is hypothesized that flexion toward either side is an attempt to relieve tension on the nerve root from the herniated fragment. A foot drop in a patient may be associated with an L4 or L5 paresis.

The patient's pelvic tilt with walking should also be assessed. A positive Trendelenburg sign occurs with L5 nerve root compression resulting in weakened hip abductors, gluteus medius, and gluteus minimus. As a result, during gait, the pelvis will tilt downward on the unaffected side when the heel plants on the affected side. Another common test used to elicit the patient's symptoms is the straight-leg raise or Lesegue test. If the patient develops symptoms on the ipsilateral side with the straight leg raised to 30 degrees or more the test is positive. If the patients develops symptoms on the contralateral side the test is referred to as a crossed straight leg raise test. The straight leg raise test has high sensitivity and low specificity for LDH, while the crossed straight leg raise test has high specificity with low sensitivity for LDH [56]. If patients present with bowel or bladder symptoms and/or loss of continence, saddle anesthesia, and diminished genital sensation, this may be cauda equina syndrome and warrants immediate decompression.

IMAGING

MRI is the preferred diagnostic modality for LDH. MRI enables delineation of the soft tissue elements more than CT. One study correlated clinical outcomes with the size of the herniated disc fragments on MRI [57]. The results demonstrated discs > 6mm were more likely to have a positive straight leg raise on examination, and in the operative group, the larger discs (>6mm) were predictive of improved surgical outcomes, whereas discs < 6mm had fair and poor outcomes [57].

MRI is also the preferred diagnostic modality for post-operative imaging. Studies have shown that post-op imaging should be delayed for 6 months in order to fully assess the operative site, free from edema and hematoma [58]. Furthermore, post-operative scar tissue and fibrosis will enhance with gadolinium contrast.

If the patient is unable to undergo an MRI, a CT myelogram provides useful imaging to localize areas of stenosis and herniation.

TREATMENT OPTIONS

Natural History of Lumbar Disc Herniation

In order to understand and inform patients of the best treatment paradigms, physicians should be knowledgeable about the natural course of LDH. There are many studies in the literature, albeit with several limitations, describing the natural history of LDH. The literature suggests that larger disc herniations tend to resorb or regress more readily than smaller disc herniations. Larger herniations penetrate the annulus or PLL thus exposing disc material to the systemic circulation of the epidural space eliciting an inflammatory response [92- 94]. Phagocytic mechanisms and neovascularization of the outermost layer of herniated disc material result in disc resorption [95- 97]. Also, degradation of proteoglycans in the NP results in dehydration of the herniated disc fragment, followed by a decrease in overall disc volume [98, 99].

A recent study by Kjaer et. al [89] followed patients for 8 years with LDH, the majority of which were at L4-5 and L5-S1. The authors performed a prospective population-based observational study on a Danish population. The authors invited a random sample of 40 year olds to participate in the study, thus this population did not necessarily have back pain or disc herniations. 412 participated and received a baseline MRI, a 4 year follow up MRI, and an 8 year follow up MRI. The data demonstrated that over 8 years for those patients with LDH; 65% of herniations remained unchanged, 17.5% decreased, 12.5% increased, and 5% had a fluctuating pattern.

Chun et. al, [90] performed a meta-analysis of the recent literature to determine the probability of spontaneous disc regression among each type of herniated disc in patients that underwent conservative management with: bed rest, analgesics, non-steroidal anti-inflammatory drugs (NSAIDs), exercise, physical therapy, and steroid injections. The authors found a spontaneous regression rate of 96% for sequestered discs, 70% for extruded disc, 41% for protrusions, and 13% for disc bulges. The rate of complete resolution was 43% for sequestered discs and 15% for extruded discs.

Seo et. al., [91] reviewed volumetric changes in LDH using three-dimensional measurements obtained from MRI. The authors performed MRIs on initial visit and 6 months later in patients with LDH who received conservative management. They found that the extent of disc containment and migration, the initial size of the herniated disc, and the degree of intactness of the posterior longitudinal ligament [PLL) were all significantly correlated with resorption and increased disc volume. The risk of volumetric increment in LDH appeared to be high in patients with small, contained disc herniations. Furthermore, 88% of transligamentous-type LDH patients exhibited resorption, compared with only 41.9% of those with subligamentous-type LDH.

Another prospective study by Saal et al. [100] followed patients treated conservatively for LDH for a mean of 25 months. Disc extrusions were measured with MRI imaging at presentation and upon follow-up. The largest disc extrusions were noted to decrease the most in size from initial visit to time of follow-up.

The natural history of LDH:

- Phagocytic mechanisms, neovascularization of the outermost layer of herniated disc material, and degradation of proteoglycans in the NP, all result in decreased fragment size.
- Larger herniations tend to resorb more readily than smaller herniations.
- Transligamentous herniations resorb more than subligamentous herniations.

- Sequestered discs resorb more than extruded, protruded, or bulging discs.
- Overall, most studies show that LDH tend to reduce in size over time [90-93].

Non-Surgical/Conservative Management

The initial treatment of LDH is typically, conservative, non-surgical management. However, conservative management is only applicable when patients *do not have* progressive neurologic deficits, severe unremitting pain, or cauda equina syndrome (discussed later in this chapter).

Medication

Initial management of LDH consists of treatment of the pain symptoms with non-steroidal anti-inflammatory drugs (NSAIDs), cyclooxygenase-2 inhibitors (COX-2), narcotics, muscle relaxants, and modification of activities. Clinicians must evaluate a patient's past medical history before prescribing NSAIDs and COX-2 inhibitors. These medications are typically contraindicated in patients with a history of GI bleeding, peptic ulcers, and renal disease. Acetaminophen has been shown to be efficacious in patients with mild to moderate pain [102], but NSAIDs are typically the first line medication of choice. Tramadol has also shown efficacy in pain control as compared to placebos [103].

Physical Therapy

Physical therapy (PT) is often prescribed in conjunction with pain medication. The focus of PT varies depending on practice preference, but the program usually entails: core strengthening, paraspinal flexibility, extension maneuvers, and stretching. PT has been shown to produce good and excellent outcomes, less health care utilization, and increased return to work rates in those patients that exhibit "centralization" [106- 110]. Centralization is operationally defined as when a patient's symptoms move distally from the appendicular skeleton to a more central location in the axial lumbar spine with specific end range extension movements of the lumbar spine [111].

Chiropractic manipulation is controversial for treatment of LDH, with no evidence showing that chiropractic manipulation alters disc physiology. Also of note, bed rest is not recommended for more than 2 days; with longer periods of bed rest potentiating adverse effects [101].

Epidural Steroid Injections

Some practitioners will also initially recommend epidural (ESI) or transforaminal (TFESI) steroid injections for pain relief. Studies have shown the efficacy of ESI/TFESI in early relief of radicular pain from LDH when compared to controls [104, 105]. It is important to note that patients without prior surgery receive better pain relief from ESIs than those with prior surgery [115]. Patients with prior microdiscectomies may have pain from epidural scarring or fibrosis which an ESI will not ameliorate. Complications from ESIs are rare but can include headaches (from intra-dural puncture), epidural hematomas, arachnoiditis, meningitis, and retroperitoneal hematomas [102, 112, 113].

Contraindications to ESIs include:

- Patients that are on anticoagulants or have coagulopathies. There is a substantial risk for epidural hematomas in these patients.
- The American Society of Regional Anesthesia recommends that patients stop Ticlopidine for 14 days and Clopidogrel for 7 days prior to ESI [114].
- Aspirin recommendations vary but most practitioners will hold the ASA for 5 to 7 days [115].
- Uncontrolled diabetes is a relative contraindication, but can be performed with increasing glucose medications prior to ESI and close blood sugar monitoring afterward is recommended [115].
- Patients with systemic or local active infections [115].

Surgical Management

Several techniques are available for treatment of lumbar disc herniations and ultimately, the decision on which technique to use lies with the surgeon and which procedure he/she is most comfortable with. Though the techniques vary, there are only a few conventions of LDH surgery and the objective of the operation is the same; regardless of technique.

The objective of the surgery is to decompress the affected nerve root in an atraumatic fashion and to maintain the stability of the axial lumbar spine i.e., maintain the structural integrity of the pars and lateral facet joints. If the surgeon is too aggressive with bony removal of the lateral facets or pars, this may result in overt or micro-instability which would necessitate a fusion procedure in the future. Some surgeons will remove the entire disc at the affected level, whereas the authors of this chapter prefer a more minimally invasive approach and mostly perform fragmentectomies. The surgeon should remember that minimizing scar formation during the procedure is always essential in case reherniation does occur at a later point and re-operation is necessary.

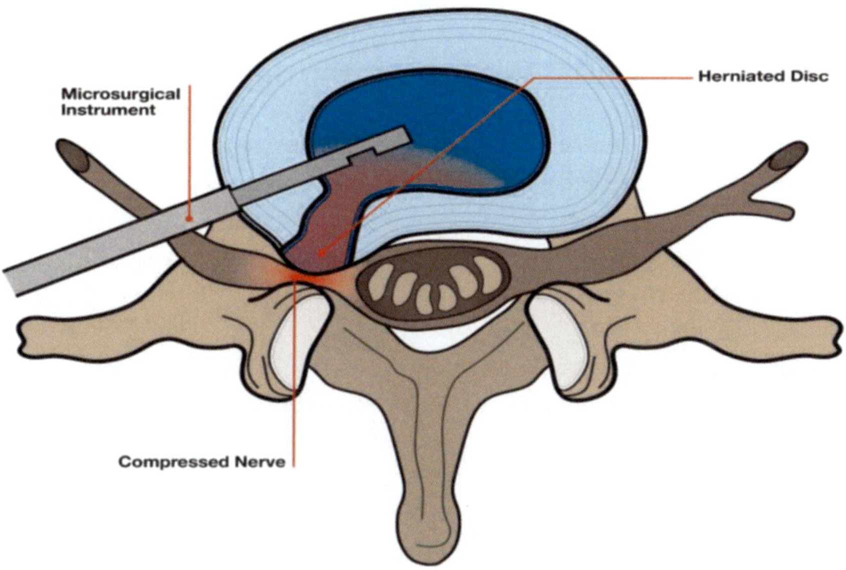

Figure 5. Laminectomy.

Surgical Techniques

The patient is brought to the operating room and general endotracheal anesthesia is induced. The patient is typically intubated on a stretcher in the operating room and flipped prone onto the surgical table. Different tables can be used depending on the procedure and surgeon preference. The authors prefer a Jackson (OSI) table with a Wilson frame attachment. However, an Andrews frame can be attached to a standard Mizuho table to facilitate a prone kneeling position. A C-arm or X-ray is then utilized to localize the appropriate level.

Open Laminectomy and Disc Removal

Once prepped and draped, a 3-5 cm midline incision is made, which may be longer for obese patients. The subcutaneous tissue is dissected down to the spinous process in standard fashion and subperiosteal dissection technique thereafter (Figure 5). At this point, the authors recommend the use of a surgical microscope for improved visualization. The laminectomy is performed in the standard fashion with care to preserve the lateral facets and pars. Subsequently, the flavectomy is performed and epidural fat and thecal sac can be seen. Of note, the wide interlaminar space at L5-S1 enables adequate access to the disc without the need for a laminectomy. At this point, the surgeon should find the exiting nerve root and carefully bipolar epidural vessels as necessary. The medial facet is typically drilled in order to expose the exiting nerve root. The surgeon then can mobilize the nerve root with a Penfield

4 and then retract the nerve medially to expose the disc. If the disc herniation is transligamentous, the fragment can be removed with a pituitary rongeur. Whereas if the herniation is subligamentous, A No. 15 or No. 11 blade is used to create a small annulotomy to remove the herniated fragment. The nerve root is examined to ensure that it is decompressed. The area is irrigated and meticulous hemostasis should be achieved. The wound is closed in a standard fashion. Typically, a subcutaneous or epidural JP is not needed.

Microlaminotomy/Microdiscectomy (MID)

Microlaminotomy and Tubular Microdiscectomy are now considered the gold standard operation for removal of lumbar disc herniations. Microlaminotomy is performed with a 2-3 cm incision in the midline and the subcutaneous dissection is carried out in the standard fashion of the open laminectomy. Once the fascia is exposed, the subperiosteal dissection is performed only on the side ipsilateral to the herniation. Most surgeons will use a McCulloch or Caspar retractors at this point. There is no difference between the open and microlaminotomy from this point forward and the discectomy is performed in a similar fashion.

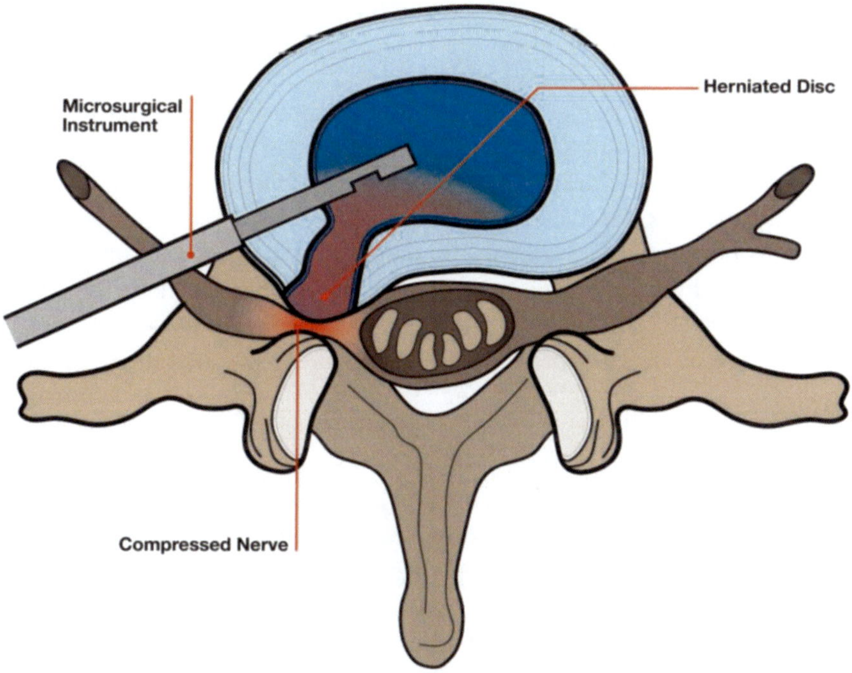

Figure 6. Microdiscectomy.

Tubular Microdiscectomy

The authors prefer the tubular microdiscectomy technique for LDH operations (Figure 6). After intubation, the patient is positioned on a Jackson table with a Wilson frame, with the tubular retractor arm placed opposite the surgeon. Once localized and draped, a 1.5-2 cm incision is made on the ipsilateral side of the herniation, 1 cm lateral to the midline. The subcutaneous tissue is separated with monopolar cauterization down to the thoracolumbar fascia. Once reached, the fascia is incised with a 15 mm blade and the dilator tubes are introduced sequentially under fluoroscopic guidance, ultimately docking a 15mm tube on the lamina overlying the disc space of interest. As a technical note, the lamina of the superior vertebra typically overlaps in the intervertebral disc space. The microscope is brought into the field and utilized until completion of the procedure. The hemi-laminotomy is performed in the standard fashion described above.

Endoscopic Surgery

Endoscopic spine surgery is a newer technique that has gained traction with some surgeons (Figure 7). The technique can be performed from various approaches, either transforaminally from a posterolateral or lateral approach, and interlaminar from a posterior approach. The endoscopic technique allows surgeons to perform these procedures under local anesthesia. Thus, patients can be awake for the procedure and comment on if their radicular pain is better during surgery.

Depending on surgeon preference, patients are positioned prone or lateral on an x-ray permeable table with bolstering under the hips and thorax for support in the prone position. For the transforaminal approach the appropriate levels are localized and with the use of AP and Lateral fluoroscopy and an atraumatic spinal needle is inserted into the appropriate disc space through Kambin's triangle, between the exiting nerve root and the traversing root. Sequential reamers are used to enlarge the foramen and to remove the ventral aspect of the superior facet. An 8-10 mm working cannula is then inserted over the dilators and a drill is used to enlarge the foramen to expose the exiting nerve root and the pedicle. Different degree endoscopes can be used to fully visualize the exiting and traversing nerve roots for areas of compression. The discectomy is performed in a similar fashion as described above, with the exception of endoscopic instruments and visualization provided via endoscope as opposed to microscopy. Again, the procedure can be performed with local anesthesia, so the patient can comment on pain relief during the surgery. If the patient still has pain after the fragment is removed, the surgeon can further investigate the operative area for further disc material or other areas of nerve root compression. For further elaboration on the technical aspects of the procedure, Jasper et. al [116] provides a detailed case report of an endoscopic transforaminal approach for removal of a lumbar disc herniation.

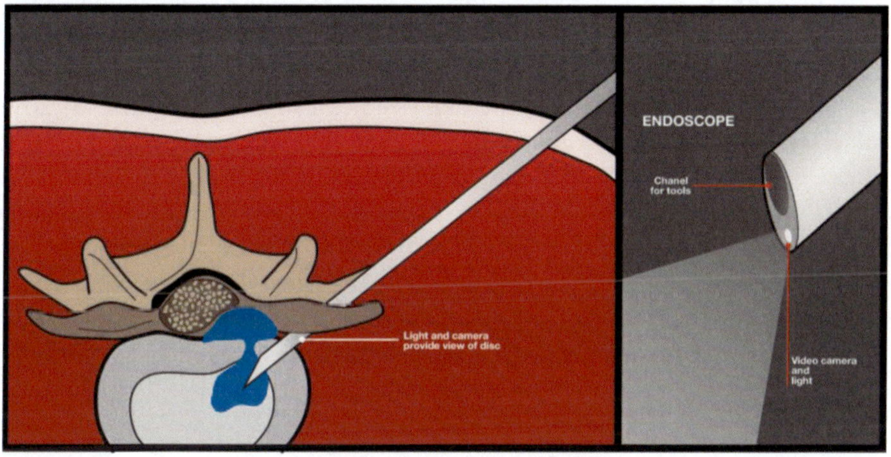

Figure 7. Endoscopic Spine Surgery.

Percutaneous Laser Disc Decompression

Percutaneous Laser Disc Decompression (PLDD) was approved by the FDA in 1991 and is a relative new procedure for treatment of LDH. Contraindications to the procedure are:

- Central stenosis
- Bony spurs that prevent percutaneous entry into disc space
- Sequestered fragments
- Ruptured PLL
- (relative contraindication) Neurologic deficit
- (relative contraindication) Significant facet arthropathy

This procedure can be performed under local anesthesia. After the patient is anesthetized, he is flipped prone onto an open Jackson table or flat x-ray permeable table. With fluoroscopy, an 18-gauage 7 inch needle is introduced into the NP, parallel to the endplates, by means of a standard posterolateral approach. The end point of the needle on AP projection should be halfway between the lateral border of the spinous process and the medial border of the pedicle (Figure 8). Lateral films should demonstrate the needle tip at the junction of the posterior ¼ of the disc with the anterior ¾. There is variability depending on technique after needle insertion. There is a LASE system, Laser fiber or Modified Choy Technique, and rigid-scope endoscopic laser technique. The modified Choy Technique is described below:

The technique involves inserting a Nd:YAG fiber through the needle tip and subsequently removing the insertion needle. Typically, lesioning at 20W with 5 seconds between 1-second pulses is used. The total energy used is 1000 J or up to 1500J is the patient is great than 165cm in height. The patient is able to alert the physician if there is any new radicular pain during the ablative period.

It is important to note that during the PLDD procedure there is no direct visualization of the nerve roots, disc material, or thecal sac. The extent of neurologic decompression cannot be determined by this procedure.

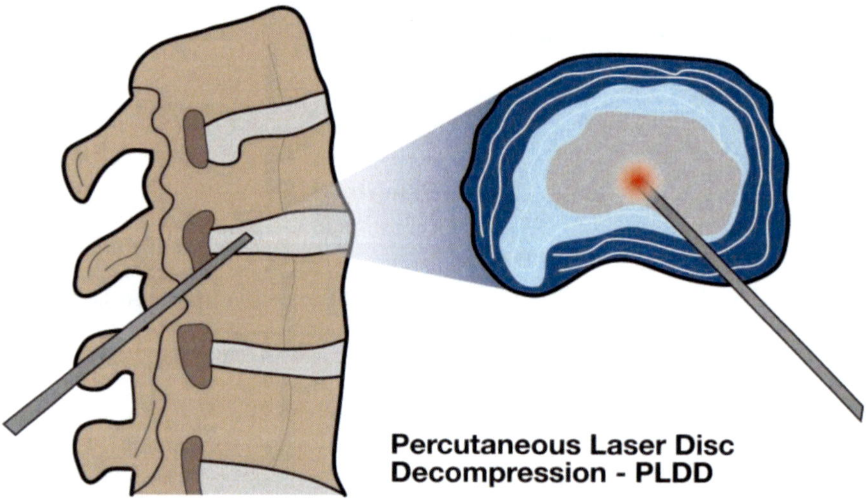

Figure 8. Percutaneous Laser Disc Decompression.

Post-Operative Management

The senior authors of the chapter typically discharge a patient the same day after an uncomplicated discectomy. If the patient has significant co-morbidities then the patient will be admitted for overnight observation. Post-operatively, patients are instructed to not lift objects more than 5 lbs and to limit bending and lifting for 4 weeks. Patients will normally return to work, depending on the type of occupation, after 1 week and will start rehabilitation, if needed, after 4 weeks.

There is varying data on the efficacy of early rehabilitation. A Cochrane database review by Oosterhuis [132] demonstrated that exercise programs starting 4-6 weeks post-op seem to lead to a faster decrease in pain and disability as compared to no treatment, with small to medium effect sizes. Also, high intensity programs lead to a slightly faster decrease in pain and disability versus low intensity regimens. Of note, the quality of the studies reviewed in the analysis varied drastically. Large randomized controlled trials are still needed on the subject.

Non-Operative Treatment Versus Operative Treatment

There have been several trials delineating outcomes of patients that underwent non-operative vs operative management of lumbar disc herniations. Much of the data presented demonstrates that there is a role for surgical intervention for the treatment of LDH and radiculopathy. Operative patients have earlier recoveries than would have otherwise occurred spontaneously.

One classic study was performed by Weber [117]. The study performed was a prospective, randomized study analyzing surgery vs non-operative care. The patients were placed into 3 study groups: one group had definitive indications for surgery, another group had no indications for surgery, and the last group could be treated with or without surgery. The last group was randomly assigned to operative or non-operative management.

The data demonstrate that at 1 year good results occurred in 33% of the non-operative group vs. 66% in the operative group; at 4 years, 51% of the non-operative group reported good results vs. 66% in the operative, and at 10 years 55% of the non-operative group reported good results vs. 57% in the operative group. The study demonstrates that initially, the operative group did better than the non-operative group, but over a 10 year period the outcome data appeared to converge [117].

The MAINE lumbar study was a long term prospective cohort analyzing 507 patients with LDH referred to a neurosurgeon or orthopaedic surgeon [118]. Of the 507 patients 275 were treated surgically and 232 non-surgically. At 1 year follow-up 71% of surgically treated patients reported that their predominant symptom was better or completely gone compared with 43% non-surgically treated patients. At 10 years, 69% of patients initially treated with surgery reported improvement in their predominant symptoms versus

61% treated non-surgically [119]. Also, 56% of surgical patients vs 40% non-surgical reported that their low back pain and leg pain were completely gone and were more satisfied with their current status (71% vs. 56%). [119]. However, at 10 years, there were no differences in work or disability status between both groups.

The spine patient outcomes research trial, (SPORT) is another large, recent, trial comparing operative vs. non-operative patients with LDH [120-122]. The trial was conducted in 11 states at 13 medical centers and included men and women who had symptoms and confirmatory signs of lumbar radiculopathy that persisted for at least six weeks, who had disc herniation at a corresponding level and side on imaging, and who were considered surgical candidates were eligible. Participants were offered enrollment in one of 2 groups, a randomized trial or an observational cohort prospective randomized [501 participants) and observational cohorts [743 participants) at 13 spine clinics in 11 US states. Interventions were standard open discectomy versus usual non-operative care which entailed active physical therapy, education/counseling with home exercise instruction, and non-steroidal anti-inflammatory. Main outcome measures were changes from baseline in the SF-36 Bodily Pain (BP) and Physical Function (PF) scales and the modified Oswestry Disability Index (ODI - AAOS/Modems version) assessed at 6 weeks, 3 and 6 months, and annually thereafter [120-122].

In the observational cohort, at 3 months, those patients who chose surgery had larger improvements in the primary outcome measures of bodily pain (mean change: surgery, 40.9 vs non-operative care, 26.0; treatment effect, 14.8; 95% confidence interval, 10.8-18.9), physical function (mean change: surgery, 40.7 vs non-operative care, 25.3; treatment effect, 15.4; 95% CI, 11.6-19.2), and Oswestry Disability Index (mean change: surgery, −36.1 vs non-operative care, −20.9; treatment effect, −15.2; 95% CI, −18.5. to −11.8).

These differences narrowed somewhat at 2 years. At 4 years, the combined data, in both randomized and observational cohorts, those patients who underwent surgery for LDH had greater improvement than non-operative patients in all primary and secondary outcome measures except work status [122]. In the 8 year follow-up, combining the randomized and observational cohorts demonstrated a significant improvement in pain, function, satisfaction, and self-rated progress over 8 years in the surgical cohort vs the non-operative one [126].

Finally, looking at cost-effectiveness data from the SPORT analysis [125], the authors noted that surgery was more initially more costly than non-operative management, however health outcomes in the first 2 years were better with surgical management. Furthermore, when looking at costs per quality-adjusted life years (QALY) gained with surgery as compared to non-operative management, the totals were $34,355 vs $69,403 for surgery and non-operative management, respectively. Thus, surgery is ultimately a more cost-effective treatment modality than conservative management for the treatment of symptomatic LDH patients [125].

Key Points:

- Most LDH respond well to conservative management within the first 3 months of symptom onset.
- Patients with progressive neurologic deficits or cauda equina are absolute indications for surgery.
- The ideal surgical patient for LDH is one with severe unilateral radicular pain who has tried and failed conservative management and whose imaging correlates with the clinical findings.
- Discectomy in patients appears to provide faster symptomatic relief in appropriately selected patients as opposed to the natural history of the disease.
- Over the course of several years the differences between outcomes in the operative patients and non-operative patients narrows, but surgical patients still report better outcomes than non-operative patients.
- Improvement in back pain, paresthesias, and weakness, are less reliable outcomes than improvement in radicular pain.
- Surgical management of LDH is more cost-effective than non-operative management for treatment of symptomatic LDH patients.

Surgical Outcome Data

Outcomes for surgical intervention have been well documented and produce reliable results as demonstrated in the non-operative vs. operative treatment section of the chapter. Also described earlier in the chapter, a study performed by Carragee et. al [57], found that operations on larger discs (>6mm) produced better results than patients with disc < 6mm. However, disc size is a less reliable predictor of outcome in the non-operative group. In another study by Knop-Jergas [123] found that patients with paracentral and intraforaminal discs had the best outcomes with 80% of patients yielding good or excellent results.

The post-hoc analysis of the SPORT data [124] found that patients with lateral disc herniations had the greatest improvement from surgery vs non-operative management. Furthermore, the data demonstrated that the level of disc herniation or morphology did not influence outcome in either the surgical or non-surgical groups.

Of note, social and psychological factors have a strong influence on outcomes after LDH surgery. A study by Sorensen found that the outcome of LDH surgery could be predicted correctly in 86% of patients based on pre-operative psychological assessment [127]. Another study analyzing personality factors and results of LDH surgery found that patients that were self-confident, concerned with their illness, only mildly depressed, optimistic regarding their outcome, and able to withstand setbacks without resorting to emergency reactions had good outcomes [128]. An analysis performed by Johansson [129] found that low expectations for work return within 3 months after surgery was also significantly predictive for residual leg pain.

Return to Play Outcomes

A study from the Professional Athlete Spine Initiative (PASI) in 342 players with LDH from baseball, football, hockey, and basketball returned to play 82% of the time with 81% of surgically treated patients returning to play for an average of 3.3 more years [130]. Another recent study by Minhas et al. [131], studied 61 players in the NBA with an LDH. 34 players underwent discectomy, 27 were managed conservatively. Return to play did not differ between the groups, player efficiency in the operated group was lower than the non-operative group in the first year post-op, but no difference was seen 2 and 3 years after surgery [131]. In another recent study by Watkins [133] determining return to play in MLB, NBA, NFL and NHL athletes after lumbar discectomy, found no significant differences in return to play after level of surgery. Although, L5-S1 discectomies were the most common procedure and L3-4 discectomies were the least common. No discectomies were performed at L1-2, or L2-3. This study accounted for off-seasons in the individual sports and found that 89.3% returned to play after surgery with an average off time of 5.8 months. Furthermore, 50% of players returned to sport at 3 months, 72% at 6 months and 84% at 12 months [133].

Key Points:

- > 6mm disc herniations produce better post-operative outcomes than disc herniations < 6mm.
- Paracentral and intra-foraminal disc herniations produce good post-operative outcomes, whereas patients with lateral disc herniations do better with surgery as opposed to non-operative treatment.
- Location of disc herniation does not influence post-surgical outcome
- Social and psychological factors do influence post-operative outcomes, namely depression and desire to return to work.
- 50% of athletes will return to play at 6 months and 84% at 1 year post lumbar discectomy.
- The athlete may not be at his peak performance during the 1st year post-op, but will return to his baseline during subsequent years.

Comparison of Different Surgical Techniques

There is debate in the literature regarding which procedure yields the best outcomes when comparing standard open discectomy (SOD), minimally invasive lumbar discectomy (MLD), tubular microdiscectomy (MTD), endoscopic discectomy (ED) and percutaneous laser disc decompression (PLDD). The authors of the chapter have a personal preference for the tubular microdiscectomy technique.

A study by Ryang et. al [134] compared standard open discectomy (SOD) versus tubular/trocar microdiscectomy (MTD). The authors found small, non-significant, differences that favored MTD over SOD in regard to decreased operative time, blood loss, and complication rate. However, at follow up of 16 months, there were no differences in clinical outcomes as measured by CAS pain, Oswestry Disability Index (ODI), or SF-36 scales [134]. Another randomized prospective trial comparing SOD vs MLD found that: size of incision, and length of hospital stay were greater in the SOD group, and operative time was greater in the MLD group. Overall patient outcome was comparable between the 2 groups [135].

A meta-analysis of the literature comparing minimally invasive (MIS) techniques (MLD and MTD) versus SOD for LDH found moderate-quality evidence that failed to show an advantage of MIS techniques over SOD in terms of short and long-term pain outcomes. There was also low-quality evidence that suggested higher rates of nerve root injury, durotomy, and re-operation with the minimally invasive techniques when compared to the standard open surgery [136]. However, the authors did not consider blood loss, radiation exposure, operating time, and muscle injury when performing the meta-analysis [136].

Arts et al., performed a double-blind randomized controlled trial comparing MTD versus MLD for LDH in 328 patients. They found no significant differences in clinical or functional outcomes for either group. The study followed patients for 2 years and noted small differences with MTD patients reporting more leg pain and low back pain, however the differences did not achieve statistical significance or clinical relevance [137].

However, when considering the complications associated with obese patients MIS procedures afford benefits over SOD. In a retrospective review Tomasino et al. [138], studied 115 obese and nonobese patients that underwent a 1 level lumbar laminectomy or microdiscectomy via MTD. The outcomes were comparable between both groups and when compared to SOD, MTD offered smaller incisions, and decreased operative time, blood loss, and length of stay [138].

Another recent study comparing microsurgical, endoscopic, and endoscopically assisted discectomies in both a randomized prospective cohort and a retrospective cohort found all procedures were effective in relieving acute radicular symptoms. The study found no significant differences in outcome at 1 year follow-up. However, recurrent disc herniation occurred more frequently after endoscopic discectomy as compared to MTD and MLD [140].

In another prospective randomized study comparing full-endoscopic interlaminar and transforaminal lumbar discectomy versus conventional MLD, the authors found no difference in clinical outcomes between both groups and similar recurrent disc herniation rates (6.2%). The authors reported benefits of ED over MLD and MTD to include: expanded fields of view, shorter operative times, reduced anatomic trauma, and facilitation of revision operations. Possible disadvantages of ED over MLD and MTD include the limited possibility of extending the approach in the event of unforeseen complications, and in the trans-foraminal technique, there is an elevated risk of exiting nerve root injury. Furthermore, the learning curve is steeper in the ED technique as compared to the MIS techniques [141].

Percutaneous laser discectomy was compared to conventional MLD for treatment of sciatica in a randomized controlled trial performed by Brouwer et. al, [142]. The goal of the study was to demonstrate non-inferiority of PLDD to

MLD. 115 surgical candidates with sciatica from a disc herniation smaller than one-third of the spinal canal were included. Patients were randomly assigned to either the PLDD (n = 57) or MLD (n = 58) group. It is important to note that the following patients were excluded from the study: patients with cauda equina syndrome, previous spinal surgery at the same disc level, lytic or degenerative spondylolisthesis, sequestered disc herniation, disc height less than 7 mm, and patients with central canal stenosis. The results showed non-inferiority of PLDD compared to MLD at 52 weeks using the Roland-Moriss Disability Questionnaire. There was a higher speed of recovery in favor of MLD and the number of reoperations was significantly less in the MLD group (38% vs 16%).

Minimally invasive and endoscopic techniques are technically demanding and require significant expertise. There is a well-documented learning curve associated with these procedures [139, 141], however; the benefits over standard open techniques include: decreased blood loss, operative time, incision length, and length of stay [134-138]. The differences between the MIS and ED techniques are negligible and preference should depend on the surgeons comfort with the procedure and their level of training. PLDD has limited indications and may provide benefit for some patients with small disc bulges or herniations that are in direct continuity with the NP.

Comparisons of the different procedures, with the exception of the PLDD, are provided in Table 1 and 2. Table 3 demonstrates comparisons between open discectomy versus microdiscectomy, and microdiscectomy versus tubular microdiscectomy.

Key Points:

- Standard open discectomy has similar patient outcomes when compared to minimally invasive techniques e.g., tubular microdiscectomy, microdiscectomy, and endoscopic techniques.
- MIS techniques compared to open techniques offers decreased blood loss, operative time, incision size, and length of stay.
- Differences in outcomes between MLD, MTD, and ED are negligible.
- PLDD has very limited proven indications: only for small disc bulges or protrusions.
- PLDD has been associated with a higher need for re-operation.

Table 1. Comparison of Operative Techniques

	Standard discectomy	Microsurgical tubular discectomy (MTD)	Microsurgical discectomy (MLD)	Microendoscopic discectomy (MED)	Percutaneous endoscopic discectomy (PED)
Procedural factors					
Retractor		Tubular retractor	Eg, Caspar	Tubular retractor	None
Surgical instruments		Bayonetted microinstruments	Microsurgical instruments	Endoscope	Endoscope
Navigation	Preoperative x-ray/image intensification	Preoperative x-ray/image intensification	Preoperative x-ray/image intensification	Preoperative x-ray/image intensification	Preoperative x-ray/image intensification
Surgical exposure	1. Wide exposure 2. Good visualization of surrounding structures	1. Small skin incision 2. Surrounding structures protected by retractors	1. Small skin incision 2. Surrounding structures protected by retractors	1. Small skin incision 2. Surrounding structures protected by tubes	1. Percutaneous stab incision 2. Structures traversed by endoscope
Paraspinal muscles	Injured during surgical exposure	Potentially less damage to muscles due to muscle-splitting technique	• Minimal damage to paravertebral muscles • Preservation of muscle insertions and segmental innervation	Potentially less damage to muscles due to muscle-splitting technique	• Least muscle damage • Segmental muscle of erector spine is not violated
Bony window	Laminotomy needed		Obviates need for laminectomy and avoids damage to facet joint	Laminotomy, potential damage to medial facet joints	Facet joints are protected
Magnification and illumination of the surgical field	–	+++ (microscope)	++++ (microscope)	++ (endoscope)	++
Ligamentum flavum flap	Not possible	Possible	Ligamentum flavum can be raised as a flap and preserved	Very difficult to raise a flap	Flavum not violated at all

Table 1. (Continued)

	Standard discectomy	Microsurgical tubular discectomy (MTD)	Microsurgical discectomy (MLD)	Microendoscopic discectomy (MED)	Percutaneous endoscopic discectomy (PED)
Hemostasis	• Hemostasis is very difficult • Blood loss is more	• Hemostasis around the tube is difficult to access and control • Blood loss is less	• Better hemostasis due to identification, coagulation of epidural veins • Blood loss is less	• Hemostasis around the tube is difficult to access and control • Blood loss is less	• Laser discectomy causes very less bleeding • Blood loss is least
Annulus repair	Very difficult	Possible	Possible	Not possible	Not possible
Surgical technique	Easy to perform	Significant learning curve	Significant learning curve	Significant learning curve	Significant learning curve
Wound infection	Less chance	Minimal	Potential risks ++	Minimal	Less chances
Surgical limitations	–	Tubular retractor may need to be angled to optimize visualization	–	Tubular retractor may need to be angled to optimize visualization	• Difficult to treat central disc herniations, those associated with foraminal stenosis • Movement of the instruments is limited inside the foramen • If the disc has migrated cranially or caudally, the transforaminal approach is not possible • At L5–S1 it is impossible to gain adequate access and at the upper levels, the procedure is quite demanding

The "+" symbol indicates the strength of association of a particular feature with the type of surgery. The more "+" symbols, the stronger the association.

Reprint from: [174] Härtl R. Andreas K. Minimally Invasive Spine Surgery—Techniques, Evidence, and Controversies. 2012 ed. Switzerland, Davos Platz: Thieme; 2012. p. 294.

Table 2. Comparison of Operative Techniques

	Standard discectomy	Microsurgical tubular discectomy (MTD)	Microsurgical discectomy (MLD)	Microendoscopic discectomy (MED)	Percutaneous endoscopic discectomy (PED)
Patient factors					
Surgical Incision	• Long incision • Painful (++++)	• Good cosmesis (2.5 cm long scar) • Less painful (++) • Advantageous in obese patients (good retraction with minimal skin incision)	• Good cosmesis (2.5 cm long scar) • Less painful (++)	• Good cosmesis (2.5 cm long scar) • Less painful (++) • Advantageous in obese patients (good retraction with minimal skin incision)	• Excellent cosmesis • Stab wound incisions much less painful
Hospitalization	Longer hospitalization and delayed rehabilitation	• Earlier return to work • Day care procedure in most cases	Shorter hospitalization period, quicker rehabilitation, earlier return to work	• Earlier return to work • Day care procedure in most cases	• Least period of inactivity • Outpatient procedure in most cases
Anesthesia	Always under general anesthetic	Usually under general anesthetic, but can also be performed under local anesthetic	Usually under general anesthetic	Usually under general anesthetic, but can also be performed under local anesthetic	Carried out under local anesthetic
Surgeon factors					
Teaching aid	Not possible for two people to visualize simultaneously	Optimal teaching aid to assistants	Optimal teaching aid to assistants	Only the surgeon can see, feel, and do at the same time	Only the surgeon can see, feel, and do at the same time
Handling of instruments	Direct visualization of field and instruments	Needs hand-eye coordination with microscope	Needs hand-eye coordination with microscope	Needs hand-eye coordination with monitor	Needs hand eye-coordination with monitor

Surgery in recurrent discs	Difficult surgery in recurrent discs	In surgery for recurrent disc herniations, safe dissection of epidural adhesions and/or scar tissue is possible	In surgery for recurrent disc herniations, safe dissection of epidural adhesions and/or scar tissue is possible	Difficult surgery in recurrent discs	The posterolateral approach does not cause fibrosis along the simply muscle-dilating approach. Recurrent surgeries are easier and safe to do
Visualization of field	Unmagnified 3-D view	3-D view through microscope	3-D view through microscope	2-D view but angled endoscope can also see medially displaced fragments	Only 2-D view possible

The "+" symbol indicates the strength of association of a particular feature with the type of surgery. The more "+" symbols, the stronger the association.

Reprint from: [175] Härtl R. Andreas K. Minimally Invasive Spine Surgery—Techniques, Evidence, and Controversies. 2012 ed. Switzerland, Davos Platz: Thieme; 2012. p. 295.

Table 3. Evidence based Results of 3 prospective trials comparing standard discectomy vs. microdiscectomy, and microdiscectomy vs. microsurgical tubular discectomy

Procedure	Standard discectomy versus micro-surgical discectomy (MLD) (a)		Standard discectomy versus micro-surgical discectomy (MLD) (b)		Microsurgical tubular discectomy (MTD) versus microdiscectomy (c)	
Study design	Prospective randomized		Prospective, nonrandomized		Multicenter prospective randomized	
Parameters	Standard	MLD	Standard	MLD	MTD	MLD (loupe magnification)
Patients per group	62	57	225	36	167	161
Surgical duration (minutes)	40±12	45±8 (S)	NS		47 ± 22	36 ±16 (S)
Blood loss	39±11 g	25±9 g (S)	Significantly less in microdiscectomy		150 ± 90ml	135 ± 85 ml (NS)
Hospital stay (days)	8.3±0.8	8.5±2.3 (S)	5.9 ± 3	6.0± 2.8 (NS)	3.3± 1.2	3.3 ± 1.1 (NS)
Analgesic need	NS		Not assessed		Not assessed	
Muscle damage/need for analgesics	NS		Not assessed		Not assessed	
Postoperative back pain	Significantly more in standard discectomy		VAS 4.4 ± 2.7	4.5 ± 2.9 (NS)	Significantly less pain in MLD	
Leg pain improvement	Significantly better in microdiscectomy		VAS 7.6 ± 1.7	6.9 ± 2.5 (NS)	Significantly more improvement in MLD	
Complications	NIL	2 recurrences	2.8%	2.2% (NS)	20	13 (NS)
Short-term results	Not assessed		No significant difference		No significant difference	
Long-term results	77% good	77% good	Leg pain significantly better		69%	79% (S)

Evidence-based results of three prospective trials comparing standard discectomy, microdiscectomy, and microendoscopic discectomy techniques.

S: statistically significant, NS: not statistically significant, VAS: visual analog scale.

a) Katayama Y, Matsuyama Y, Yoshihara H (2006). Comparison of surgical outcomes between macrodisectomy and microdisectomy for lumbar disc herniation: a prospective randomized study with surgery performed by the same spine surgeon. *J Spinal Discrd Tech;* 19(5):344-347.

b) Porchet F, Bartanusz V, Kleinstueck FS (2009). Microdiscectomy compared with standard discectomy: an old problem revisited with new outcome measures with the framework of a spine surgical registry. *Eur Spine J;* 18 Suppl 3:S360-S366.

c) Arts MP, Brand R, Akker ME, et al. (2009). Tubular discectomy vs conventional microdiskectomy for sciatica: a randomized controlled trial. *JAMA;* 302(2):149-158.

Reprint from: [176] Härtl R. Andreas K. Minimally Invasive Spine Surgery—Techniques, Evidence, and Controversies. 2012 ed. Switzerland, Davos Platz: Thieme; 2012. p. 307.

EXTRA FORAMINAL (FAR LATERAL) DISC HERNIATIONS

Extra foraminal or, far lateral, lumbar disc herniations (FLLDH) account for 2.6 to 11.7% of all lumbar disc herniations resulting in nerve root compression [143-146], the majority of which occur at L4-5 [148, 151]. Far lateral disc herniations are classically lateral to the neural foramen (Figure 2). Of note, these herniations compress the exiting nerve root as opposed to the descending nerve root which is typically compressed by central disc herniations. Accessing FLLDH without destabilizing the lumbar spine or injuring the nerve root is challenging. Earlier techniques to approach FLLDH required a unilateral facetectomy, which ultimately resulted in fusion surgery for these patients [147].

Standard open techniques can be used without a facetectomy to access the far-lateral herniations. However, as described by Virk et al., [148] standard open techniques require long midline incisions (4-8cm) and wide sub-periosteal dissections resulting in significant muscle retraction and post-operative morbidity. To minimize muscle trauma with open techniques, the Wiltse paraspinal muscle-splitting approach has been used with success. Weiner et al., [149] accessed far lateral herniations using the Wiltse technique and followed patients for an average of 5.5 years after surgery. They found that 85% of patients were satisfied with their post-op results, pain was eliminated in 60% of patients, while 50% reported still having some degree of low back pain.

Liu et at., [150] performed an investigation using ED, MTD, and a minimally invasive transforaminal lumbar interbody fusion (TLIF), techniques for treating FLLDH. The authors characterized the herniations as type I (foraminal), type II (extra-foraminal), and type III (mixed). The authors found ED was associated with the shortest operation time and simplest anesthesia and least trauma, especially for type I herniations. MTD was particularly useful for type II herniations and TLIF produced the best outcomes for type III herniations because the authors need to remove the ipsilateral facet joint to access the herniations.

The authors prefer to approach FLLDH using MTD as described by Virk and Elowitz (Figure 9) [148]. The authors describe their approach by making a 2 cm incision, 2 cm lateral to midline, ipsilateral to the pathology. The thoracolumbar fascia is opened with a stab incision (1 cm) by scalpel or bovie electrocautery. The initial dilator is introduced through the fascial incision and docked on the lateral aspect of the pars interarticularis under fluoroscopic guidance. K-wires and Steinmann pins are not used in order to lower the risk of durotomy or nerve root injury. Serial dilation occurs until an 18 mm tubular retractor placed. An operative microscope is utilized to identify the bony landmarks; defined medially as the lateral aspect of the pars and caudally by the inferior facet. The lateral pars is drilled to maximize medial exposure. The ligament is opened to expose Kambin's triangle. The nerve root is gently retracted supero-laterally to remove the extruded disc. The authors reported excellent results with complete resolution of symptoms in all patients; with none returning after 6 week follow up with recurrent or new symptoms or the need for re-operation or fusion [148].

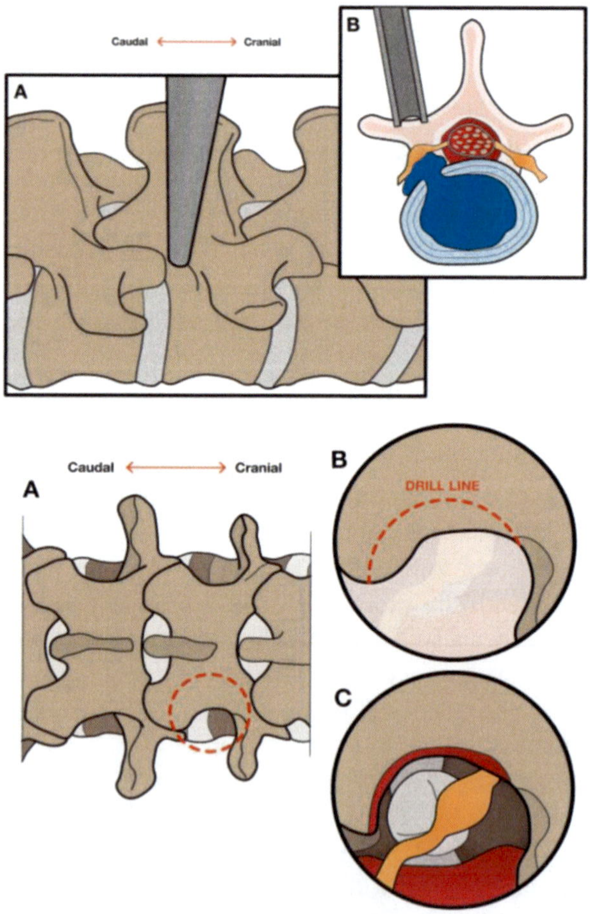

Figure 9. Virk and Elowitz Approach.

Key points:

- Surgery for far lateral disc herniations is more complicated than other types of LDH.
- Care must be taken to preserve the bony architecture to prevent instability.
- If the facet joint must be taken, fusion surgery is indicated and produces good outcomes.
- MIS techniques produce excellent results and most surgeries can be performed by MTD without destabilizing the lumbar spine.

RECURRENT DISC HERNIATION

Recurrent disc herniation (RDH) is defined as reherniation of disc material at the level of a prior lumbar discectomy. The frequency of RDH herniations varies in the literature, but rates are generally reported as 5 to 15% [152-156]. Patients who have RDH may present with the same symptomatology as their initial herniation. It is important to distinguish whether the recurrence of symptoms is due to scar tissue or RDH. As described previously in this chapter, post-operative scar tissue and fibrosis will enhance with gadolinium contrast, whereas RDH will not.

A prospective study was performed by McGirt et al. [157] studying whether aggressive disc space removal was associated with increased risk of RDH. The study observed 100 patients which underwent lumbar discectomy surgery that were followed for 2 years. 11 patients experienced RDH. The authors found that patients experiencing symptomatic RDH requiring re-operation had a greater mean annular defect area and lower percentage of their disc volume removed (46 +/- 18 vs. 32 +/- 14mm^2). Furthermore, larger annular defects were associated with earlier symptomatic reherniation (4 months after surgery). Thus, the authors concluded that large annular defects with less aggressive disc space removal is associated with increased risk of reherniation. It was also demonstrated that aggressive disc space removal was associated with loss of disc height, which ultimately, may exacerbate lumbar disc degeneration. Conversely, Thorne et al., [158] found no correlation between amount of disc removed and risk of RDH. McGirt et. al., [157] explained the contradiction stating that it is the residual proportion of disc left after discectomy, rather than absolute volume removed, that carries prognostic significance of RDH.

Another retrospective review by Moliterno et. al [162] noted a recurrence rate of 9.5% in patients undergoing MTD for LDH, with the most common level involved being L5-S1. The mean length to recurrence was 12 weeks and lower body mass index (BMI) was significantly associated with recurrence. A recent large meta-analysis investigated age, gender, BMI, smoking, level of herniation, herniation type, and BMI as of risk factors for RDH. The authors found that smoking, lumbar disc protrusion without a herniated fragment, and diabetes were all correlated with RDH [161]. Interestingly, obesity was not correlated with increased risk of RDH.

The authors of this chapter evaluate each patient on a case-by-case basis but generally recommend fusion surgery when more than 2 discectomies are performed at the same level for RDH.

Annular Repair

As described above, large annular defects are associated with reherniation and progressive disc degeneration. Newer techniques and research have focused on annular repair and biologic glues to prevent RDH after discectomy.

A large prospective, randomized, multicenter trial studying annular repair in lumbar discectomy found that using the Xclose annular repair system (Anulex Technologies, Minnetonka, MN) reduced RDH at 3 and 6 months post op [172]. There was also a trend toward reduced risk of RDH through 2 years, but these values did not achieve significance.

Yu et al. [169], performed a comprehensive review of the literature on techniques available for annular and disc repair. The authors found that approaches involving mechanical treatments such as suturing, i.e., Xclose, and annulopasty, failed to improve annular healing strength in long-term clinical trials [170-172].

In contrast to mechanical AF repair, Grunert et al., reported promising data from their current trials on biologic glue for AF repair. They successfully demonstrated the in vivo efficacy of riboflavin cross-linked high-density collages gels to facilitate annular repair in a needle-punctured rat-tail model. Their results demonstrated preservation of NP size, hydration and prevention of further degeneration [173].

Key Points:

- Large annular defects and less aggressive disc removal may be associated with increased risk of RDH.
- Volume of disc material removed is associated with decreased disc height and possibly increased degeneration.
- Smoking, disc protrusion, and diabetes were correlated with increased risk of RDH.
- Lower BMI may be a risk factor for RDH.
- Annular repair is a promising new technique to prevent RDH.
- The authors recommend fusion surgery when more than 2 discectomies are performed at the same level for RDH.

Cauda Equina Syndrome

Cauda equine syndrome (CES) is caused by compression of the lumbar and sacral roots which results in bowel or bladder incontinence and/or saddle anesthesia. There can be associated weakness in the lower extremities, paresthesias in a dermatomal distribution, and absent/decreased reflexes [163]. Acute CES is usually caused by LDH where the herniated fragment occupies the whole canal [164]. CES is more common with a central disc herniation, but can occur with lateral or paracentral herniations as well [166, 167]. When acute CES occurs, it is a surgical emergency and immediate imaging should be performed followed by surgical decompression. MRI is the standard for imaging, however a CT with contrast can be performed if the patient cannot undergo an MRI.

The data has shown that CES should be treated within 48 hours as opposed to later than 48 hours, due to improved outcomes in resolution of sensory and motor deficits, rectal function, and urinary function [165]. Furthermore, studies have also shown the presence of preoperative chronic low back pain is associated with poorer outcomes in urinary and rectal function and older patients are less likely to fully regain sexual function after surgery [165]. Post-void residual should be measured in CES patients pre-operatively and should be followed post-operatively as well.

There is considerable debate in the literature on which surgical technique is optimal for decompression in patients with CES. Either MIS or open techniques can be employed and studies have demonstrated that either technique is appropriate and result in comparable outcomes [163, 167, 168]. Some studies favor MIS techniques over SOD for CES, with improved VAS,

ODI, and Frankel scores in MIS techniques [168]. Ultimately the type of surgical approach should be determined by the experience of the surgeon and the nature of the injury resulting in CES.

Key Points:

- CES is a surgical emergency.
- MRI is the optimal imaging modality.
- CES surgery should be performed within 48 hours of presentation.
- Open or MIS techniques can be used for decompression.

CONCLUSION

Given their prevalence, lumbar disc herniations present challenges and a set of options for conservative and surgical remedy. Although it is not essential to know the details of every procedure outlined here, spine surgeons must possess mastery of several different techniques while also generally aware of alternatives.

REFERENCES

[1] Schiller JS, Lucas JW, Ward BW, Peregoy JA. Summary health statistics for U.S. adults: *National Health Interview Survey*, 2010. National Center for Health Statistics. Vital Health Stat 10(252); 2012. Available at: http://www.cdc.gov/nchs/data/ series/sr_10/sr10_252.pdf.

[2] Dagenais S, Caro J, Haldeman S. A systematic review of low back pain cost of illness studies in the United States and internationally. *Spine J* 2008;8(1):8–20.

[3] Hart LG, Deyo RA, Cherkin DC. Physician office visits for low back pain. Frequency, clinical evaluation, and treatment patterns from a U.S. national survey. *Spine* (Phila Pa 1976) 1995;20(1):11–19.

[4] Alexander RM. Elasticity in human and animal backs. In: Vleeming A, Mooney V, Dorman T, Snijders CJ, Stoeckart R, eds. *Movement, Stability and Low Back Pain.* Edinburgh, UK: Churchill Livingstone; 1997.

[5] Choi K. S., Cohn M. J., and Harfe B. D., 2008, "Identification of Nucleus Pulposus Precursor Cells and Notochordal Remnants in the

Mouse: Implications for Disk Degeneration and Chordoma Formation," *Dev. Dyn.,* 2008; 237(12), pp. 3953–3958.

[6] Peacock A., 1951, Observations on the Prenatal Development of the Intervertebral Disc in Man," *J. Anat.,* 85(3), pp. 260–274.

[7] Walmsley R., 1953, The Development and Growth of the Intervertebral Disc, *Edinburgh Med. J.*, 60(8), pp. 341–364.

[8] Ellis K., Bagwell J., and Bagnat M., 2013, "Notochord Vacuoles are Lysosome-Related Organelles That Function in Axis and Spine Morphogenesis," *J. Cell. Biol.,* 200(5), pp. 667–679.

[9] Hwang PY, Chen J, Jing L, Hoffman BD, Setton LA, The role of extracellular matrix elasticity and composition in regulating the nucleus pulposus cell phenotype in the intervertebral disc: a narrative review. *J Biomech Eng.* 2014 Feb;136(2):021010.

[10] Marchand F, Ahmed AM. Investigation of the laminate structure of lumbar disc anulus fibrosus. *Spine* 1990;15:402–410.

[11] Tsantrizos A, Ito K, Aebi M, et al. Internal strains in healthy and degenerated lumbar intervertebral discs. *Spine* 2005;30:2129–2137.

[12] Diagnosis, Management, and Treatment of Discogenic Pain Volume 3: A Volume in the Interventional and Neuromodulatory Techniques for Pain Management Series; Expert Consult Premium Edition -- Enhanced Online Features and Print Leonardo Kapural, MD, PhD, Philip Kim, MD Timothy Deer, MD Chapter 11 Disc herniations 113-129. Larkin, Demarco, Suros, Cohen.

[13] Elves MW, Bucknill T, Sullivan MF: In vitro inhibition of leucocyte migration in patients with intervertebral disc lesions. *Orthop Clin North Am* 6(1):59-65, 1975.

[14] Zhao F, Pollintine P, Hole BD, Adams MA, Dolan P. Vertebral fractures usually affect the cranial endplate because it is thinner and supported by less-dense trabecular bone. *Bone* 2009;44(2):372–379.

[15] Grant JP, Oxland TR, Dvorak MF. Mapping the structural propertiesof the lumbosacral vertebral endplates. *Spine* 2001;26(8):889–896.

[16] Coventry M., Ghormley R., and Kernohan J.: The intervertebral disc: its microscopic anatomy and pathology. Part II: Changes in then intervertebral disc concomitant with age. *J Bone Joint Surg* 1945; 27: pp. 233.

[17] Raj P.: Intervertebral disc: anatomy-physiology-pathophysiology-treatment. *Pain Pract* 2008; 8: pp. 18.

[18] Urban J., Smith S., and Fairbank J.: Nutrition of the intervertebral disc. *Spine* (Phila Pa 1976) 2004; 29: pp. 2700.

[19] Coventry M., Ghormley R., and Kernohan J.: The intervertebral disc: its microscopic anatomy and pathology. Part II: Changes in then intervertebral disc concomitant with age. *J Bone Joint Surg* 1945; 27: pp. 233.

[20] Rudert M., and Tillmann B.: Detection of lymph and blood vessels in the human intervertebral disc by histochemical and immunohistochemical methods. *Ann Anat* 1993; 175: pp. 237.

[21] Rudert M., and Tillmann B.: Detection of lymph and blood vessels in the human intervertebral disc by histochemical and immunohistochemical methods. *Ann Anat* 1993; 175: pp. 237.

[22] Hassler O.: The human intervertebral disc: a micro-angiographical study on its vascular supply at various ages. *Acta Orthop Scand* 1969; 40: pp. 765.

[23] Genuario JW, Mehta S, Nunley RM, The Washington Health Policy Fellows. Discrepancy in healthcare utilization: Is more better in orthopedic surgery? The American Academy of Orthopedic Surgeons web site. Available at: http://www.aaos.org/news/bulletin/jun07/reimbursement2.asp. Accessed August 23, 2007.

[24] Katz JN. Lumbar disc disorders and low-back pain: socioeconomic factors and consequences. *J Bone Joint Surg Am* 2006;88(Suppl 2):21–24.

[25] Asch H.L., Lewis P.J., Moreland D.B., et al: Prospective multiple outcomes study of outpatient lumbar microdiscectomy: should 75 to 80% success rates be the norm? *J Neurosurg* 2002; 96: pp. 34.

[26] Koebbe C.J., Maroon J.C., Abla A., et al: Lumbar microdiscectomy: a historical perspective and current technical considerations. *Neurosurg Focus* 2002; 13: pp. E3.

[27] Mattila V.M., Saarni L., Parkkari J., et al: Early risk factors for lumbar discectomy: an 11-year follow-up of 57,408 adolescents. *Eur Spine J* 2008; 17: pp. 1317.

[28] Ramirez L.F.: Thisted R: Complications and demographic characteristics of patients undergoing lumbar discectomy in community hospitals. *Neurosurgery* 1989; 25: pp. 226.

[29] Bogduk N, Long DM. The anatomy of the so-called "articular nerves" and their relationship to facet denervation in the treatment of low back pain. *J Neurosurg* 1979;51:172–7.

[30] Bogduk N, Tynan W, Wilson AS. The nerve supply to the human lumbar intervertebral discs. *J Anat* 1981;132:39–56.

[31] Bogduk N. The innervation of the lumbar spine. *Spine* 1983;8:286–93.

[32] Brena SF, Wolf SL, Chapman SL, Hammonds WD. Chronic back pain: Electromyographic, motion and behavioral assessments following sympathetic blocks and placebos. *Pain* 1980;8:1–10.
[33] Edgar MA, Nundy S. Innervation of spinal dura mater. *J Neurol Neurosurg Psychiatry* 1966;29:530–4.
[34] Groen GJ, Baljet B, Drukker J. Nerves and nerve plexuses of the human vertebral column. *Am J Anat* 1990:188:282–96.
[35] Kimmel DL. Innervation of spinal dura mater and dura mater of the posterior cranial fossa. *Neurology* 1961;11:800–9.
[36] Kojima Y, Maeda T, Arai R, Shichikawa K. Nerve supply to the posterior longitudinal ligament and the intervertebral disc of the rat vertebral column as studied by acetylcholinesterase histochemistry. *J Anat* 1990;169:237–55.
[37] Ohtori S et al: Sensory innervation of the dorsal portion of the lumbar intervertebral disc in rats. *Spine* 24:2295-2299, 1999.
[38] Frei H, Oxland TR, Rathonyi GC, et al: The effect of nucleotomy on lumbar spine mechanics in compression and shear loading. *Spine* (Phila Pa 1976) 26:2080-2089, 2001.
[39] Heliovaara M.: *Epidemiology of sciatica and herniated lumbar intervertebral disc*. The Social Insurance Institution, Finland, ML: 76, Helsinki, 1988.
[40] Hirsh c., Jonsson B., Lewin T.: Low back symptoms in a Swedish female population. *Clin. Orthop*. 63: 171-176, 1969.
[41] Cherkin DC, Deyo RA, Loeser JD, Bush T, Waddell G. An international comparison of back surgery rates. *Spine* 1994; 19:1201-6.
[42] Pouriesa M, Fouladi RF and Mesbahi S. Disproportion of end plates and the lumbar intervertebral disc herniation. *Spine J* 2013; 13: 402-407.
[43] Frymoyer JW, Pope MH, Clements JH, Wilder DG, MacPherson B, Ashikaga T (1983) Risk factors in low-back pain. An epidemiological survey. *J Bone Joint Surg Am* 65:213–218.
[44] Friberg S, Hirsch C. Anatomical and clinical studies on lumbar disc degeneration. *Acta Orthop Scand* 1949;19:222–242.
[45] Schultz A, Andersson G, Ortengren R, et al. Loads on the lumbar spine. *J Bone Joint Surg Am* 1982;64:713–720.
[46] Postacchini F. Lumbar Disc Herniations. *Etiopathogenesis. Springer* 1999; pp 153-154.
[47] Spengler DM, Ouellette EA, Battie M, et al: Elective discectomy for herniation of a lumbar disc: Additional experience with an objective method. *J Bone Joint Surg Am* 72:320-327, 1990.

[48] McCulloch JA, Transfelt EE: *Macnab's Backache. Baltimore,* Williams and Wilkins, 1997.
[49] Dang L, Liu Z (2010) A review of current treatment for lumbar disc herniation in children and adolescents. *Eur Spine J* 19:205–214. doi:10.1007/s00586-009-1202-7.
[50] Epstein JA, Lavine LS (1964) Herniated lumbar intervertebral discs in teen-age children. *J Neurosurg* 21:1070–1075.
[51] Grobler LJ, Simmons EH, Barrington TW (1979) Intervertebral disc herniation in the adolescent. *Spine* 4:267–278.
[52] Garrido E, Humphreys RP, Hendrick EB, Hoffman HJ (1978) Lumbar disc disease in children. *Neurosurgery* 2:22–26.
[53] Zitting P, Rantakallio P, Vanharanta H (1998) Cumulative incidence of lumbar disc diseases leading to hospitalization up to the age of 28 years. *Spine* 23:2337–2343 (discussion 2334–2343).
[54] Palmgren T, Gronblad M, Virri J, et al: An immunohistochemical study of nerve structures in the annulus fibrosus of human normal lumbar intervertebral discs. *Spine* 2001; 24: pp. 2075-2079.
[55] Rengachary SS, and Balabhadra RSV: Black disc disease: a commentary. *Neurosurg Focus* 2002; 13: pp. E14.
[56] Devillé WL, van der Wint DA, Dzaferagic A, et al: The test of Lasègue: systematic review of the accuracy in diagnosing herniated discs. *Spine* 2000; 25: pp. 1140-1147.
[57] Carragee EJ, Kim D: A prospective analysis of magnetic resonance imaging findings in patients with sciatica and lumbar disc herniation: Correlation of outcomes with disc fragment and canal morphology. *Spine* (Phila Pa 1976) 22:1650-1660, 1997.
[58] Heithoff KB: Recurrent disc herniation and gadolinium. *Spine-Line* Sept/Oct:23-26, 2002.
[59] Nygaard OP, Mellgren SI, Osterud B. The inflammatory properties of contained and noncontained lumbar disc herniation. *Spine* 1997;22 (21):2484–2488.
[60] Hasegawa T, An HS, Inufusa A, Mikawa Y, Watanabe R. The effect of age on inflammatory responses and nerve root injuries after lumbar disc herniation: an experimental study in a canine model. *Spine* 2000;25 (8):937–940.
[61] Gronblad M, Virri J, Tolonen J, et al. A controlled immunohistochemical study of inflammatory cells in disc herniation tissue. *Spine* 1994;19(24):2744–2751.

[62] Habtemariam A, Gronblad M, Virri J, Seitsalo S, Karaharju E. A comparative immunohistochemical study of inflammatory cells in acute-stage and chronic-stage disc herniations. *Spine* 1998;23(20): 2159–2165.

[63] Yoshida M, Nakamura T, Sei A, Kikuchi T, Takagi K, Matsukawa A. Intervertebral disc cells produce tumor necrosis factor alpha, interleukin-1beta, and monocyte chemoattractant protein-1 immediately after herniation: an experimental study using a new hernia model. *Spine* 2005;30(1):55–61.

[64] Anderson DG, Tannoury C. Molecular pathogenic factors in symptomatic disc degeneration. *Spine J* 2005;5(6, Suppl):260S–266S.

[65] Mundt DJ, Kelsey JL, Golden AL, et al. An epidemiologic study of sports and weight lifting as possible risk factors for herniated lumbar and cervical discs: the Northeast Collaborative Group on Low Back Pain. *Am J Sports Med.* 1993;21(6):854-860.

[66] Mundt D. J., Kelsey J. 1., Golden A. N. et a!.: An epidemiologic study of non-occupational lifting as a risk factor for herniated lumbar intervertebral disc. *Spine* 18: 595-602, 1993.

[67] Anderson CK, Chaffin DB: A biomechanical evaluation of five lifting techniques. *Applied Ergonomics* 17:2-8, 1986.

[68] Andersson BJG, Ortengren R, Nachemson A: Quantitative studies of back loads in lifting. *Spine* 1:178-185, 1976.

[69] Andersson G, Ortengren R, Nachemson A: Quantitative studies of the load on the back in different working postures. *Scand J Rehabil Med* (Suppl) 6:173-181, 1978.

[70] Bendix T, Eid SE: The distance between the load and the body with three bi-manuallifting techniques. *Applied Ergonomics* 14:185-192,1983.

[71] Kelsey J. L., Hardy R: Driving of motor vehicles as a risk factor for acute herniated lumbar intervertebral disc. *Am. J. Epidemiol.* 102: 63-73, 1975.

[72] Kamijo K., Tsujimara H., Obara H. et al.: Evaluation of seating comfort. *Society of Automotive Engineers technical paper series* 820761: 1-6, 1982.

[73] Porter R w., Thorp 1.: Familial aspects of disc protrusion. *Orthop. Trans.* 10: 524, 1986.

[74] Sward 1., Hellstrom M., Jacobsson B. et a!.: Disc degeneration and associated abnormalities of the spine in elite gymnast. A magnetic resonance imaging study. *Spine* 16: 437-443,1991.

[75] Wilder D. G., Woodworth B. B., Frymoyer J. w. et al.:Vibration and the human spine. *Spine* 7: 243, 1982.
[76] Heliövaara M. Occupation and risk of herniated lumbar intervertebral disk and sciatica leading to hospitalization. *J Chron Dis* 1987; 40: 259–64.
[77] Jensen MV, Tüchsen F, Ørhedem E. Prolapsed cervical intervertebral disc in male professional drivers in Denmark, 1981–90: a longitudinal study of hospitalizations. *Spine* 1996; 21: 2352–55.
[78] Battié MC, Videman T, Laura E, et al. Occupational driving and lumbar disc degeneration: a case control study. *Lancet* 2002; 360: 1369 – 74.
[79] Kelsey J. L., Githens P. B., 0' Conner T. et al.: Acute prolapsed lumbar intervertebral disc. An epidemiologic study with special reference to driving automobiles and cigarette smoking. *Spine* 9: 608-613, 1984.
[80] Saftic R, Grgic M, Ebling B, Splavski B. Case-control study of risk factors for lumbar intervertebral disc herniation in Croatian island populations. *Croat Med J.* 2006;47:593-600.
[81] An HS, Silveri CP, Simpson JM, et al. Comparison of smoking habits between patients with surgically confirmed herniated lumbar and cervical disc disease and controls. *J Spinal Disord.* 1994;7:369-373.
[82] Heliövaara M, Knekt P, Aromaa A. Incidence and risk factors of herniated lumbar intervertebral disc or sciatica leading to hospitalization. *J Chronic Dis.* 1987;40:251-258.
[83] Wang D, Nasto LA, Roughley P, et al. Spine degeneration in a murine model of chronic human tobacco smokers. *Osteoarthritis Cartilage.* 2012;20(8):896-905.
[84] Akmal M, Kesani A, Anand B, Singh A, Wiseman M, Goodship A. Effect of nicotine on spinal disc cells: a cellular mechanism for disc degeneration. *Spine* (Phila Pa 1976). 2004;29:568-575.
[85] Uematsu Y, Matuzaki H, Iwahashi M. Effects of nicotine on the intervertebral disc: an experimental study in rabbits. *J Orthop Sci.* 2001;6:177-182.
[86] Oda H, Matsuzaki H, Tokuhashi Y, Wakabayashi K, Uematsu Y, Iwahashi M. Degeneration of intervertebral discs due to smoking: experimental assessment in a rat-smokingmodel. *J Orthop Sci.* 2004;9:135-141.
[87] Nemoto Y, Matsuzaki H, Tokuhasi Y, et al. Histological changes in intervertebral discs after smoking and cessation: experimental studying using a rat passive smoking model. *J Orthop Sci.* 2006;11:191-197.

[88] Battié MC, Videman T, Kaprio J, Gibbons LE, Gill K, Manninen H, et al. The Twin Spine Study: contributions to a changing view of disc degeneration. *Spine J.* 2009;9:47–59.

[89] Kjaer P, Tunset A, Boyle E, Jensen T. Progression of lumbar disc herniations over an eight year period in a group of adult Danes from the general population longitudinal MRI study using quantitative measures. *BMC Musculoskelet Disord.* 2016 Jan 15;17(1):26.

[90] Chiu CC, Chuang TY, Chang KH, Wu CH, Lin PW, Hsu WY. The probability of spontaneous regression of lumbar herniated disc: a systematic review. *Clin Rehabil.* 2015;29(2):184–95.

[91] Seo JY, Roh YH, Kim YH, Ha KY. Three-dimensional analysis of volumetric changes in herniated discs of the lumbar spine: does spontaneous resorption of herniated discs always occur? *Eur Spine J.* 2014;1–10.

[92] Komori H, Shinomiya K, Nakai O, Yamaura I, Takeda S, Furuya K (1996) The natural history of herniated nucleus pulposus with radiculopathy. *Spine* 21:225–229.

[93] Teplick JG, Haskin ME (1985) Spontaneous regression of herniated nucleus pulposus. *AJR Am J Roentgenol* 145:371–375.

[94] Maigne JY, Rime B, Deligne B (1992) Computed tomographic follow-up study of forty-eight cases of nonoperatively treated lumbar intervertebral disc herniation. *Spine* (Phila Pa 1976) 17:1071–1074.

[95] Haro H, Kato T, Komori H, Osada M, Shinomiya K (2002) Vascular endothelial growth factor (VEGF)-induced angiogenesis in herniated disc resorption. *J Orthopaedic Res* 20:409–415.

[96] Arai Y, Yasuma T, Shitoto K, Yamauchi Y, Suzuki F (2000) Immunohistological study of intervertebral disc herniation of lumbar spine. *J Orthop Sci* 5:229–231.

[97] Yasuma T, Arai K, Yamauchi Y (1993) The histology of lumbar intervertebral disc herniation. The significance of small blood vessels in the extruded tissue. *Spine* (Phila Pa 1976) 18:1761–1765.

[98] Autio RA, Karppinen J, Niinimaki J, Ojala R, Kurunlahti M, Haapea M, Vanharanta H, Tervonen O (2006) Determinants of spontaneous resorption of intervertebral disc herniations. *Spine* 31:1247–1252.

[99] Henmi T, Sairyo K, Nakano S, Kanematsu Y, Kajikawa T, Katoh S, Goel VK (2002) Natural history of extruded lumbar intervertebral disc herniation. *J Med Invest* 49:40–43.

[100] Saal JA, Saal JS, Herzog RJ. The natural history of lumbar intervertebral disc extrusions treated nonoperatively. *Spine* (Phila Pa 1976). 1990;15(7):683–6.
[101] Deyo RA, Diehl AK, Rosenthal M: How many days of bedrest for acute low back pain? A randomized clinical trial. *N Engl J Med* 315:1064-1070, 1986.
[102] Shen FH, Samartzis BS, Andersson GB. Nonsurgical management of acute and chronic low back pain. *J Am Acad Orthop Surg* 2006;14(8): 477–487.
[103] Schnitzer TJ, Ferraro A, Hunsche E, Kong SX. A comprehenxive review of clinical trials on the efficacy and safety of drugs for the treatment of low back pain. *J Pain Symptom Manage* 2004;28(1):72–95.
[104] Rhee JM, Schaufele M, Abdu WA. Radiculopathy and the herniated lumbar disc: controversies regarding pathophysiology and management. *J Bone Joint Surg Am* 2006;88(9):2070–2080.
[105] DePalma MJ, Bhargava A, Slipman CW. A critical appraisal of the evidence for selective nerve root injection in the treatment of lumbosacral radiculopathy. *Arch Phys Med Rehabil* 2005;86(7): 1477–1483.
[106] Werneke M, Hart DL, Cook D. A descriptive study of the centralization phenomenon. A prospective analysis. *Spine* 1999;24(7):676–683.
[107] Donelson R, Silva G, Murphy K. The centralization phenomenon: its usefulness in evaluating and treating referred pain. *Spine* 1990;15: 211–213.
[108] Karas R, McIntosh G, Hall H, et al. The relationship between nonorganic signs and centralization of symptoms in the prediction of return to work for patients with low back pain. *Phys Ther* 1997;77: 354–360.
[109] Long A. The centralization phenomenon: its usefulness as a predictor of outcome in conservative treatment of chronic low back pain. *Spine* 1995;20:2513–2521.
[110] Sufka A, Hauger B, Trenary M, et al. Centralization of low back pain and perceived functional outcome. *J Orthop Sports Phys Ther* 1998;27:205–212.
[111] Delitto A, Cibulka M, Erhard R, et al. Evidence for an extension mobilization category in acute low back syndrome: a prescriptive validation pilot study. *Phys Ther* 1993;73:216–228.
[112] Armon C, Argoff CE, Samuels J, Backonja MM. Assessment: use of epidural steroid injections to treat radicular lumbosacral pain. Report of

the Therapeutics and Technology Assessment Subcommittee of the American Academy of Neurology. *Amer Acad Neuro* 2007;68:723–729.

[113] Hooten MW, Mizerak A, Carns PE, Huntoon MA. Discitis after lumbar epidural corticosteroid injection: a case report and analysis of the case report literature. *Pain Med* 2006;7(1):46–51.

[114] Mathis JM. Epidural steroid injections. *Neuroimaging Clin N Am.* 2010;20(2):193–202.

[115] Horlocker T.T., Wedel D.J., Benzon H., et al: Regional anesthesia and the anticoagulated patient: defining the risks (the second ASRA Consensus Conference on Neuraxial Anesthesia and Anticoagulation). *Reg Anesth Pain Med* 2003; 28: pp. 172-197.

[116] Jasper GP, Francisco GM, Telfeian AE. Endoscopic transforaminal discectomy for an extruded lumbar disc herniation. *Pain Physician.* 2013;16:E31–5.

[117] Weber H: Lumbar disc herniation: A controlled, prospective study with ten years of observations. *Spine* (Phila Pa 1976) 8:131-140, 1983.

[118] Atlas SJ, Deyo RA, Keller RB, et al. The Maine lumbar spine study, II: One-year outcomes of surgical and nonsurgical treatment of sciatica. *Spine* 1996;21:1777-86.

[119] Long-term outcomes of surgical and nonsurgical management of sciatica secondary to a lumbar disc herniation: 10 year results from the maine lumbar spine study. Atlas SJ, Keller RB, Wu YA, Deyo RA, Singer DE. *Spine* (Phila Pa 1976) 2005;30:927–935.

[120] Weinstein JN, Lurie JD, Tosteson TD, et al. Surgical vs nonoperative treatment
for lumbar disk herniation: the Spine Patient Outcomes Research Trial (SPORT) observational cohort. *JAMA*. 2006;296:2451–2459.

[121] Weinstein JN, Tosteson TD, Lurie JD, Tosteson AN, Hanscom B, Skinner JS, et al. Surgical vs nonoperative treatment for lumbar disk herniation: the Spine Patient Outcomes Research Trial (SPORT): a randomized trial. *JAMA*. 2006;296(20):2441–50.

[122] Weinstein JN, Lurie JD, Tosteson TD, et al. Surgical versus nonoperative treatment for lumbar disc herniation: four-year results for the Spine Patient Outcomes Research Trial (SPORT*). Spine.* 2008; 33:2789–2800.

[123] Knop-Jergas BM, Zucherman JF, Hsu KY, et al: Anatomic position of a herniated nucleus pulposus predicts the outcome of lumbar discectomy. *J Spinal Disord* 9:246-250, 1996.

[124] Pearson AM, Blood EA, Frymoyer JW, et al: SPORT lumbar intervertebral disk herniation and back pain: Does treatment, location, or morphology matter? *Spine* (Phila Pa 1976) 33:428-435, 2008.

[125] Tosteson AN, Skinner JS, Tosteson TD, et al. The cost effectiveness of surgical versus nonoperative treatment for lumbar disc herniation over two years: evidence from the Spine Patient Outcomes Research Trial (SPORT). *Spine.* 2008; 33(19):2108–15.

[126] Lurie JD, Tosteson TD, Tosteson AN, et al. Surgical versus nonoperative treatment for lumbar disc herniation: Eight-year results for the spine patient outcomes research trial. *Spine* (Phila Pa 1976) 2014;39:3–16.

[127] Sorensen LV, Mors O, Skovlund O: A prospective study of the importance of psychological and social factors for the outcome after surgery in patients with slipped lumbar disk operated upon for the first time. *Acta Neurochir* (Wien) 88:119-125, 1987.

[128] Cashion EL, Lynch WJ: Personality factors and results of lumbar disc surgery. *Neurosurgery* 4:141-145, 1979.

[129] Johansson AC, Linton SJ, Rosenblad A, Bergkvist L, Nilsson O. A prospective study of cognitive behavioural factors as predictors of pain, disability and quality of life one year after lumbar disc surgery. *Disabil Rehabil.* 2010;32:521–529.

[130] Hsu WK, McCarthy KJ, Savage JW, Roberts DW, Roc GC, Micev AJ, et al. The Professional Athlete Spine Initiative: outcomes after lumbar disc herniation in 342 elite professional athletes. *Spine J.* 2011;11(3): 180–6.

[131] Minhas SV, Kester BS, Hsu WK. Outcomes After Lumbar Disc Herniation in the National Basketball Association. *Sports Health.* 2016 Jan;8(1):43-9.

[132] Oosterhuis T, Costa LOP, Maher CG, de Vet HCW, van Tulder MW, Ostelo RWJG. Rehabilitation after lumbar disc surgery. *Cochrane Database of Systematic Reviews* 2014, Issue 3 Art. No.: CD003007.

[133] Watkins RG IV., Hanna R, Chang D, Watkins RG III. Return-to-play outcomes after microscopic lumbar diskectomy in professional athletes. *Am J Sports Med.* 2012;40:2530-2535.

[134] Ryang YM, Oertel MF, Mayfrank L, et al. Standard open microdiscectomy versus minimal access trocar microdiscectomy: results of a prospective randomized study. *Neurosurgery* 2008;62:174-81, discussion 181-2.

[135] Righesso O, Falavigna A, Avanzi O.. Comparison of open discectomy with microendoscopic discectomy in lumbar disc herniations: results of a randomized controlled trial. *Neurosurgery* 2007; 61:545-9, discussion 549.

[136] Evaniew N, Khan M, Drew B, Kwok D, Bhandari M, Ghert M. Minimally invasive versus open surgery for cervical and lumbar discectomy: a systematic review and meta-analysis. *CMAJ Open.* 2014 Oct 1;2(4):E295-305.

[137] Arts MP, Brand R, van den Akker ME, et al. Tubular diskectomy vs conventional microdiskectomy for the treatment of lumbar disk herniation: 2-year results of a double-blind randomized controlled trial. *Neurosurgery* 2011;69:135,44.

[138] Tomasino A, Parikh K, Steinberger J, Knopman J, Boockvar J, Härtl R. Tubular microsurgery for lumbar discectomies and laminectomies in obese patients: operative results and outcome. *Spine* 2009; 34(18).

[139] Parikh K, Tomasino A, Knopman J, Boockvar J, Härtl R. Operative results and learning curve: microscope-assisted tubular microsurgery for 1- and 2-level discectomies and laminectomies. *Neurosurg Focus.* 2008;25:E14.

[140] Belykh E, Giers MB, Preul MC, Theodore N, Byvaltsev V. Prospective comparison of microsurgical, endoscopic, and endoscopically assisted discectomies: Clinical effectiveness and complications in railway workers. *World Neurosurg.* 2016 Feb 17. pii: S1878-8750(16)00292-8.

[141] Ruetten S, Komp M, Merk H, Godolias G. Full-endoscopic interlaminar and transforaminal lumbar discectomy versus conventional microsurgical technique: a prospective, randomized, controlled study. *Spine* (Phila Pa 1976) 2008;33:931–939.

[142] Brouwer PA, Brand R, van den Akker-van Marle ME, Jacobs WC, Schenk B, van den Berg-Huijsmans AA, et al. Percutaneous laser disc decompression versus conventional microdiscectomy in sciatica: a randomized controlled trial. *Spine J.* 2015;15:857–865.

[143] Maroon JC, Kopitnik TA, Schulhof LA, Abla A, Wilberger JE. Diagnosis and microsurgical approach to far-lateral disc herniation in the lumbar spine. *J Neurosurg* 1990; 72: 378-382.

[144] Benini A. Der Zugang zu den lateralen lumbalen Diskushernien am Beispiel einer Hernie L4/L5. *Oper Orthop Traumatol* 1998; 10: 103-116.

[145] Abdullah AF, Wolber PG, Warfield JR, Gunadi IK. Surgical management of extreme lateral lumbar disc herniations: review of 138 cases. *Neurosurgery* 1988; 22: 648-653.

[146] O'Hara LJ, Marshall RW. Far lateral lumbar disc herniation. The key to the intertransverse approach. *J Bone Joint Surg Br* 1997; 79: 943-947.

[147] Garrido E, Connaughton PN: Unilateral facetectomy approach for lateral lumbar disc herniation. *J Neurosurg* 74:754-756, 1991.

[148] Virk MS, Elowitz E (2015) A Minimally Invasive Approach to the Lumbar Neural Foramen and Extraforaminal Compartment: Modified Surgical Technique. J Spine 4:203.

[149] Weiner BK, Dabbah M. Lateral lumbar disc herniations treated with a paraspinal approach: an independent assessment of longer-term outcomes. *J Spinal Disord Tech.* 2005;18:519–521.

[150] Liu T, Zhou Y, Wang J, et al. Clinical efficacy of three different minimally invasive procedures for far lateral lumbar disc herniation. *Chinese Medical Journal.* 2012;125:1082–8.

[151] O'Brien MF, Peterson D, Crockard HA. A posterolateral microsurgical approach to extreme-lateral lumbar disc herniation. *J Neurosurg* 1995; 83: 636-640.

[152] Connolly ES. Surgery for recurrent lumbar disc herniation. *Clin Neurosurg* 1992;39:211-6.

[153] Fandino J, Botana C, Viladrich A, Gomez-Bueno J. Reoperation after lumbar disc surgery: results in 130 cases. *Acta Neurochir* (Wien) 1993;122:102-4.

[154] Swartz KR, Trost GR. Recurrent lumbar disc herniation. *Neurosurg Focus.* 2003;15:E10.

[155] Carragee EJ, Han MY, Suen PW, et al. Clinical outcomes after lumbar discectomy for sciatica: the effects of fragment type and anular competence. *J Bone Joint Surg Am.* 2003;85:102–108.

[156] Leven DM, Passias PG, Errico TJ, et al. Risk factors for reoperation in patients treated surgically for intervertebral disc herniations: a subanalysis of the eight-year data from the sport trial. *Spine J.* 2014; 14:S95–S96.

[157] McGirt MJ, Eustacchio S, Varga P, Vilendecic M, Trummer M, Gorensek M, et al. A prospective cohort study of close interval computed tomography and magnetic resonance imaging after primary lumbar discectomy: factors associated with recurrent disc herniation and disc height loss. *Spine* (Phila Pa 1976)2009;34(19):2044–2051.

[158] Thome C, Barth M, Scharf J, et al. Outcome after lumbar sequestrectomy compared with microdiscectomy: a prospective randomized study. *J Neurosurg Spine* 2005;2:271–8.

[159] Gill CS, Sandell LJ, El-Zawawy HB, et al. Effects of cigarette smoking on early medial collateral ligament healing in a mouse model. *J Orthop Res.* 2006;24:2141–2149.

[160] Nemoto Y, Matsuzaki H, Tokuhasi Y, et al. Histological changes in intervertebral discs after smoking and cessation: experimental study using a rat passive smoking model. *J Orthop Sci.* 2006;11:191–197.

[161] Huang W, Han Z, Liu J, Yu L, Yu X. Risk Factors for Recurrent Lumbar Disc Herniation: A Systematic Review and Meta-Analysis. *Medicine* (Baltimore). 2016 Jan;95(2):e2378.

[162] Moliterno JA, Knopman J, Parikh K, Cohan JN, Huang QD, Aaker GD, Grivoyannis AD, Patel AR, Hartl R, Boockvar JA. Results and risk factors for recurrence following single-level tubular lumbar microdiscectomy. *J Neurosurg Spine.* 2010;12:680–686.

[163] Shih P, Smith TR, Fessler RG, Song JK. Minimally invasive discectomy for the treatment of disc herniation causing cauda equina syndrome. *Clin Neurosci.* 2011 Sep;18(9):1219-23.

[164] Olivero WC, Wang H, Hanigan WC, et al. Cauda equina syndrome (CES) from lumbar disc herniations. *J Spinal Disord Tech* 2009; 22:202–6.

[165] Ahn UM, Ahn NU, Buchowski JM, Garrett ES, Sieber AN, Kostuik JP. Caudaequina syndrome secondary to lumbar disc herniation: a meta-analysis of surgical outcomes. *Spine* (Phila Pa 1976)2000;25: 1515–1522.

[166] Walker JL, Schulak D, Murtagh R: Midline disk herniations of the lumbar spine. *South Med J* 86:13-17, 1993.

[167] Tay ECK, Chacha PB: Midline prolapse of a lumbar intervertebral disc with compression of the cauda equina. *J Bone Joint Surg Br* 61:43-46, 1979.

[168] Shen L, Fang C, Qiu Y, Xing S, Chen D, He X, Wang J, Lai J, Shi G, Zhang J, Liao T, Tan J. Study on different surgical approaches for acute Lumber disk protrusion combined with Cauda Equina Syndrome. *Int J Clin Exp Pathol* 2014;7(12):8875-8880.

[169] Moriguchi, Y, Alimi, M, Khair, T, Manolarakis, G, Berlin, C, Bonassar, L, Härtl, Roger. Biological Treatment Approaches for Degenerative Disk Disease: A Literature Review of In Vivo Animal and Clinical Data. *Global Spine Journal.* 2016. EPRINT.

[170] Ahlgren BD, Lui W, Herkowitz HN, Panjabi MM, Guiboux JP. Effect of anular repair on the healing strength of the intervertebral disc: a sheep model. *Spine* (Phila Pa 1976) 2000;25(17): 2165–2170.

[171] Chiang CJ, Cheng CK, Sun JS, Liao CJ, Wang YH, Tsuang YH. The effect of a new anular repair after discectomy in intervertebral disc degeneration: an experimental study using a porcine spine model. *Spine* (Phila Pa 1976) 2011;36(10):761–769.

[172] Bailey A, Araghi A, Blumenthal S, Huffmon GV; Anular Repair Clinical Study Group. Prospective, multicenter, randomized, controlled study of anular repair in lumbar discectomy: two-year follow-up. *Spine* (Phila Pa 1976) 2013;38(14):1161–1169.

[173] 7 Grunert P, Borde BH, Hudson KD, Macielak MR, Bonassar LJ, Härtl R. Annular repair using high-density collagen gel: a rat-tail in vivo model. *Spine* (Phila Pa 1976) 2014;39(3):198–206.

[174] Härtl R. Andreas K. *Minimally Invasive Spine Surgery—Techniques, Evidence, and Controversies.* 2012 ed. Switzerland, Davos Platz: Thieme; 2012. p. 294.

[175] Härtl R. Andreas K. *Minimally Invasive Spine Surgery—Techniques, Evidence, and Controversies.* 2012 ed. Switzerland, Davos Platz: Thieme; 2012. p. 295.

[176] Härtl R. Andreas K. *Minimally Invasive Spine Surgery—Techniques, Evidence, and Controversies.* 2012 ed. Switzerland, Davos Platz: Thieme; 2012. p. 307.

In: Intervertebral Disc Degeneration
Editors: A. L. Ho and A. M. Desai

ISBN: 978-1-63485-829-8

Chapter 9

LUMBAR DEGENERATIVE SPONDYLOLISTHESIS

Sam Cartmell, B. A., Eric S. Sussman, MD and John K. Ratliff*[*]*, MD
Stanford University School of Medicine,
Department of Neurological Surgery,
Stanford University School of Medicine, Stanford, California, US

ABSTRACT

Lumbar Degenerative Spondylolisthesis (LDS) is a common condition affecting the lumbar spine characterized by chronic arthritis and bony remodeling of the facet joints. Epidemiologic studies have revealed that LDS is a relatively common condition among older patients, and may be asymptomatic in many affected individuals. While conservative treatment measures are often utilized initially, the mainstay of management for persistently symptomatic LDS is surgical decompression. Despite a number of recent well-designed randomized clinical trials, there remains no consensus regarding the optimal method of surgical treatment, including whether or not lumbar spinal fusion provides added clinical benefit beyond decompression alone. This chapter reviews the epidemiology and clinical presentation of LDS, as well as the

---

[*] Corresponding Author address Correspondence to: John K. Ratliff (jratliff@stanford.edu), Department of Neurosurgery. Stanford University School of Medicine. 300 Pasteur Drive, R281. Stanford, CA 94303-5327.

existing evidence for the range of surgical treatments that have been utilized in patients suffering from this condition.

Keywords: lumbar disc degeneration, decompression, fusion, spondylolisthesis

Introduction

Spondylolisthesis (Greek *spondylos* "vertebrae" + *oliothesis* "dislocation, slipping") is defined as the anterior translation of one vertebral body relative to the next caudad vertebrae. Spondylolisthesis has numerous etiologies, and most commonly affects the lumbar spine. Since the first description of this clinical syndrome in the late 18th century, several classification systems have been proposed. The most widely used schema is the Wiltse Classification system, which identifies five forms of spondylolisthesis based on the location and character of the defect (Table 1). Type 1, or *dysplastic* spondylolisthesis, is due to congenital abnormalities of the superior sacral and/or inferior L5 facet. Type II, or *isthmic* spondylolisthesisis is due to a defect in the pars interarticularis, and is further divided into three subtypes: IIa due to a stress fracture of the pars, IIb due to elongation of the pars, and IIc due to acute or traumatic fracture of the pars. Type III, or *degenerative* spondylolisthesis, is due to intersegmental instability at the location of the facet joints secondary to chronic arthritis and bony remodeling. Type IV, or *traumatic* spondylolisthesis, is due to fractures of elements of the neural arch aside from the pars. Finally, Type V, or *pathological* spondylolisthesis, is due to generalized or localized destruction of the posterior elements, as may occur in the setting of underlying malignancy, infection or another secondary process (Wiltse, Newman, and Macnab 1976). Another important schema is the Meyerding Classification system, which assigns a grade (I–IV) based on the extent of anterior migration of the cephalad vertebral body on the caudad vertebral body (Meyerding 1933) (Table 2). This chapter will focus on Wiltse Type III spondylolisthesis, or lumbar degenerative spondylolisthesis (LDS).

Epidemiology and Risk Factors

Given the underlying degenerative etiology of this disease, LDS typically occurs in older patients. It rarely occurs before age 40, and the prevalence increases in a stepwise fashion from the 5th to the 7th decade of life. There is a distinct female gender predominance, with some sources citing a six-fold increased incidence in females. In addition, black individuals are affected as much as three times as frequently as Caucasians (ROSENBERG 1976; Jacobsen et al. 2007; Kalichman, Kim, et al. 2009).

The majority of available epidemiologic data regarding LDS comes from two large longitudinal regional health studies. A cross-sectional analysis of a subgroup of patients from the Framingham Heart Study investigated the relationship between lower back pain and LDS. Among 188 patients aged 40-80 who underwent CT imaging to assess for aortic calcification, 13.6% had radiographic evidence of LDS on CT imaging, with a 1:3 male-to-female ratio. The vast majority of these patients were classified as Meyerding Grade I (0-25%) (Kalichman, Kim, et al. 2009). In a cohort of patients from the Copenhagen Osteoarthritis Study, approximately 2.7% of males and 8.4% of females demonstrated radiographic evidence of LDS, for an overall prevalence of 6.3% (Jacobsen et al. 2007).

A variety of risk factors for LDS have been identified. Chief among these risk factors is increased age, which is consistent with the known chronic degenerative etiology of this subtype of spondylolisthesis (Herkowitz 1995). Both the Framingham and Copenhagen cohorts discussed above identified a significant association between LDS prevalence and age, with a peak prevalence in the 7th decade of life (Kalichman, Kim, et al. 2009; Jacobsen et al. 2007). Other epidemiologic studies have reaffirmed that LDS is most prevalent in geriatric patients, with an overall prevalence of roughly 29% in white women over the age of 65 (Vogt et al. 1998).

Table 1. Wiltse Classification

WILTSE CLASSIFICATION	
Type	Nature of Defect
Dysplastic (I)	Congenital abnormality of Sacrum/arch of L5
Isthmic (II)	Lesion of Pars Interarticularis
Degenerative (III)	Long-standing intersegmental instability
Traumatic (IV)	Fractures in areas other than pars
Pathological (V)	Generalized or localized bone disease

Table 2. Meyerding Classification. Slippage refers to [Extent of migration of rostral body] / [A/P length of caudal vertebral body] * 100. Although Grade V was not part of Meyerding's original classification, providers may refer to it when using this system

MEYERDING CLASSIFICATION	
Grade	Slippage
I	<25%
II	26-50%
III	51-75%
IV	76-100%
V	>100% (Spondyloptosis)

As mentioned previously, it is well-established that women are at an increased risk for LDS. Estimates vary, but have placed the overall male-to-female ratio in the range of 1:3 – 1:6 (Jacobsen et al. 2007; Kalichman, Kim, et al. 2009; Rosenberg 1975). It has been speculated that this gender difference may be due to hormonal effects on the laxity of the joint. Indeed, LDS is more common among patients who have undergone oophorectomy (Imada, Matsui, and Tsuji 1995); however, the data concerning the effect of parity on LDS are equivocal (Jacobsen et al. 2007; Sanderson and Fraser 1996). Interestingly, the gender disparity in LDS appears to be dependent on the spinal level, such that women are significantly more likely to have slips of L3 and L4 vertebral bodies, but not of L5 (Jacobsen et al. 2007).

With regard to the racial differences mentioned previously, an early study of 200 patients and 20 cadavers noted the prevalence of LDS among black patients was roughly three times that of white patients (Rosenberg 1975). Whether other ethnicities are also at higher risk of LDS is not yet known, but a recent study examining variation in lumbar facet orientation among several Asian ethnic groups found no association with ethnicity (Williams et al. 2016). Numerous anatomic and biomechanical risk factors have also been identified, including decreased disc height, increased lumbar index, hyperlordotic sagittal balance, sagittally-oriented facet joints, and ligamentous laxity (Bird et al. 1980; Grobler et al. 1993; BODEN et al. 1996; Love, Fagan, and Fraser 1999; I.-R. Chen and Wei 2009; Fujiwara et al. 2001; Dai 2001; Kalichman, Suri, et al. 2009; Devine, Schenk-Kisser, and Skelly 2012; Jacobsen et al. 2007). A wide range of other variables, including physical activity, occupation, BMI, and smoking have been examined in relation to LDS, but evidence supporting the role of these factors is equivocal or absent. While some studies have reported increased prevalence of LDS among those with higher levels of physical activity (Denard et al. 2010; Mariconda et al. 2007) and professional seniority among taxi drivers (J.-C. Chen et al. 2004), others have found no association with physical activity or occupation (Jacobsen et al. 2007). BMI and smoking have been consistently reported to be unrelated to LDS incidence (Devine, Schenk-Kisser, and Skelly 2012), with the exception of a single study, which noted a correlation between BMI and LDS incidence *only among women* (Jacobsen et al. 2007).

Clinical Presentation and Natural History

There is significant variation in the predominant clinical features and the severity of symptoms among patients with LDS. Patients may be asymptomatic despite radiographic spondylolisthesis, whereas other patients may present with significant neurogenic claudication, characterized by leg pain, weakness and/or paresthesias associated with back extension and ambulation (Porter 1996; Katz and Harris 2009). Isolated back *pain* is a less common manifestation of LDS (Kalichman, Kim, et al. 2009).

Observation of patients who elected for conservative rather than operative management offers insight into the natural history of LDS. In one such cohort of 145 patients followed for a minimum of 10 years, Matsunaga et al. noted radiographic progression (≥5% increase in degree of slip) in roughly a third of patients. A relationship between radiographic progression and changes in clinical symptoms was not present, but initial clinical presentation may offer insight into subsequent disease course. That is, 76% of those without neurologic symptoms on initial presentation remained symptom-free on follow-up, whereas 83% of patients with neurogenic claudication or vesicoureteral dysfunction experienced further decline in their symptoms in the absence of surgical intervention (Matsunaga, Ijiri, and Hayashi 2000). An earlier report from a similar cohort of 40 patients followed for a minimum of 5 years indicated that severity of radiographic disease on initial presentation did not predict subsequent progression (Matsunaga et al. 1990). Instead, factors deemed important in progression related to the presence of mechanical stress and stability of the intervertebral joints. Among the earlier cohort, repetitive occupation-related anterior flexion of the spine was present in 75% of those that progressed as opposed to 10% of those that did not. In addition to mechanical factors, general joint laxity was observed in 65% of all patients, and no progression of disease was noted in patients who showed evidence of spur formation, subcartilaginous sclerosis, increased intervertebral disk narrowing, or ossification of the ligaments (Matsunaga et al. 1990). Longer-term follow up similarly revealed that no patients with significant narrowing of the intervertebral disk demonstrated radiographic progression of disease, whereas 96% of those *without* disc-space narrowing *did* progress (Matsunaga, Ijiri, and Hayashi 2000). This suggests that while disk degeneration may be an important step in the initial pathogenesis of LDS, subsequent degeneration and narrowing may be a mechanism of natural re-stabilization. Re-stabilization may also help to resolve symptoms, as the degree of intervertebral disk narrowing correlated with a decrease in the severity of lower back pain (Matsunaga, Ijiri, and Hayashi 2000).

Pathophysiology and Biomechanics

LDS results from the degeneration of the facet joints without an associated defect or disruption in the neural arch (Watters et al. 2009). As described previously, a variety of anatomic and morphologic factors have been implicated in LDS, including decreased disc height, increased lumbar index, hyperlordotic sagittal balance, sagittally-oriented facet joints, and ligamentous laxity. The diagnosis of LDS is typically made radiographically when a vertebral body is seen to have migrated greater than or equal to 5% anterior to the vertebral body below (Denard et al. 2010). Importantly, the extent of migration rarely exceeds 25-30% in LDS (Herkowitz 1995). In contrast to isthmic (Type II) spondylolisthesis, which typically affects the L5-S1 interspace, LDS occurs at the L4-5 interspace in the majority of patients (Kalichman, Suri, et al. 2009).

Patients with LDS typically have chronic and often diffuse degenerative spine disease – including intervertebral disc bulging, ligamentum flavum and facet joint hypertrophy and prominent osteophyte complexes – which results in a baseline narrowing of the spinal canal (Figure 1). Spondylolisthesis further decreases the cross-sectional area of the canal, and also compromises the neural foramina, where spinal nerves traverse to exit the spinal canal (Katz and Harris 2009). Biomechanically, lumbar extension as seen with standing upright and ambulation results in a decrease in the cross-sectional, mid-sagittal and sub-articular diameters of the canal, as well as neuro-foraminal narrowing. This narrowing may lead to compression of peri-medullary venous complexes, which in turn causes venous engorgement and ischemia (OLMARKER, RYDEVIK, and HOLM 1989; OLMARKER et al. 1989; OLMARKER et al.

1991; Porter 1996). This is the likely pathophysiologic mechanism underlying the typical neurogenic claudication experienced by LDS patients, as described above.

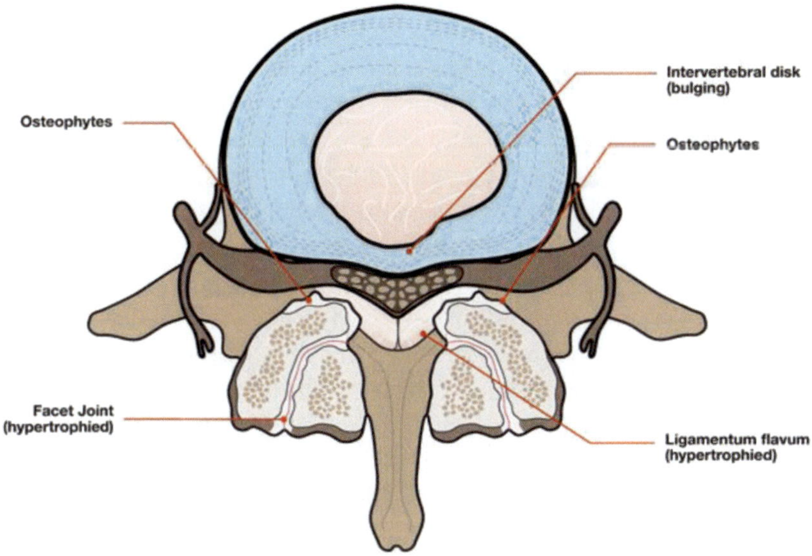

Figure 1. Various Types of Disc Degeneration.

Treatments

Treatment options for patients with LDS span the gamut, from conservative non-operative therapy to multi-level decompression and instrumented fusion operations. With the exception of the Spine Patient Outcomes Research Trial (SPORT), the literature is largely lacking in well-designed randomized controlled trials of LDS treatment. Thus, the literature reviewed here is predominantly Class II and III.

Non-Operative

Non-operative therapy for LDS consists of activity modification, anti-inflammatory medication, physical therapy, or corticosteroid injections. It is well accepted that these conservative interventions should be offered to most patients as an initial treatment; however, there are no clear guidelines that specify the precise regimen or duration of conservative management.

In the absence of a well-validated program, a reasonable approach to non-operative management includes patient education on ergonomic lifting technique and lifestyle modification to minimize inappropriate or excessive mechanical stress on the lumbar spine. Physical therapy is also an essential component of non-operative management and should focus on stabilization of the trunk and lumbar spine. In particular, flexion-based exercises, as well as those targeting deep abdominal muscles, are preferred over extension-based exercises (Gramse, Sinaki, and Ilstrup 1980; Sinaki et al. 1989; O'Sullivan et al. 1997). Sparse evidence exists to support the benefit of lumbar orthotics in LDS patients, however this may be attempted in conjunction with other conservative measures described above (Spratt et al. 1993). Symptomatic relief and pain control may be achieved with use of NSAIDs or epidural corticosteroid injections; however, no evidence exists to suggest these measures address the underlying cause or reverse the course of the disease (van Tulder et al. 2000; Cuckler et al. 1985; Kraiwattanapong et al. 2014). These measures may be most appropriate in patients who present without neurologic signs or symptoms, as the majority of these patients will not experience disease progression.

Operative

In the case of debilitating or persistent symptoms despite the above mentioned conservative measures, surgical intervention should be strongly considered (Kovacs, Urrútia, and Alarcón 2011). In fact, while operative treatment has not been found to be uniformly superior to non-operative treatment (Garet et al. 2013), the SPORT Trial did report substantially improved outcomes with regard to both pain and function at 2- and 4-year follow-up in the surgical arm (Weinstein et al. 2009; Weinstein et al. 2007). Unfortunately, the methodology of the SPORT Trial did not standardize the surgical arm of the study, and thus did not provide Class I evidence regarding the optimal surgical intervention for LDS patients. The spectrum of surgical options, and the available evidence for each, will be discussed in the following sections.

Indications for surgical treatment are not clearly defined, but a general consensus is that surgery is appropriate in patients who continue to experience debilitating symptoms after 3-4 months of non-operative treatment (Steiger et al. 2014). Patients with predominantly leg pain secondary to LDS-associated stenosis may experience better symptomatic relief from surgery as compared with those patients presenting with predominantly back pain (Pearson et al. 2011). As with all surgical procedures, the indications for surgery must be considered in the context of operative risk, which was estimated to be 9.2% in one relatively recent series of 10,242 patients with either Type II or Type III spondylolisthesis. Importantly, the rate of surgical complications in this study – which included durotomy, wound infection, hardware infection or failure, neurological sequalae, and mortality - was noted to increase with increasing Meyerding grade (Charles A Sansur et al. 2010).

Surgical Decompression

At the time of this publication, the cornerstone of operative management for LDS is surgical decompression, either with or without fusion. Laminectomy is the most commonly performed decompressive procedure in these patients, and allows for decompression of the central canal, lateral recesses and neural foramina (Figure 2). However, fenestrated procedures, including laminotomy and foraminotomy, may be considered to preserve the integrity of the posterior elements and thereby minimize the stress on adjacent levels (Eismont, Norton, and Hirsch 2014). Several studies, including a meta-analysis of 11 papers, have demonstrated satisfactory outcomes in roughly 70% of patients treated with decompression without fusion (Mardjetko, Connolly, and Shott 1994; Epstein 1998; Kristof et al. 2002). Despite this, the general bias in spinal surgery has been one of increasing complexity of operative intervention and increased utilization of surgical fusion (Deyo et al. 2010), and the operative management of LDS patients has not been immune to this trend. Nonetheless, it is important to note that decompression without fusion is a valid surgical option in LDS patients, particularly in those with a "stable" slip and minimal translation and/or angulation, as well as in elderly patients in whom the increased morbidity and mortality of fusion procedures cannot be justified (Epstein 1998; Rudolf A Kristof et al. 2009; Joaquim et al. 2015).

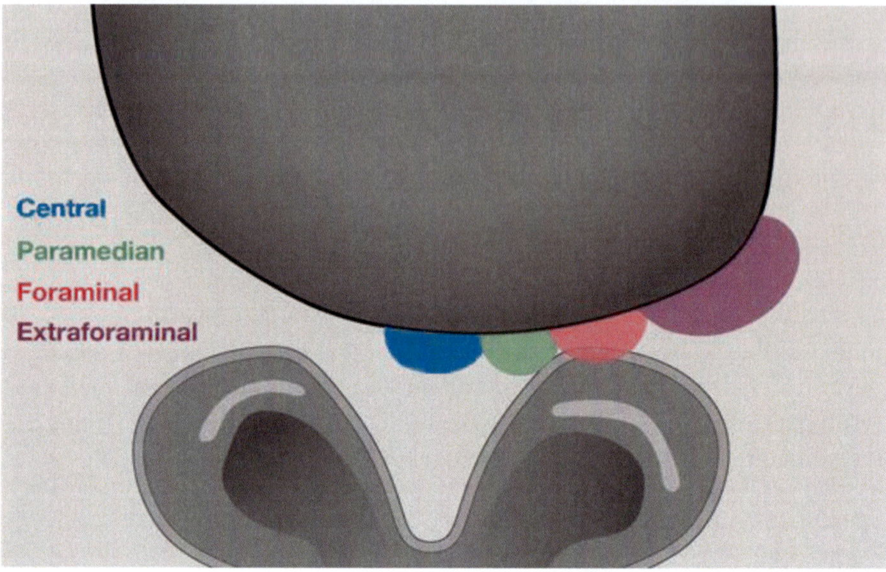

Figure 2. Relative Locations of Disc Herniation.

Fusion

The role of fusion in LDS treatment remains controversial. In theory, fusion may prevent progression of the inherent instability associated with spondylolisthesis and subsequent decompression (Resnick et al. 2014). In one of the first studies to tackle the question of fusion and decompression versus decompression alone, Herkowitz and Kurz enrolled 50 patients in a prospective, randomized trial and found the addition of fusion led to a significant improvement clinical outcomes and reduction in pain (Herkowitz and Kurz 1991). A more recent meta-analysis examined the role of fusion and similarly found superior clinical outcomes in patients who underwent fusion (Martin et al. 2007). Although instrumented fusion has not been shown to further improve clinical outcomes, the use of instrumentation does lead to a more robust and durable fusion, making this the standard of care when a fusion is desired (Fischgrund et al. 1997; Gibson and Waddell 2005; Kimura et al. 2001; Eismont, Norton, and Hirsch 2014).

Two recent randomized controlled trials published in the New England Journal of Medicine provide conflicting Class I evidence regarding the benefit of lumbar spinal fusion in patients with LDS (Försth et al. 2016; Ghogawala et al. 2016). In both studies, patients aged 50-80 with degenerative spondylolisthesis and symptomatic lumbar spinal stenosis were randomized to either decompressive laminectomy alone, or laminectomy with fusion. The Swedish Spinal Stenosis Study (Försth et al. 2016) included both spinal stenosis patients with LDS and those without LDS, however the stratification of these two subgroups allowed for the selective analysis of the LDS cohort. In the Ghogawala et al. study, laminectomy plus fusion was associated with a statistically significant improvement in overall physical health-related quality of life as compared with laminectomy alone, and this difference remained significant at four-year follow-up. In contrast, the Swedish Study did not identify a difference between the two groups with regard to patient-reported outcome measures or 6-minute walk test at two-year follow-up. Importantly, the fusion technique was not specified or standardized in the Swedish Study, but was instead left to the discretion of the surgeon. In contrast, all patients randomized to the fusion arm in the Ghogawala Study underwent posterolateral instrumented fusion. In both studies, the fusion group was associated with longer operating times and increased intra-operative blood loss.

As with most aspects of surgical management of LDS, there is no consensus regarding the optimal technique of surgical fusion in this patient population. A stratified subgroup analysis of the SPORT data found no significant difference in clinical outcome between those patients treated by conventional posterolateral fusion versus those who underwent anterior and posterior (360°) fusion operations (Abdu et al. 2009). Interbody fusions – including anterior lumbar interbody fusion (ALIF), posterior lumbar interbody fusion (PLIF), and transforaminal lumbar interbody fusion (TLIF) – have been utilized in LDS patients (Figure 3). According to one study, 76% of LDS patients treated with ALIF had a positive outcome at 10 years (Takahashi et al. 1990). A separate study showed that ALIF compared favorably with posterior decompression (Satomi et al. 1992). PLIF and TLIF have similarly been shown to be effective treatments of LDS (Yan et al. 2008), and have the additional benefit of avoiding morbidity associated with the anterior approach. However, a notable complication of the interbody fusion technique is the development of adjacent segment disease (ASD), which can require surgical revision. Of note, some surgeons advocate for a reduction of the spondylolisthesis at the time of decompression and fusion, however the evidence for this technique is inconclusive (Watters et al. 2009).

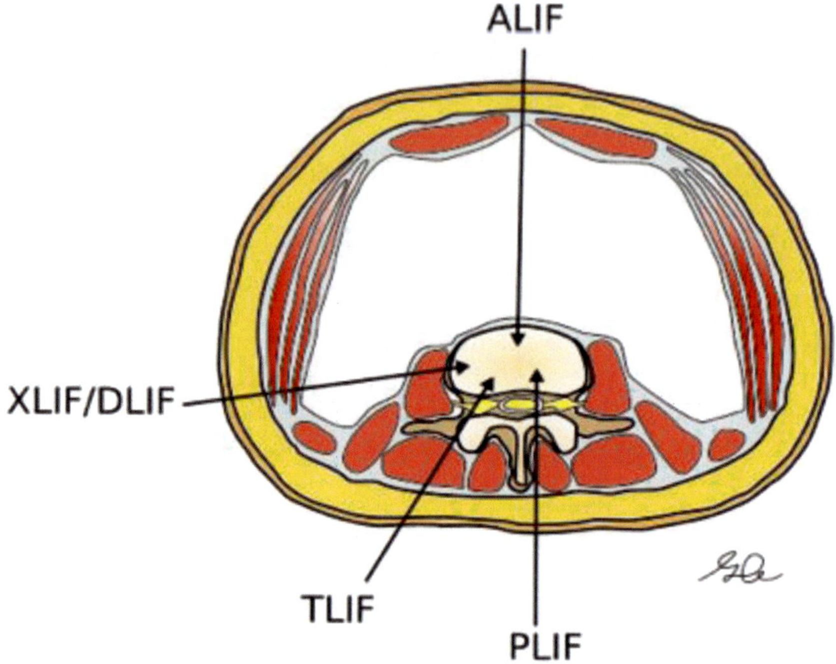

Figure 3. Interbody Fusion Approaches.

Alternative Surgical Approaches

Classic operative management of LDS consists of the above-described procedures, but other techniques have been attempted experimentally in the setting of LDS. Minimally invasive surgery (MIS) in the treatment of LDS aims to achieve similar clinical outcomes while avoiding complications related to extensive muscular and ligamentous dissection. The feasibility of a percutaneous microendoscopic approach (Figure 4) was demonstrated in the early 2000's in cadaver studies, and some of the first human MIS surgeries for LDS were described shortly thereafter (S. Palmer, Turner, and Palmer 2002; Guiot, Khoo, and Fessler 2002). Due to the relatively recent development of these techniques, long-term follow up studies are still needed to determine efficacy relative to traditional open approaches. Nonetheless, a handful studies indicate a minimally invasive approach to decompression alone achieves positive clinical outcomes in the treatment of LDS (Jang et al. 2012; Kelleher et al. 2010; Mori et al. 2016). Moreover, because MIS minimizes the risk of direct destabilization, it has the theoretical advantage of preserving the re-stabilization process observed in the natural history of LDS, and may therefore reduce the need for fusion in some patients (Mori et al. 2016).

That being said, minimally invasive approaches may also be employed for performance of fusion procedures, as in the case of an MIS-TLIFrr. Kim et al. examined MIS-TLIF in 44 patients, 19 of whom had LDS. At 5-year follow up, statistically significant improvements in back and leg pain were observed (Kim, Jung, and Lee 2012). Two other studies compared minimally invasive TLIF to open TLIF and reported shorter hospital stays and decreased blood loss with similar long-term outcomes with the MIS approach (Jang et al. 2012; Wong et al. 2014).

In light of the well-described drawbacks of fusion procedures, there has been a concerted effort to develop novel surgical techniques that achieve similar stabilization without causing the adjacent segment disease or motion limitation characteristic of spinal fusion. Disk arthroplasty, or total disk replacement (TDR) is intended primarily for use in patients with discogenic back pain, and became FDA approved for this indication in the mid-2000s. It has been suggested that TDR is contraindicated in patients with LDS >3mm due to additional destabilization caused by obligatory discectomy (Berg et al. 2009). Nonetheless, a pilot study of seven subjects suggested that TDR may be an effective approach for treating the symptoms of LDS, and there is some evidence to support the role TDR for symptomatic treatment in patients with a spondylolisthesis <3mm (Hähnle et al. 2008; Berg et al. 2009).

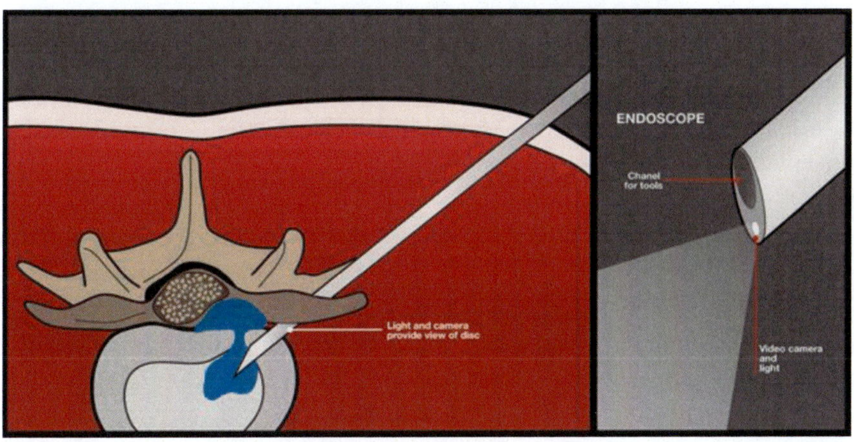

Figure 4. Percutaneous Microendoscopic Approach.

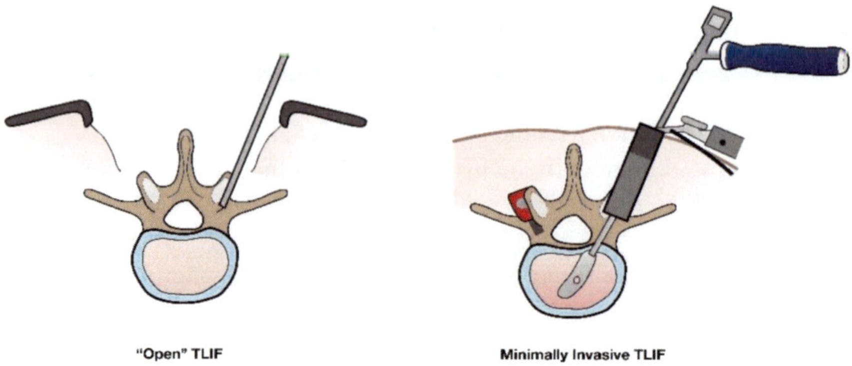

Figure 5. Comparison of "Open" TLIF to MIS-TLIF.

Conclusion

LDS is a common condition characterized by anterior migration of the lumbar vertebral body due to gradual destabilization of the intervertebral joints, occurring most often at the L4 vertebral body. LDS almost exclusively affects patients older than 40 years of age, is more common in women, and occurs with a higher incidence in black patients. The clinical presentation of LDS may be asymptomatic, but low back pain and neurogenic claudication are the most common symptoms, when present. Natural history studies have demonstrated that the majority of patients who present without neurologic symptoms will experience no further neurologic decline, whereas those presenting *with* neurologic symptoms can be expected to undergo further clinical deterioration.

Strong evidence exists to suggest that patients with persistent symptoms referable to LDS experience better clinical outcomes with surgical management, as compared with patients treated conservatively. While many surgical options exist, the cornerstone of surgical management is decompression. The addition of lumbar spinal fusion may be considered to provide further stabilization, however the existing evidence is ambiguous regarding the clinical benefit of this procedure. There is also no consensus in the literature to support a particular fusion technique in this patient population.

REFERENCES

Abdu, William A, Jon D Lurie, Kevin F Spratt, Anna N A Tosteson, Wenyan Zhao, Tor D Tosteson, Harry Herkowitz, et al. 2009. "Degenerative Spondylolisthesis: Does Fusion Method Influence Outcome? Four-Year Results of the Spine Patient Outcomes Research Trial." *Spine* 34 (21): 2351–60. doi:10.1097/BRS.0b013e3181b8a829.

Berg, Svante, Tycho Tullberg, Björn Branth, Claes Olerud, and Hans Tropp. 2009. "Total Disc Replacement Compared to Lumbar Fusion: a Randomised Controlled Trial with 2-Year Follow-Up." *European Spine Journal: Official Publication of the European Spine Society, the European Spinal Deformity Society, and the European Section of the Cervical Spine Research Society* 18 (10): 1512–19. doi:10.1007/s00586-009-1047-0.

Bird, H A, C J Eastmond, A Hudson, and V Wright. 1980. "Is Generalized Joint Laxity a Factor in Spondylolisthesis?" *Scandinavian Journal of Rheumatology* 9 (4): 203–5.

Boden, Scott D, K Daniel Riew, Ken Yamaguchi, Thomas P Branch, Dieter Schellinger, and Sam W Wiesel. 1996. "Orientation of the Lumbar Facet Joints: Association with Degenerative Disc Disease*." *J Bone Joint Surg Am* 78 (3). The American Orthopedic Association: 403–11. doi:10.1097/00007632-198105000-00006.

Charles A Sansur, Davis L Reames, Justin S Smith, D Kojo Hamilton, Sigurd H Berven, Paul A Broadstone, Theodore J Choma, et al. 2010. "Morbidity and Mortality in the Surgical Treatment of 10,242 Adults with Spondylolisthesis." *Dx.Doi.org*, November. American Association of Neurological Surgeons. doi:10.3171/2010.5.SPINE09529.

Chen, I-Ru, and Ta-Sen Wei. 2009. "Disc Height and Lumbar Index as Independent Predictors of Degenerative Spondylolisthesis in Middle-Aged Women with Low Back Pain." *Spine* 34 (13): 1402–9. doi:10.1097/BRS.0b013e31817b8fbd.

Chen, J-C, W P Chan, J N Katz, W P Chang, and D C Christiani. 2004. "Occupational and Personal Factors Associated with Acquired Lumbar Spondylolisthesis of Urban Taxi Drivers." *Occupational and Environmental Medicine* 61 (12): 992–98. doi:10.1136/oem.2003.011775.

Cuckler, J M, P A Bernini, S W Wiesel, R E Booth, R H Rothman, and G T Pickens. 1985. "The Use of Epidural Steroids in the Treatment of Lumbar Radicular Pain. a Prospective, Randomized, Double-Blind Study." *J Bone Joint Surg Am* 67 (1): 63–66.

Dai, L Y. 2001. "Orientation and Tropism of Lumbar Facet Joints in Degenerative Spondylolisthesis." *International Orthopaedics* 25 (1). Springer: 40–42. doi:10.1007/s002640000201.

Denard, Patrick J, Kathleen F Holton, Jessica Miller, Howard A Fink, Deborah M Kado, Jung U Yoo, Lynn M Marshall, Osteoporotic Fractures in Men (MrOS) Study Group. 2010. "Lumbar Spondylolisthesis Among Elderly Men: Prevalence, Correlates, and Progression." *Spine* 35 (10): 1072–78. doi:10.1097/BRS.0b013e3181bd9e19.

Devine, John G, Jeannette M Schenk-Kisser, and Andrea C Skelly. 2012. "Risk Factors for Degenerative Spondylolisthesis: a Systematic Review." *Evidence-Based Spine-Care Journal* 3 (2): 25–34. doi:10.1055/s-0031-1298615.

Deyo, Richard A, Sohail K Mirza, Brook I Martin, William Kreuter, David C Goodman, and Jeffrey G Jarvik. 2010. "Trends, Major Medical Complications, and Charges Associated with Surgery for Lumbar Spinal Stenosis in Older Adults." *Jama* 303 (13). American Medical Association: 1259–65. doi:10.1001/jama.2010.338.

Eismont, Frank J, Robert P Norton, and Brandon P Hirsch. 2014. "Surgical Management of Lumbar Degenerative Spondylolisthesis." *The Journal of the American Academy of Orthopaedic Surgeons* 22 (4): 203–13. doi:10.5435/JAAOS-22-04-203.

Epstein, N E. 1998. "Decompression in the Surgical Management of Degenerative Spondylolisthesis: Advantages of a Conservative Approach in 290 Patients." *Journal of Spinal Disorders* 11 (2): 116–22–discussion123.

Fischgrund, J S, M Mackay, H N Herkowitz, R Brower, D M Montgomery, and L T Kurz. 1997. "1997 Volvo Award Winner in Clinical Studies. Degenerative Lumbar Spondylolisthesis with Spinal Stenosis: a Prospective, Randomized Study Comparing Decompressive Laminectomy and Arthrodesis with and Without Spinal Instrumentation." *Spine* 22 (24): 2807–12.

Försth, Peter, Gylfi Ólafsson, Thomas Carlsson, Anders Frost, Fredrik Borgström, Peter Fritzell, Patrik Öhagen, Karl Michaëlsson, and Bengt Sandén. 2016. "A Randomized, Controlled Trial of Fusion Surgery for Lumbar Spinal Stenosis." *The New England Journal of Medicine* 374 (15): 1413–23. doi:10.1056/NEJMoa1513721.

Fujiwara, A, K Tamai, H S An, T H Lim, H Yoshida, A Kurihashi, and K Saotome. 2001. "Orientation and Osteoarthritis of the Lumbar Facet Joint." *Clinical Orthopaedics and Related Research*, no. 385 (April): 88–94.

Garet, Matthew, Michael P Reiman, Jessie Mathers, and Jonathan Sylvain. 2013. "Nonoperative Treatment in Lumbar Spondylolysis and Spondylolisthesis: a Systematic Review.." *Sports Health* 5 (3): 225–32. doi:10.1177/1941738113480936.

Ghogawala, Zoher, James Dziura, William E Butler, Feng Dai, Norma Terrin, Subu N Magge, Jean-Valery C E Coumans, et al. 2016. "Laminectomy Plus Fusion Versus Laminectomy Alone for Lumbar Spondylolisthesis." *The New England Journal of Medicine* 374 (15): 1424–34. doi:10.1056/NEJMoa1508788.

Gibson, J N Alastair, and Gordon Waddell. 2005. "Surgery for Degenerative Lumbar Spondylosis: Updated Cochrane Review." *Spine* 30 (20): 2312–20.

Gramse, R R, M Sinaki, and D M Ilstrup. 1980. "Lumbar Spondylolisthesis: a Rational Approach to Conservative Treatment." *Mayo Clinic Proceedings* 55 (11): 681–86.

Grobler, Leon J, Peter A Robertson, John E Novotny, and Malcolm H Pope. 1993. "Etiology of Spondylolisthesis: Assessment of the Role Played by Lumbar Facet Joint Morphology." *Spine* 18 (1): 80.

Guiot, Bernard H, Larry T Khoo, and Richard G Fessler. 2002. "A Minimally Invasive Technique for Decompression of the Lumbar Spine." *Spine* 27 (4): 432–38.

Hähnle, Ulrich R, Karen Sliwa, Malan de Villiers, Ian R Weinberg, Barry M B E Sweet, and Geoffrey P Candy. 2008. "Is Degenerative Spondylolisthesis a Contraindication for Total Disc Replacement? Kineflex Lumbar Disc Replacement in 7 Patients with 24-Month Follow-Up." *SAS Journal* 2 (2): 92–100. doi:10.1016/SASJ-2007-0125-NT.

Herkowitz, H N. 1995. "Spine Update. Degenerative Lumbar Spondylolisthesis." *Spine* 20 (9): 1084–90.

Herkowitz, H N, and L T Kurz. 1991. "Degenerative Lumbar Spondylolisthesis with Spinal Stenosis. a Prospective Study Comparing Decompression with Decompression and Intertransverse Process Arthrodesis." *J Bone Joint Surg Am* 73 (6): 802–8.

Imada, K, H Matsui, and H Tsuji. 1995. "Oophorectomy Predisposes to Degenerative Spondylolisthesis." *Journal of Bone and Joint Surgery - British Volume* 77 (1): 126–30.

Jacobsen, Steffen, Stig Sonne-Holm, Hans Rovsing, Henrik Monrad, and Peter Gebuhr. 2007. "Degenerative Lumbar Spondylolisthesis: an Epidemiological Perspective: the Copenhagen Osteoarthritis Study." *Spine* 32 (1): 120–25. doi:10.1097/01.brs.0000250979.12398.96.

Jang, Jun-Won, Jin-Hun Park, Seung-Jae Hyun, and Seung-Chul Rhim. 2012. "Clinical Outcomes and Radiologic Changes Following Microsurgical Bilateral Decompression via a Unilateral Approach in Patients with Lumbar Canal Stenosis and Grade I Degenerative Spondylolisthesis with a Minimum 3-Year Follow-Up." *Journal of Spinal Disorders and Techniques*, October, 1. doi:10.1097/BSD.0b013e31827566a8.

Joaquim, Andrei F, Jeronimo B Milano, Enrico Ghizoni, and Alpesh A Patel. 2015. "Is There a Role for Decompression Alone for Treating Symptomatic Degenerative Lumbar Spondylolisthesis?: a Systematic Review." *Journal of Spinal Disorders and Techniques*, December, 1. doi:10.1097/BSD.0000000000000357.

Kalichman, Leonid, David H Kim, Ling Li, Ali Guermazi, Valery Berkin, and David J Hunter. 2009. "Spondylolysis and Spondylolisthesis: Prevalence and Association with Low Back Pain in the Adult Community-Based Population." *Spine* 34 (2). NIH Public Access: 199–205. doi:10.1097/BRS.0b013e31818edcfd.

Kalichman, Leonid, Pradeep Suri, Ali Guermazi, Ling Li, and David J Hunter. 2009. "Facet Orientation and Tropism: Associations with Facet Joint Osteoarthritis and Degeneratives." *Spine* 34 (16): E579–85. doi:10.1097/BRS.0b013e3181aa2acb.

Katz, Jeffrey N, and Mitchel B Harris. 2009. "Lumbar Spinal Stenosis." *Dx.Doi.org* 358 (8). Massachusetts Medical Society: 818–25. doi:10.1056/NEJMcp0708097.

Kelleher, Michael O, Marcus Timlin, Oma Persaud, and Yoga Raja Rampersaud. 2010. "Success and Failure of Minimally Invasive Decompression for Focal Lumbar Spinal Stenosis in Patients with and Without Deformity." *Spine* 35 (19): E981–87. doi:10.1097/BRS.0b013e3181c46fb4.

Kim, Jin-Sung, Byungjoo Jung, and Sang-Ho Lee. 2012. "Instrumented Minimally Invasive Spinal-Transforaminal Lumbar Interbody Fusion (MIS-TLIF); Minimum 5-Years Follow-Up with Clinical and Radiologic

Outcomes." *Journal of Spinal Disorders and Techniques*, September, 1. doi:10.1097/BSD.0b013e31827415cd.

Kimura, I, H Shingu, M Murata, and H Hashiguchi. 2001. "Lumbar Posterolateral Fusion Alone or with Transpedicular Instrumentation in L4--L5 Degenerative Spondylolisthesis." *Journal of Spinal Disorders* 14 (4): 301–10.

Kovacs, Francisco M, Gerard Urrútia, and José Domingo Alarcón. 2011. "Surgery Versus Conservative Treatment for Symptomatic Lumbar Spinal Stenosis: a Systematic Review of Randomized Controlled Trials." *Spine* 36 (20): E1335–51. doi:10.1097/BRS.0b013e31820c97b1.

Kraiwattanapong, Chaiwat, Supaporn Wechmongkolgorn, Bangon Chatriyanuyok, Patarawan Woratanarat, Umaporn Udomsubpayakul, Pongsathorn Chanplakorn, Gun Keorochana, and Wiwat Wajanavisit. 2014. "Outcomes of Fluoroscopically Guided Lumbar Transforaminal Epidural Steroid Injections in Degenerative Lumbar Spondylolisthesis Patients." *Asian Spine Journal* 8 (2): 119–28. doi:10.4184/asj.2014.8.2.119.

Kristof, Rudolf A, Ales F Aliashkevich, Michael Schuster, Bernhard Meyer, Horst Urbach, and Johannes Schramm. 2002. "Degenerative Lumbar Spondylolisthesis-Induced Radicular Compression: Nonfusion-Related Decompression in Selected Patients Without Hypermobility on Flexion-Extension Radiographs." *Journal of Neurosurgery* 97 (3 Suppl): 281–86.

Love, T W, A B Fagan, and R D Fraser. 1999. "Degenerative Spondylolisthesis." *Bone and Joint Journal* 81-B (4). Bone and Joint Journal: 670–74.

Mardjetko, S M, P J Connolly, and S Shott. 1994. "Degenerative Lumbar Spondylolisthesis. a Meta-Analysis of Literature 1970-1993." *Spine* 19 (20 Suppl): 2256S–2265S.

Mariconda, Massimo, Olimpio Galasso, Luigi Imbimbo, Giovanni Lotti, and Carlo Milano. 2007. "Relationship Between Alterations of the Lumbar Spine, Visualized with Magnetic Resonance Imaging, and Occupational Variables." *European Spine Journal: Official Publication of the European Spine Society, the European Spinal Deformity Society, and the European Section of the Cervical Spine Research Society* 16 (2): 255–66. doi:10.1007/s00586-005-0036-1.

Martin, C Ryan, Adam T Gruszczynski, Heike A Braunsfurth, Salah M Fallatah, Joseph O'Neil, and Eugene K Wai. 2007. "The Surgical Management of Degenerative Lumbar Spondylolisthesis: a Systematic Review." *Spine* 32 (16): 1791–98. doi:10.1097/BRS.0b013e3180bc219e.

Matsunaga, S, K Ijiri, and K Hayashi. 2000. "Nonsurgically Managed Patients with Degenerative Spondylolisthesis: a 10- to 18-Year Follow-Up Study." *Journal of Neurosurgery* 93 (2 Suppl): 194–98.

Matsunaga, S, T Sakou, Y Morizono, A Masuda, and A M Demirtas. 1990. "Natural History of Degenerative Spondylolisthesis. Pathogenesis and Natural Course of the Slippage." *Spine* 15 (11): 1204–10.

Meyerding, Henry W. 1933. "Diagnosis and Roentgenologic Evidence in Spondylolisthesis 1." *Radiology* 20 (2): 108–20. doi:10.1148/20.2.108.

Mori, Gen, Yasuo Mikami, Yuji Arai, Takumi Ikeda, Masateru Nagae, Hitoshi Tonomura, Ryota Takatori, Koshiro Sawada, Hiroyoshi Fujiwara, and Toshikazu Kubo. 2016. "Outcomes in Cases of Lumbar Degenerative Spondylolisthesis More Than 5 Years After Treatment with Minimally Invasive Decompression: Examination of Pre- and Postoperative Slippage, Intervertebral Disc Changes, and Clinical Results." *Journal of Neurosurgery. Spine* 24 (3): 367–74. doi:10.3171/2015.6.SPINE141298.

O'Sullivan, P B, G D Phyty, L T Twomey, and G T Allison. 1997. "Evaluation of Specific Stabilizing Exercise in the Treatment of Chronic Low Back Pain with Radiologic Diagnosis of Spondylolysis or Spondylolisthesis." *Spine* 22 (24): 2959–67.

Olmarker, Kjell, Björn Rydevik, and Sten Holm. 1989. "Edema Formation in Spinal Nerve Roots Induced by Experimental, Graded Compression: an Experimental Study on the Pig Cauda Equina with Special Reference to Differences in Effects Between Rapid and Slow Onset of Compression." *Spine* 14 (6): 569.

Olmarker, Kjell, Björn Rydevik, Sten Holm, and Ulf Bagge. 1989. "Effects of Experimental Graded Compression on Blood Flow in Spinal Nerve Roots. a Vital Microscopic Study on the Porcine Cauda Equina." *Journal of Orthopaedic Research* 7 (6). Wiley Subscription Services, Inc., A Wiley Company: 817–23. doi:10.1002/jor.1100070607.

Olmarker, Kjell, Sten Holm, Anna-Lena Rosenqvist, and Björn Rydevik. 1991. "Experimental Nerve Root Compression: a Model of Acute, Graded Compression of the Porcine Cauda Equina and an Analysis of Neural and Vascular Anatomy." *Spine* 16 (1): 61.

Palmer, Sylvain, Robert Turner, and Rosemary Palmer. 2002. "Bilateral Decompressive Surgery in Lumbar Spinal Stenosis Associated with Spondylolisthesis: Unilateral Approach and Use of a Microscope and Tubular Retractor System." *Neurosurgical Focus* 13 (1): E4.

Pearson, Adam, Emily Blood, Jon Lurie, William Abdu, Dilip Sengupta, John W Frymoyer, and James Weinstein. 2011. "Predominant Leg Pain Is Associated with Better Surgical Outcomes in Degenerative Spondylolisthesis and Spinal Stenosis: Results From the Spine Patient Outcomes Research Trial (SPORT)." *Spine* 36 (3): 219–29. doi:10.1097/BRS.0b013e3181d77c21.

Porter, Richard W. 1996. "Spinal Stenosis and Neurogenic Claudication." *Spine* 21 (17): 2046.

Resnick, Daniel K, William C Watters, Alok Sharan, Praveen V Mummaneni, Andrew T Dailey, Jeffrey C Wang, Tanvir F Choudhri, et al. 2014. "Guideline Update for the Performance of Fusion Procedures for Degenerative Disease of the Lumbar Spine. Part 9: Lumbar Fusion for Stenosis with Spondylolisthesis." *Journal of Neurosurgery. Spine* 21 (1): 54–61. doi:10.3171/2014.4.SPINE14274.

Rosenberg, N J. 1975. "Degenerative Spondylolisthesis. Predisposing Factors." *J Bone Joint Surg Am* 57 (4): 467–74.

Rosenberg, Norman J. 1976. "Degenerative Spondylolisthesis: Surgical Treatment." *Clinical Orthopaedics and Related Research* 117 (June): 112.

Rudolf A Kristof, Ales F Aliashkevich, Michael Schuster, Bernhard Meyer, Horst Urbach, Johannes Schramm. 2009. "Degenerative Lumbar Spondylolisthesis—Induced Radicular Compression: Nonfusion-Related Decompression in Selected Patients Without Hypermobility on Flexion—Extension Radiographs." *Dx.Doi.org* 97 (3). Journal of Neurosurgery Publishing Group: 281–86. doi:10.3171/spi.2002.97.3.0281.

Sanderson, P L, and R D Fraser. 1996. "The Influence of Pregnancy on the Development of Degenerative Spondylolisthesis." *Journal of Bone and Joint Surgery - British Volume* 78 (6): 951–54.

Satomi, K, K Hirabayashi, Y Toyama, and Y Fujimura. 1992. "A Clinical Study of Degenerative Spondylolisthesis. Radiographic Analysis and Choice of Treatment." *Spine* 17 (11): 1329–36.

Sinaki, M, M P Lutness, D M Ilstrup, C P Chu, and R R Gramse. 1989. "Lumbar Spondylolisthesis: Retrospective Comparison and Three-Year Follow-Up of Two Conservative Treatment Programs." *Archives of Physical Medicine and Rehabilitation* 70 (8): 594–98.

Spratt, K F, J N Weinstein, T R Lehmann, J Woody, and H Sayre. 1993. "Efficacy of Flexion and Extension Treatments Incorporating Braces for Low-Back Pain Patients with Retrodisplacement, Spondylolisthesis, or Normal Sagittal Translation." *Spine* 18 (13): 1839–49.

Steiger, F, H-J Becker, C J Standaert, F Balague, J-P Vader, F Porchet, and A F Mannion. 2014. "Surgery in Lumbar Degenerative Spondylolisthesis: Indications, Outcomes and Complications. a Systematic Review." *European Spine Journal: Official Publication of the European Spine Society, the European Spinal Deformity Society, and the European Section of the Cervical Spine Research Society* 23 (5): 945–73. doi:10.1007/s00586-013-3144-3.

Takahashi, K, H Kitahara, M Yamagata, M Murakami, K Takata, K Miyamoto, M Mimura, Y Akahashi, and H Moriya. 1990. "Long-Term Results of Anterior Interbody Fusion for Treatment of Degenerative Spondylolisthesis." *Spine* 15 (11): 1211–15.

van Tulder, M W, R J Scholten, B W Koes, and R A Deyo. 2000. "Nonsteroidal Anti-Inflammatory Drugs for Low Back Pain: a Systematic Review Within the Framework of the Cochrane Collaboration Back Review Group." *Spine* 25 (19): 2501–13.

Vogt, M T, D Rubin, R S Valentin, L Palermo, W F Donaldson, M Nevitt, and J A Cauley. 1998. "Lumbar Olisthesis and Lower Back Symptoms in Elderly White Women. the Study of Osteoporotic Fractures." *Spine* 23 (23): 2640–47.

Watters, William C, Christopher M Bono, Thomas J Gilbert, D Scott Kreiner, Daniel J Mazanec, William O Shaffer, Jamie Baisden, et al. 2009. "An Evidence-Based Clinical Guideline for the Diagnosis and Treatment of Degenerative Lumbar Spondylolisthesis." *The Spine Journal: Official Journal of the North American Spine Society*. doi:10.1016/j.spinee.2009.03.016.

Weinstein, James N, Jon D Lurie, Tor D Tosteson, Brett Hanscom, Anna N A Tosteson, Emily A Blood, Nancy J O Birkmeyer, et al. 2007. "Surgical Versus Nonsurgical Treatment for Lumbar Degenerative Spondylolisthesis." *The New England Journal of Medicine* 356 (22): 2257–70. doi:10.1056/NEJMoa070302.

Weinstein, James N, Jon D Lurie, Tor D Tosteson, Wenyan Zhao, Emily A Blood, Anna N A Tosteson, Nancy Birkmeyer, et al. 2009. "Surgical Compared with Nonoperative Treatment for Lumbar Degenerative Spondylolisthesis. Four-Year Results in the Spine Patient Outcomes Research Trial (SPORT) Randomized and Observational Cohorts." *J Bone Joint Surg Am* 91 (6): 1295–1304. doi:10.2106/JBJS.H.00913.

Williams, Richard, Jason Pui Yin Cheung, Ben Goss, Shanmuganathan Rajasekaran, Yoshiharu Kawaguchi, Shankar Acharya, Mamoru Kawakami, et al. 2016. "An International Multicenter Study Assessing the

Role of Ethnicity on Variation of Lumbar Facet Joint Orientation and the Occurrence of Degenerative Spondylolisthesis in Asia Pacific: a Study From the AOSpine Asia Pacific Research Collaboration Consortium." *Global Spine Journal* 6 (1): 35–45. doi:10.1055/s-0035-1555655.

Wiltse, L L, P H Newman, and I Macnab. 1976. "Classification of Spondylolisis and Spondylolisthesis." *Clinical Orthopaedics and Related Research*, no. 117 (June): 23–29.

Wong, Albert P, Zachary A Smith, James A Stadler, Xue Yu Hu, Jia Zhi Yan, Xin Feng Li, Ji Hyun Lee, and Larry T Khoo. 2014. "Minimally Invasive Transforaminal Lumbar Interbody Fusion (MI-TLIF): Surgical Technique, Long-Term 4-Year Prospective Outcomes, and Complications Compared with an Open TLIF Cohort." *Neurosurgery Clinics of North America* 25 (2): 279–304. doi:10.1016/j.nec.2013.12.007.

Yan, Deng-lu, Fu-xing Pei, Jian Li, and Cheng-long Soo. 2008. "Comparative Study of PILF and TLIF Treatment in Adult Degenerative Spondylolisthesis." *European Spine Journal: Official Publication of the European Spine Society, the European Spinal Deformity Society, and the European Section of the Cervical Spine Research Society* 17 (10): 1311–16. doi:10.1007/s00586-008-0739-1.

In: Intervertebral Disc Degeneration
Editors: A. L. Ho and A. M. Desai
ISBN: 978-1-63485-829-8

Chapter 10

EMERGING TREATMENTS FOR INTERVERTEBRAL DISC DISEASE

Gregory D. Arnone*[1]*, MD, Shivani Rangwala*[2]*, BS and Ankit I. Mehta*[1,*]*, MD

[1]Department of Neurosurgery University of Illinois at Chicago, Chicago, IL, US

[2]University of Illinois at Chicago, Chicago, IL, US

ABSTRACT

Degenerative disc disease (DDD) is a significant component of spine disorders and low back pain, and the prevalence of disc disease is increasing with an aging population. While current treatment modalities, ranging from conservative approaches to surgical interventions, are continually evolving, new therapies for intervertebral disc disease are also in development. Increased research on the cellular mechanisms underlying DDD have led to novel cell-based treatments which aim to delay rates of degeneration [1, 3]. Most of these cellular therapies remain in the research phase. Recent innovations in engineering have also pioneered several types of surgical constructs that improve the durability of treatment, while minimizing device-associated complications. Several examples include hybrid materials for intervertebral cages, zero-profile implants, expandable cages, sagittal correction implants, and disc

[*] Correspondence to: Ankit I. Mehta (ankitm@uic.edu), Department of Neurosurgery, University of Illinois at Chicago, 912 S. Wood St., M/C 799, 60612, Chicago, IL, US.

arthroplasty. Finally, surgical techniques have been refined and adapted to allow less invasive modalities such as endoscopic and percutaneous techniques to reach adequate treatment effect with less risk of adverse event and further degeneration of the incident and adjacent spinal segments. This chapter highlights several emerging non-surgical and surgical treatments for intervertebral disc disease.

Keywords: intervertebral disc disease, degenerative disc disease, treatment, emerging therapy, surgical treatment, nonsurgical treatment

INTRODUCTION

In 2005, the estimate health care expenditure for spine pathology was $86 billion, which amounts to 9% of total health care spending [1]. The annual prevalence of chronic low back pain among the adult population ranges from 15% to 45%, with a point prevalence of 30% [2]. Degenerative disc disease (DDD) is a significant component of spine disorders and low back pain, and the prevalence of disc herniation or secondary spinal stenosis increases with an aging population. Traditional treatment modalities range from conservative approaches to surgical intervention. Still, more work needs to be done to improve the quality of life for patients with DDD, as well as to address the underlying pathologial processes leading to intervertebral disc degeneration. To that effect, increased research on the cellular mechanisms underlying degenerative intervertebral disc disease have led to novel cell-based treatments which aim to delay rates of degeneration [1, 3]. Although most of these cellular therapies remain in the research phase, recent innovations in engineering have also pioneered new treatment modalities which improve surgical constructs, improve the durability of treatment, and minimize complications. Finally, surgical techniques have been refined and adapted to allow less invasive modalities to reach the same treatment effect with less risk of adverse event and further degeneration of the incident or adjacent spinal segments. This chapter highlights several emerging non surgical and surgical treatments for intervertebral disc disease.

EMERGING NONSURGICAL TREATMENT

The Concept of Directional Exercises

Low back pain is a common chief complaint seen in the physician's office, for which conservative management is the first line treatment. Recent studies show 64% of patients who present with low back pain initially still report pain symptoms at 12 months [4]. An obvious reason for poor treatment efficacy is prescribing general physical therapy for a multifactorial pathology. The optimal conservative treatment is based on the etiology of the back pain, and can take several attempts before clinical improvement is achieved. The McKenzie method, also known as Mechanical Diagnosis and Therapy (MDT), offers clinicians an evidence based assessment tool to evaluate and treat low back pain with specific directional exercises [5].

First described in 1981, the McKenzie method is a clinical tool that objectively assesses back pain to provide more directed conservative therapy. The assessment tool requires the physician to conduct a thorough history and physical exam with the goal of categorizing the level of physical impairment to three treatment groups: derangement, dysfunction and postural syndromes [5]. Patients are placed into one of these groups, and then further subclassifed based on their response to active, repetitive movements, which either increase or decrease their pain. Clare et al. observed that therapists specifically trained in the McKenzie method are able to reliably classify patients with cervical and lumbar pain into sub groups [6]. Specific movements are isolated to determine "directional preference"—position in which the pain is decreased, centralized or resolved [5]. Therapy is then guided based on the "directional preference" of patients. A systematic review of 6 studies determined the efficacy of MDT therapy for patients experiencing low back pain and who identified a specific directional preference, mainly at short term and intermediate follow up intervals [4]. Unfortunately, there is mixed evidence on MDT treatment efficacy compared to other physical therapy treatment modalities and this warrants further study [4, 5]. Still, this methodology holds promise in improving back pain symptoms through specific goal directed physical therapy.

Biological Therapies- Disc Repair and Regeneration

The normal intervertebral disc consists of an outer fibrous ring (annulus fibrosus-AF) surrounding an inner, gelatinous core (nucleus pulposus-NP), and a cartilaginous cap covering the superior and inferior surfaces (Figure 1) [1]. The AF has greater collagen content arranged concentrically at varying degrees, creating a strong structural support. The inner nucleus pulposus is a hydrophilic core composed of a greater proteoglycan (primarily aggrecan) matrix with loosely arranged collagen fibrils. Degenerative disc disease is a pathological, accelerated process of the normal age related changes to the intervertebral disc. One understanding of disc degeneration is based on gradual loss of water content from the central core causing it to lose its biomechanical properties and be more susceptible to mechanical stress. At the cellular level, there is accelerated cellular senescence compounded with increased local inflammatory response that compromises extracellular matrix integrity [3]. Understanding the biomechanical properties and cellular composition of the normal disc will allow for development of treatment targets for degenerative disc disease. Biological therapies are focused on the repair and regeneration of disc components (Figure 2). Cell based therapies aim to replace the chondrocyte- like cells of the NP and fibroblast-like cells of the AF [8].

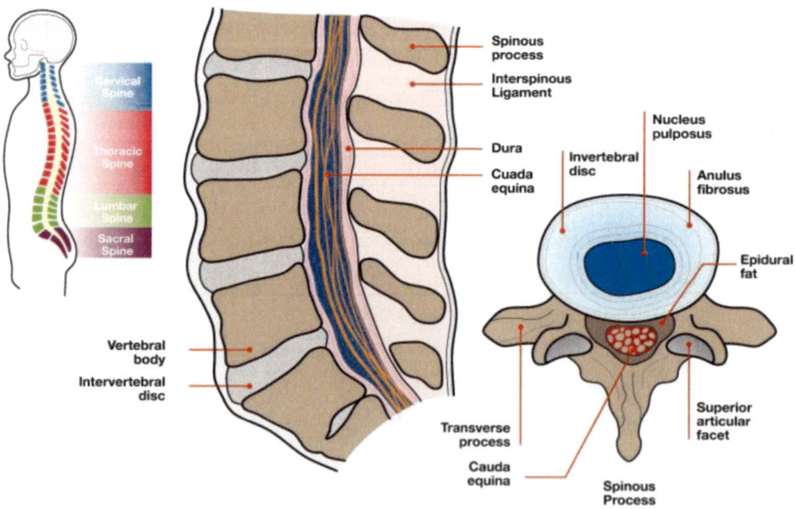

Figure 1. Intervertebral Disc Anatomy.

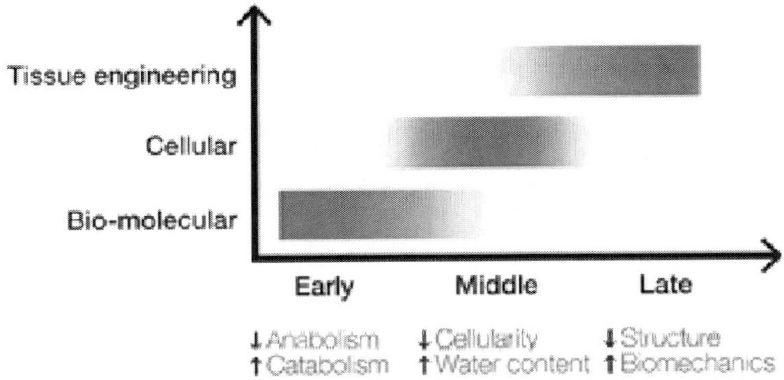

Figure 2. Biologic- and Cell-Based Therapies for IVD.

Disc innervation is restricted to the periphery and there no specific vascular supply exists for each disc—thus, each disc relies on diffusion of nutrients and oxygen from surrounding vertebrae. For this reason, the chemical milieu of each disc is low in oxygen and glucose, and fairly acidic - characteristics which present potential challenges to biological therapies [1, 7]. Risk factors for degeneration of the intervertebral disc are multifactorial, and there is increasing evidence on the genetic basis of disc degeneration from several twin studies [1]. Genetic analysis of specific receptors and extracellular matrix components are an active area of research focus. Finally, tissue engineering is being explored as another potential avenue through which disc regeneration may be prevented or reversed.

Cell-Based Therapies

Stem Cells, Chondrocytes, Intervertebral Disc Cells

The NP has low cell density and limited regenerative capacity, making disc degeneration at this level rather structurally compromising. Mesenchymal stem cells (MSC) are a natural option for cell based therapy for IVD degeneration due to their regenerative capacity. Studies with rabbit cell cultures that combined MSC and NP cells yielded greater cell proliferation, growth factor production and proteoglycan synthesis than NP cells alone [9]. A significant challenge to larger human trials is viability of stem cells in the hypoxic, acidic and nutrient deprived IVD environment [3].

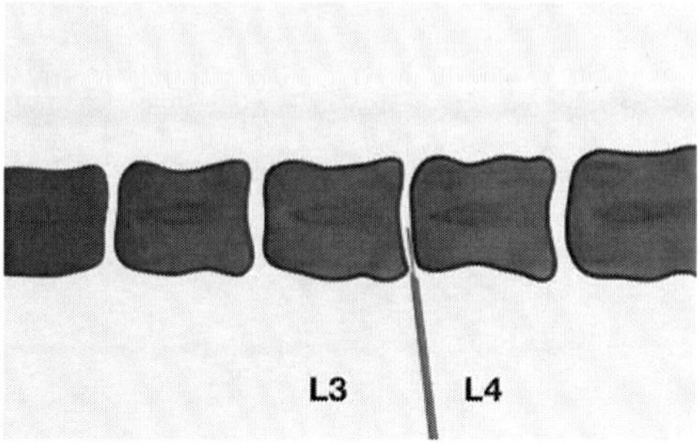

Figure 3. Chondrocyte Insertion into Disc Space.

Chondrocytic cell types are also being investigated as a potential for restorative capacity in IVD degeneration. Early trials in canine models showed disc chondrocytes could be viably transplanted into damaged IVDs and sucessfully persist in the environment, as well as produce an ECM and collagen network similar to the normal IVD tissue. Human trials have also shown promise in chondrocyte therapy. As part of the EuroDisc trial, Meisel et al. demonstrated a reduction in low back pain at 2 years (compared to control population) for patients receiving autologous disc derived chondrocyte transplant after discectomy. For the trial, harvested chondrocytes were cultured ex vivo, then inserted into the disc space and successfully shown to remain viable after transplantation, produce sufficient ECM and maintain disc dimensions on follow up imaging (Figure 3). Primary outcomes were assessed using the Oswestry low back pain disability questionnaire modified according to Hudson-Cook (OPDQ). The transplant group showed a sustained decrease in the total sum score and disability index of the OPDQ at 2 years, while the improvement in the control group leveled off after an initial effect from surgery. On evaluation of secondary MRI criteria, the transplant group was found to have significantly higher residual fluid content of their treated disc and discs at adjacent levels when compared to control [10]. Chondrocytic cell therapy shows promising results for regeneration of the IVD in symptomatic patients and continued study is warranted.

Biomolecular Therapy

Platelet Rich Plasma

Platelet rich plasma (PRP) is an autologous plasma formulation that is rich in platelets and their associated growth factors. This concentrated formulation makes the substance a source of multipotent stem cells with the potential to differentiate into targeted tissue types [3]. The use of PRP for the treatment of DDD has limited clinical evidence supporting its use, but animal studies showed promising results. In a rabbit model, introducing PRP into the intradiscal space yielded increased expression of collagen II and proteoglycans, decreased apoptotic cells and gross disc improvement on MRI relative to control disks [3]. Outside of the scope of intervertebral disc degeneration, there have been reported human trails with PRP assisted tissue regeneration with clinical success. Pak et al. reviewed 13 human studies that successfully regenerated cartilage with adipose tissue derived stem cells in human trials, 11 of which added autologus PRP to the treatment. PRP enhanced tissue regeneration by providing a source of growth factors for stem cell differentiation and a scaffold for new cartilage formation [11].

Gene Therapy

Identifying genes responsible for disc degeneration or regeneration and creating ways to target those genes is central to the conept of gene therapy. Vectors for gene delivery include viral and non viral options. Several animal studies with viral vectors have shown successful results, but human studies are still pending. In a rabbit model, TGF-β1 gene transfer via an adenovirus vector results in 5x increase in IVD expression of the gene and increased proteoglycan production relative to control discs [3]. TGF-β1 is a growth factor whose expression promotes cell growth and proliferation, making it crucial in IVD regeneration (Figure 4).

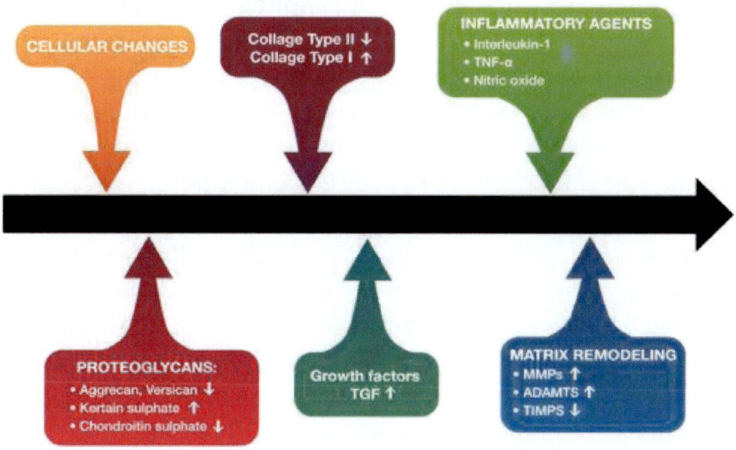

Figure 4. Role of TGF-β and ADAMTS5.

Gene therapy in other animal models have focused on stimulating other growth factors, inhibiting matrix metalloproteases (which play a role in the degradation pathway) and promoting transcription factors. A mouse model showed the role of ADAMTS5 in degradation of the NP which led to researchers designing small interference RNA targeting ADAMTS5. In a rabbit model, application of siRNA for ADAMTS5 yielded preservation of NP cells [12]. Several in vitro studies in human cells showed promising results; however, until an optimal viral vector for gene transfer is identified and an appropriate method for transferring vectors to target cells is developed, progress towards clinical application is limited at this time [3].

Immune Therapy

Growing research suggests a role of intervertebral disc immune imbalance in degnerative disc disease. The physical breakdown of the AF leads to NP herniation and exposure to immune cells. This process starts a cascade of local inflammatory response at the site of herniation, which may exacerbate IVD symptoms [13]. Further, there is some evidence to suggest decrease in FasL expression in pathological NP tissue, which will augment the local immune response after disc herniation [14, 15]. Immunotherapy techniques to control the disc environment used in conjunction with surgical discectomy could improve post operative quality of life and pain management; this is an area that warrants further investigation [13].

Nucleus Pulposus Prosthesis and Tissue Engineering

The NP core loses its mechanical properties with age as the tissue loses water content and degenerates. Hydrogels and scaffolds that can be injected into NP space to replace and regenerate local tissue are currently under investigation (Figure 5). Tsaryk, et al. demonstrate extracellular matrix production and chondrogenesis of multipotent stem cells and nasal chondrocytes *in vitro* and *in vivo* with a collagen- low molecular weight hyaluronic acid hydrogel loaded with TGF-β3 releasing microspheres [16]. Aside from hydrogel based NP replacement, nanofiber scaffolds also promote MSC differentiation into NP-like cells. Specifically, *in vitro* studies showed a combination of TGF-β1 and hypoxic growth conditions promoted maximal cell differentation on electrospun nanofiber scaffolds [17]. Much of this NP regeneration investigation is meant to promote healing and growth after nucleotomy of a degenerating disc or for early cases of degenerative IVD.

Injection of cell free polyglycolic acid-hyaluronon scaffold in the disc space after nucleotomy yielded greater tissue repair and collagen type II production compared to nucleotomy alone in rabbit models [18]. Endres et al. used this cell free implant for its porous nature, which promotes local cell migration and differentiation. Hydrogel based NP replacement requires cell implantation with growth factors to promote differentiation because gel alone cannot promote cell regeneration [16, 18].

Tissue engineering attempts to regenerate intervertebral disc tissue are still in pre-clinical stages. Based on preliminary investigation, successful scaffold constructs must have good porosity, mechanical strength properties similar to natural IVDs and be composed of non-toxic material to promote stem cell proliferation in vivo [19]. Xu et al. describe development of a biphasic scaffold which successfully cultured IVD-like tissue *in vivo* mouse models [20]. The success of this project holds promise for future in vivo three dimensional scaffolding techniques, which could replace degenerative IVD.

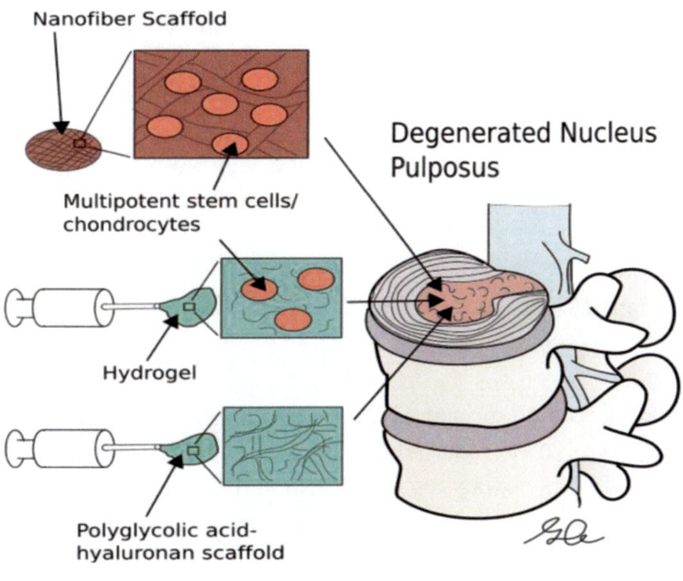

Figure 5. Hydrogel and Scaffold Injections.

EMERGING SURGICAL TREATMENT

When conservative and nonsurgical measures for DDD fail, surgery remains an effective and safe option for select patients. Surgical options for treatment of DDD range from disc removal and fusion to percutaneous and minimally invasive techniques. Improvements in each modality have led to a number of emerging products and techniques available to treating physicians.

Developments in Intervertebral Cages for Fusion Surgery

For patients with failed decompressive surgery, recurrent disc herniation, impending deformity, or loss of intervertebral disc height, removal of the interverebral disc and fusion of the adjacent vertebral segments may offer the best surgical option for treatment of their disease. In such cases, a support between the adjacent vertebral segments is used to preferentially maintain the disc height, prevent instability, and promote bony fusion. Several generations and designs of intervertebral cages using a variety of biocompatible materials have been developed and used in clinical practice. The most popular geometrical design is wedge-shaped, mimicking the end plate geometry and allowing for maximal end plate contact and incresaed implant stability in flexion, extension, and rotation. At the same time, these implants should maintain vertebral column height and restore normal lordosis. These concepts generally apply to both cervical and lumbar pathology, though several important differences in surgical technique and biomechanics of each region have led to cages designed specific to each location.

Cervical Implants

Hybrid Cages

The most common biomaterals used in cervical intervertebral implants are titanium and polymer materials, namely poly-ether-ether-ketone (PEEK). Although controversy exists regarding which material is superior, studies have shown that long-term subsidence rates may be higher with titanium implants when not used in conjunction with anterior plating [21]. PEEK as a material has a Young's modulus that is between cancellous and cortical bone and therefore is thought to decrease the rate of subsidence particularly in osteoperotic bone (Table 1) [22]. Recently, hybrid titanium/PEEK cages have been developed in an attempt to take advantage of the preferential characteristics of each materal: titanium has optimal surface characteristics and bioactivity, while the elastic modulus and radiolucency of PEEK allow for less stress shielding and easier x-ray visualization of fusion. Available examples include the A-Spine Asia Co. Combo Cervical Disc Cage (A-SPINE Asia, Taiwan) (Figure 6), and Orthofix CONSTRUX® Mini PTC™ Spacer System (Orthofix, USA); these hybrid implants have yet to be rigorously tested in the clinical arena.

Zero-Profile Implants

While standard interbody cervical fusion surgery includes concomitant placement of an anterior plate with screws, new options of low-profile plating systems have emerged. Integrated designs may address the difficulties with placing the anterior plate and quell the adverse effects of plating, namely adjacent segment degeneration and postoperative dysphagia. The designs currently available on market are the ZERO-P® VA stand-alone Spacer (DepuySynthes, USA) (Figure 7), the PEEK Prevail® Cervical Interbody Device, the COALITION® integrated plate and spacer system (Globus Medical, USA), and the ROI-C® Cervical Cage (LDR Holding Global Corporation, France). A recent meta analysis comparing the ZERO-P® system to anterior plating showed reduced operation time and blood loss, significant improvement of postoperative Japanese Orthopedic Association (JOA) score, reduction of postoperative Neck Disability Index (NDI) and Visual Analog Scale (VAS) scores, and decresaed incidence of postoperative dysphagia at early and late follow-up using the low profile implant. Important to note, however, is that the two procedures had a similar fusion rate, and that anterior plating promoted better sagittal alignment [23].

Lumbar Implants

A multitude of lumbar intervertebral cage designs are available for clinical use, tailored to the goals of treatment and specific needs of the surgery. Cages for anterior lumbar interbody fusion (ALIF) are similar to those used in cervical spine surgery, given the common anterior approach to the vertebral column and generally full exposure of the width of the disc space. Threaded cylindrical cages, titanium mesh cages, wedged structural allograft, kidney-shaped cages, and bullet shaped cages represent various design iterations over the course of the history of intervertebral cage development. Threaded cylindrical designs were shown to have inferior lateral and axial torsional resistance [24] and may be prone to subsidence when not supplemented with anterior plating or posterior fixation [25]. Those designs have largely been replaced by flat or convex shaped grafts with teeth to engage the endplates. Going further, several new cage designs for ALIF procedures are now available that incorporate the use of multiple materials as well as plate and plateless designs, similar to those of anterior cervical implants. Plateless designs eliminate the need for extensive anterior exposure in cases where illiac vessels make are difficult to mobilize on the face of the vertebral bodies.

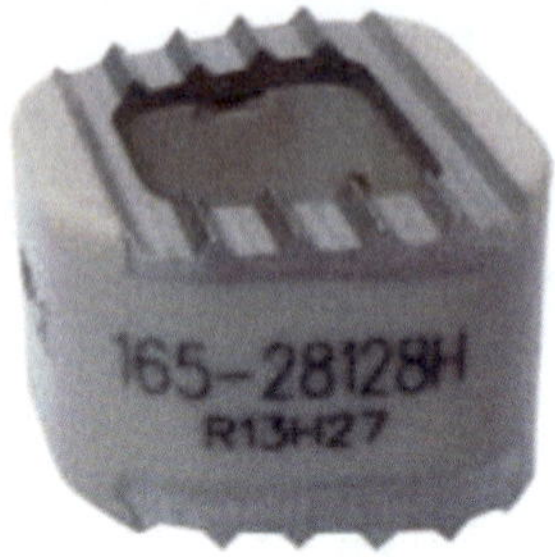

Figure 6. A-Spine Asia Co. Combo Cervical Disc Cage.

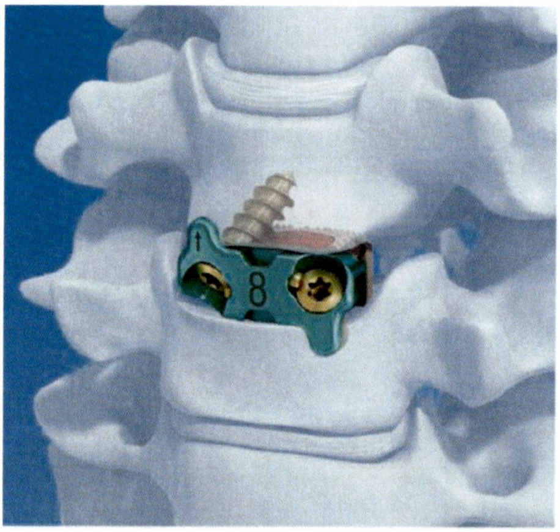

Figure 7. ZERO-P® VA stand-alone Spacer.

For patients undergoing posterior and posterolateral approach to lumbar interbody fusion, access to the disc space is obscured due to the thecal sac and cages have evolved to aid the proper placement. Kidney-shaped cages which cover a large surface area can be placed transforaminally and steered into proper position with inserter attachments at one end and implant curves that follow the end plate geometry. Some studies have shown biomechanical advantages with placement of the graft along the anterior border of the endplates, though subsequent testing has challenged the necessity of anterior graft positioning [26]. Additionally, when used in conjunction with posterior stabilization, stability seems to be consistent across all modern cage designs [27]. Nonethelesss, the kidney shape facilitates selective positioning of the graft across the width of the entire vertebral body, especially in combination with a transforaminal technique, and allows the surgeon greater control of the final construct.

Titanium Implants

Several materials have been examined for use in lumbar intervertebral implant design. Titanium was a popular initial choice in intervertebral cage design due to its widespread use as implant material in other procedures. Later, titanium use was largely supplanted by PEEK cages due to the latter material's biomechanical similarities to bone (more comparable Young's modulus of elasticity) with presumed less stress shielding. The radiolucency of PEEK also allows better visualization of bony fusion on x-rays. Despite the attractive qualities of PEEK, in vivo studies have not convincingly demonstrated superiority of PEEK implants in fusion surgeries [28], and titanium use has seen a re-emergence in many surgeons' practice. Unlike polymer implants, the surface of titanium can be modified to produce a micron-scaled roughed surface, a property which increases osteoblast maturation and induces a more osteogenic environment compared to that of PEEK materials [29, 30]. Additionally, these micro surface textures improve surface area contact between bone and implant during fusion [31]. To improve osteoinduction with polymers, these materials are often used in conjunction with biological agents, namely bone morphogenic protein (BMP), which are associated with various other risks [32]. Furthermore, PEEK materials are generally contraindicated in cases of infection and thus, titanium is favored for surgical management of discitis when medical therapy fails and the disease process renders the disc unsalvageable. Again, hybrid PEEK lumbar intervertebral implants with a surfaced titanium coating are now becoming available, though further testing is warranted to determine the true clinical benefits of the combination materials.

Lateral Interbody Implants

In addition to anterior and posterior approaches to the spine, direct lateral interbody fusion (DLIF) or extreme lateral interbody fusion (XLIF) approaches offer additional fusion options (Figure 8). Lateral approaches to the lumbar spine generally facilitate placement of a larger interbody graft and allow for coronal as well as sagittal correction. For patients with adequate bone quality, the large interbody graft may provide equivalent stability to posterior fusion techniques, while avoiding disruption or destabilization of the posterior column and musculature [33]. Laterally inserted grafts also allow for correction of coronal deformity, though only modest correction is observed in the sagittal plane [34, 35]. Sagittal correction may be further augmented in combination with the use of anterior longitudinal ligament release and lordotic cages [36, 37]. Inability to access the neural elements for direct decompression limits the use of these approaches as standalone procedures, although an adequate indirect decompression through distraction of the disc space with a large graft is achievable [38]. The lateral approach to the vertebral column can also be useful in reoperations, avoiding the posterior scar tissue. Lateral access to the spine does requires a learning curve, however, and complications related to violation of the lumbar plexus as well as the genitofemoral nerve as it traverses the lateral spine border through the psoas muscle must be avoided [39]. Neurostimulation of the psoas muscle is critical in this approach but stimulation is limited for purely sensory nerves. Similarly, risk of vascular injury to the great vessels must be weighed against the potential benefits of this approach.

Expandable Cages

Given geometric contraints of posterior or minimally invasive anterior and lateral exposures, expandable cages have been developed which facilitate safe placement of the graft through less retraction of soft tissue and neural elements, less bony removal and destabilization, and less endplate destruction during positioning. Once seated, the cage can be expanded against the endplates to ensure for enough load bearing to prevent dislodgement of the graft and generate higher endplate forces (that promote fusion) than static grafts [40]. Overdistraction remains a concern, with potential deleterious effects related to increased subsidence, though further investigation is needed to better characterize this risk [41, 42]. Such implants are perhaps most useful in more extensive procedures that span more than one disc space (such as corpectomies), but nonetheless, remain a viable option for single level fusions as well. Newer implants have incorporated the kidney-shaped cages with expandable technology (Stryker Acculif), optimizing the advantages of each design.

Laterally expandable cages are also gaining popularity as techniques shift toward more minimal exposures. These implants can be placed during minimally invasive procedures and expanded in-situ, without sacrifice of graft-endplate surface area contact. Prelminary biomechanical data suggests that these mini-expandable cages provide comparable stability in fusion procedures, and may also reduce supplemental fixation burden, facilitating minimally invasive single-position surgery [43].

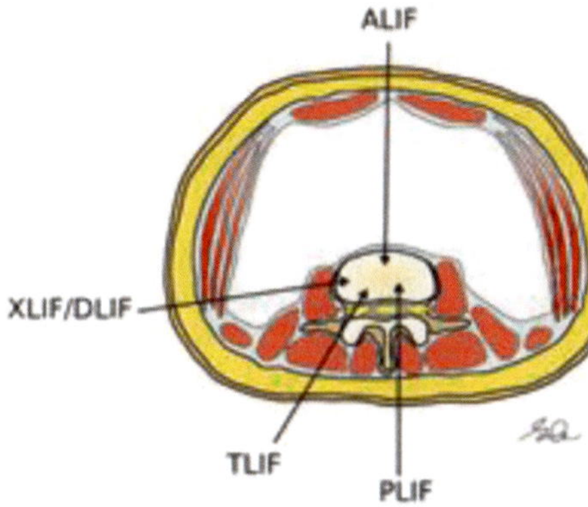

Figure 8. Lateral Body Fusion.

Sagittal Plane Correction Implants

Recent literature on spine surgery outcomes have placed an emphasis on the concept of proper sagittal vertebral alignment of the spine, inclduing its relationship to the pelvis (sagittal balance) (Figure 9). These spinopelvic parameters have subsequently been shown to correlate with level of patient disability and serve as important predictors of quality of life improvement in people undergoing spinal fusion surgery for adult spinal deformity [44-50]. As such, implants have been developed that facilitate the restoration of this sagittal alignment, adding height preferentially at the anterior spinal column, improving lumbar lordosis (Figure 10). A multitude of lordotic cage designs are now available from various vendors worldwide. The effectiveness of sagittal correction with lordotic cages varies across studies, and additional methods such as rod bending and compression across the fusion are often employed to increase lordosis [51, 52]. For multilevel TLIF surgery, the effect of lordotic cages may compound, offering a correction in the sagittal plane of greater than 5 degrees per level and possibly avoiding a more extensive and risky osteotomy operation [53]. An important caution with hyperlordotic designs is unequal loading of the endplate that may increase the chance of graft subsidence.

Disc Arthroplasty

The concept of disc arthroplasty replaces a degenerated disc with a prosthetic that most closely mimicks a physiologic state and preserves disc joint function. To that effect, one would hope to alleviate pain, eliminate the prospect of disc recurrence, and maintain or restore intervertebral disc height. Importantly, and unlike fusion procedures, arthroplasty maintains range of motion and flexibility, and prevents non-physiologic loading of adjacent segments that leads to adjacent segment degeneration. Despite the theoretical advantages of disc arthroplasty, the progress in development and acceptance of near-physiologic implants has been slowed by some early clinical setbacks and the high cost of implants. Several generations of implants have been developed for use in the cervical and lumbar spine.

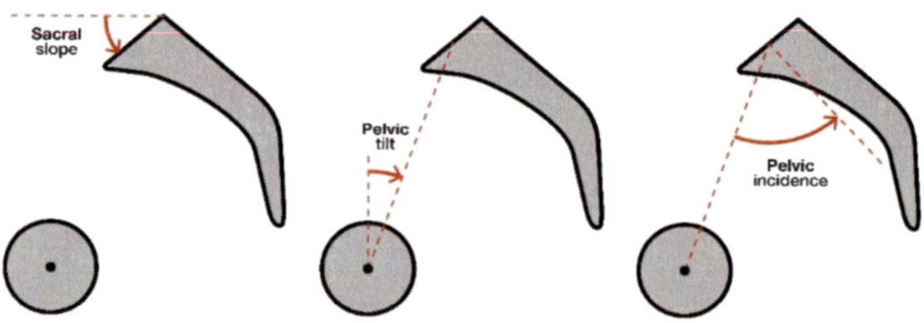

Figure 9. Sagittal Balance.

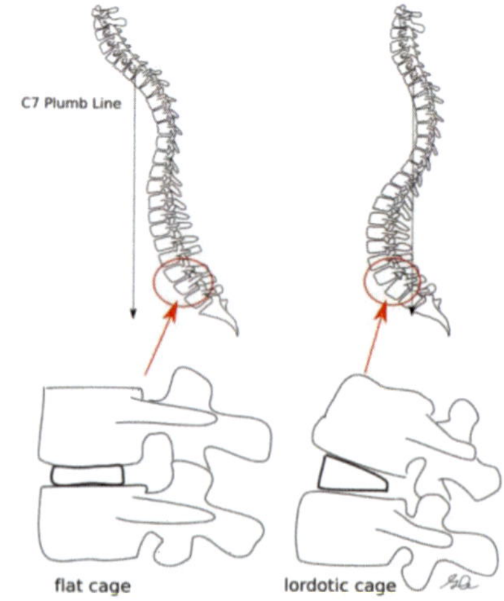

Figure 10. Implants for Sagittal Alignment.

Cervical Disc Arthroplasty

Dr. Ulf Fernstrom performed the first cervical disc arthroplasty (CDA) surgeries in patients in 1966, though this series met with generally poor results [54], and discectomy with subsequent fusion became the standard treatment for cervical degenerative disc disease. Over the past three decades, however, development of cervical disc prostheses have evolved, with numerous currently available models, including the Bryan disc (Medtronic Sofamor Danek, Memphis, TN, USA), Prestige disc (Medtronic Sofamor Danek, Memphis, TN, USA), porous coated motion (PCM) disc (NuVasive, San Diego, CA, USA), ProDisc-C disc (Synthes Spine West Chester, PA, USA), Mobi-C disc (LDR Spine, Austin, Texas, USA), and Kineflex-C disc (SpinalMotion, Mountain View, CA, USA). These designs vary in their materials and composition but are all conceptualized with the similar biomechanical goal of preserving motion and loading at the disc segement. Based on a meta-analysis of studies with 4–6 years of follow-up, patients who underwent single level disc arthroplasty showed preservation of segmental motion, a lower rate of reoperation, and greater improvements in NDI score, neck and arm pain scores, and SF 36 Health Survey physical component score than those who underwent ACDF. In a 7-year followup comparing single level disc replacement with the ProDisc-C implant to ACDF, patients treated with arthroplasty had lower rates of subsequent surgery, while clinical outcomes between the groups were similar [55]. Over the 7 year study period, disc arthroplasty was also shown to be less costly than ACDF [56]. In a separate analysis comparing single level cervcial disc arthroplasty to ACDF, arthroplasty was associated with cost savings throughout a 3-year follow up period due to lower readmission rates, fewer mechanical complications, and lower reoperation rates [57].

Two level disc arthroplasty was later compared to two level ACDF in a prospective study that included 24 centers across the United States, randomizing 330 patients to CDA with the Mobi-C device, or ACDF with corticocancellous allograft and anterior cervical plating. The authors concluded that at 48 months, the arthroplasty group had statistically significant improvements in NDI scores, SF-12 PCS scores, patient satisfaction, subsequent surgery rates, adjacent-segment degeneration, and overall success compared to the fusion group [58]. Additional cost analyses on the same patient cohort showed a greater improvement in quality of life at a lower total cost over an initial 24 month and subsequent 5 year study period, supporting the cost effectiveness of two level arthroplasty compared to ACDF [59, 60].

The use of cervical disc prosthesis implants are favored in cases of single-level disease, primary anterior or disc related pathology, preserved disc height, preserved segmental motion, absence of significant facet arthropathy, and normal sagittal alignment [61]. Practitioners should continue to exercise caution whenever adopting new technology and techniques. In a review of the literature on CDA vs ACDF, Alvin et al. found significant descrepancy in reported incidence of complications, namely adjacent segment disease and heterotopic ossification, for studies in which the authors had stated conflict of interest. Important to note, however, is that quality of life outcomes in all of these studies were unaffected by reported conflicts of interest [62]. Disc arthroplasty therefore remains a favorable option for select patients, and future data will determine the long-term complications, benefits, and cost-effectiveness of this technique.

Lumbar Disc Arthroplasty

The first lumbar disc implant, the SB Charite (Depuy), was developed in the 1980's. Early problems with migration, fatigue of the implants, and increased facet joint loading [63] led to a number of revisions and model updates. Simultaneously, a slew of other companies developed lumbar prosthetic disc implants, two of which are currently FDA approved: the Prodisc L (Synthes Spine, PA, USA) (Figure 11), and Charite (DePuy Spine, Inc., Raynham, MA, USA). These implants, however, have not caught vast clinical usage due to ongoing questions regarding the durability of outcome results of arthroplasty. A recent review of the California Office of Statewide Health Planning and Development discharge database demonstrated that total disc arthroplasty is not associated with lower rates of repeat lumbar surgery compared with lumbar fusion beyond one year [64]. A cochrane review of total disc replacement for lumbar degenerative disc disease concluded that short-term patient outcomes were equivalent to fusion surgery though prevention of adjacent level disease and facet joint degeneration was not properly assessed, cautioning the surgical community to be prudent about adopting lumbar disc replacement technology on a large scale [65]. Furthermore, mid to long-term results for multilevel lumbar disc arthroplasty show worse results in conjunction with higher complication rates, limiting the use of current designs for multilevel disc disease [66]. Nonetheless, continued long-term data will better define the complications associated with and indications for lumbar disc arthoplasty.

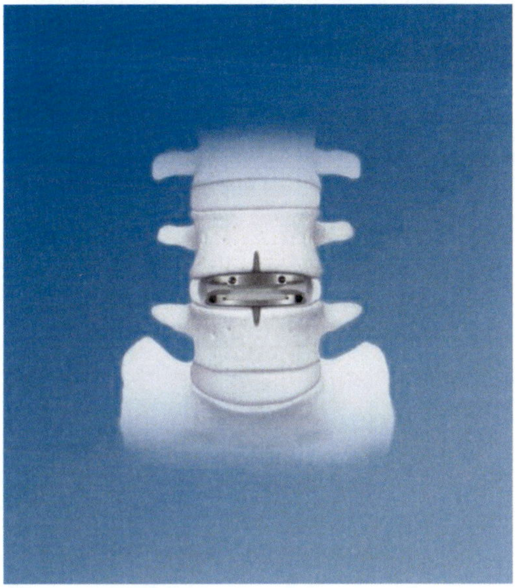

Figure 11. Prodisc Lumbar Disc Implant.

Endoscopic Techniques

Microscopic discectomy has largely supplanted open discectomy as the initial treatment of choice for refractory lumbar HNP and radiculopathy. The microscopic approach has equivalent success to open surgery, in addition to a low complication rate [67]. This procedure is also frequently done on an outpatient basis, and is often favored by patients. Spinal fusion surgeries have also been adapted with these less invasive approaches, with good outcomes and lower complication rates [68]. Moving toward the trend of less invasive techniques, endoscopic procedures have been developed through the same concept of less disruption of normal anatomy while achieving the same goals of neural decompression. Some of the earliest endoscopic techniques were developed by Dr. Parvis Kambin for percutaneous removal of the posterior third of the nuclues pulposus as a technique for indirect decompression [69]. In the modern era, endoscopic procedures are now described for anterior and posterior approaches to the cervical and lumbar spine. While these techniques have been refined for the past three decades, they are associated with additional learning curve [70] and require specialized training and familiarity with endoscopic instruments, adding a level of complexity to the procedure. While certainly not as abundant as microdiscectomy for treatment of disc disease, endoscopic approaches may play a larger part in resident training and surgical armamentarium in the future, and warrant further discussion.

Endoscopic Discectomy

Cervical Anterior

While ACDF is the mainstay operation for cervical degenerative disc disease, patients with maintenance of disc height and paracentral disc pathology may be good candidates for a less invasive discectomy without fusion. Access to the anterior cervical spine for open procedures carries risk of retraction injury. Furthermore, violation of the anterior longitudinal ligament (ALL) and entire disc space necessitates fusion after decompression; therefore, an anterior transdiscal endoscopic technique that avoids excessive tissue retraction and fusion offers many advantages. This anterior trasnsdiscal endoscopic approach can be performed percutaneously and safely [71]. Additionally, though some loss of disc height may be noted postoperatively, preservation of sagittal alignment and range of motion with good clinical outcomes is experienced in most cases [71, 72]. Important to note is that lateral disc pathology and primarily radicular symptoms are the main predictors of good outcomes with an anterior endoscopic transdiscal approach, and careful patient selection is critical [73].

Furthermore, indications for endoscopic anterior cervical approaches are being expanded, and a transcorporal endoscopic approach has recently been described for disc fragments that migrate superiorly or inferiorly away from the disc space behind the vertebral body; this may offer an alternative to a more invasive corpectomy and fusion surgery, though the technique is not yet proven [74]. Microendoscopic techniques for anterior discectomy with fusion have also been developed [75]. In a single-center prospective, randomized study, a microendoscopic group demonstrated a significantly improved early postoperative course with less laryngopharyngeal complications, and marked reduction in postoperative pain, analgesic use, and hospital stay compared to conventional ACDF [76].

Posterior

For patients with lateral disc herniation and radiculopathy, posterior microscopic foraminotomy and discectomy have become a viable alternative, eliminating the need for fusion in ACDF and maintaining the bony integrity of the posterior column by avoiding full laminectomy. Similarly, an endoscopic approach to these procedures is feasible, with outcomes equivalent to ACDF [77]. A main advantage of these approaches over conventional laminectomy is avoidance of progressive kyphotic deformity due to minimal disruption of the posterior elements. In a group of patients 24-46 months following posterior endoscopic foraminotomy, Kim et al. found that measures of cervical curvature, disk height, and segmental angle were not worsened [78].

Lumbar

Two main techniques for posterior endoscopic lumbar decompression have evolved: percutaneous endoscopic transforaminal discectomy (PETD), and percutaneous endoscopic interlaminar discectomy (PEID). PETD involves a posterolateral, transforaminal approach to the pathology using Kambin's triangle [79] (Figure 12), and is preferable for soft unilateral disc herniations with sciatica in the absence of severe neurologic deficit. PEID, on the other hand, involves a more posterior interlaminar projection and is advantageous in cases with a significant amount of canal compromise, extended disc migration, narrow neural foramen, or a high iliac crest [80]. The disadvantage of this approach is a higher risk of dural tear compared with microdiscectomy or open procedure, and thus, it is the less favored technique [81].

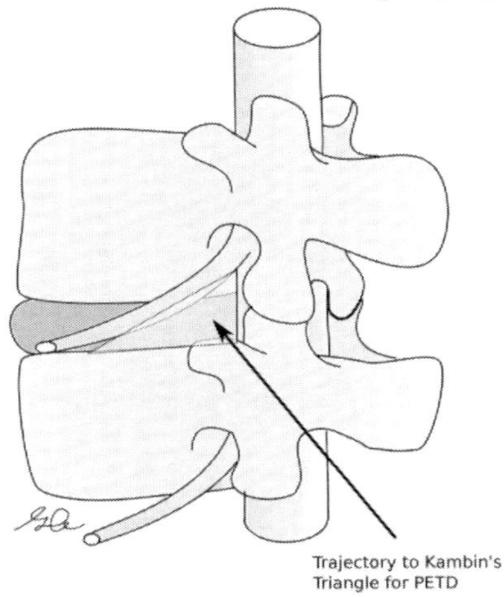

Figure 12. Kambin's Triangle Trajectory.

PETD can be used effectively for nerve root decompression in treating lateral recess stenosis, as well as for removal of herniated disc fragments [82]. PETD may also be a useful technique for recurrent disc herniation, and in a review assessing efficacy compared to redo open discectomy, had decreased operative time, blood loss, and lower complication rates with similar effect on relief of back and leg pain [80]. Furthermore, in experienced hands, the lateral endoscopic approach can be done under a local anesthetic with results equivalent to microdiscectomy [83-86]. One lingering concern over endoscopic approaches is the tendency toward higher rates of recurrent disc herniation [87, 88]. Furthermore, exiting nerve root injury leading to transient postoperative dysesthesia can be seen in 1 to 8.9 percent of cases, and can deter inexperienced surgeons from utilizing the technique [89]. Despite some limitations, endoscopic procedures are being expanded for spinal fusion as well [90], and endoscopic techniques in general may prove to be useful tools as more surgeons become familiar with the instruments and technique, and more training programs nationwide incorporate the technique into resident traning.

Percutaneous Techniques

Bridging the gap between so called "conservative" options which target symptom relief, and "surgical" options which aim to remove the pathologic process, are a variety of percutaneously performed procedures developed to address disc pathology. Similar to more invasive surgical procedures, they address the degenerated disc disease, though are done percutaneously via minimal access and are associated with less incisional pain and disruption of normal anatomy. Important to note is that these procedures are not appropriate for extruded fragments, or facet and ligamentous hypertrophy. Additionally, despite fluoroscopic guidance, the procedure itself is essentially "blind" and drawbacks include inability to directly visualize the normal anatomy to protect it, and inability to evaluate the progress and completion of decompression in real time.

Nucleotomy

Nucleotomy procedures involve fluoroscope-guided introduction of a percutaneous instrument inserted into the intervertebral disc. These percutaneous procedures have been described in the literature for its application to disc herniations in both cervical [91] and lumbar regions [92]. Various techniques can then be used to decompress the nucleus pulposus, ranging from percutaenous laser disc decompression (PLDD), radiofrequency ablation, and intradiscal electrothermal therapy (IDET), to intradiscal placement of chemically engineered products (chemonucleolysis) such as alcohols (DiscoGel®; Gelscom SAS, Caen, France), collagenase (WeiBang Biopharm, Liaoning, China), and oxygen-ozone (O_2-O_3) therapy [93]. (Figure 13) Symptom relief is dependent on an indirect effect by decreasing the intradiscal pressure and, therefore, concern over efficacy and durability of these procedures has prevented their adoption by many surgeons. In a prospective randomized trial for patients with sciatica and relatively small disc herniations, 44% of patients who had a technically successful PLDD required additional surgical intervention (re-operation) in the first year [94]. Furthermore, a systematic review of lumbar disc nucleoplasty concluded that there was only limited to fair evidence for nucleoplasty in managing radicular pain due to contained disc herniation; patients with contained disc herniation and maintained disc height may benefit most from percutaneous interventions [95].

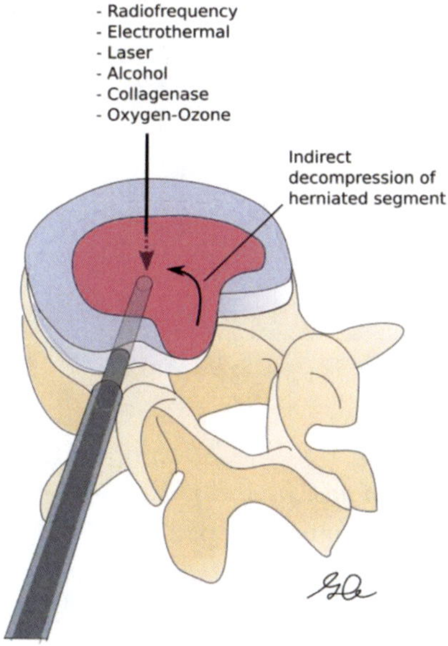

Figure 13. Percutaneous Procedure Techniques.

Automated Percutaneous Lumbar Discectomy and Dekompressor

Instruments for mechanical percutaneous disc decompression have also been developed. The Dekompressor® system (Stryker Spine, Allendale, NJ) utilizes an Archimedes' screw design to decompres the nucleus, while an automated percutaneous lumbar discectomy (APLD) system is designed with a suction/cutting probe to achieve the same result. Some authors have even described combined techniques such as APLD in conjunction with oxygen-ozone therapy to promote proteoglycan hydrolysis and fibrosis within the nucleus pulposus, leading to further disc volume reduction after mechanical decompression [96]. Similar to nucleotomy procedures, however, there exists only limited evidence for these techniques, and many of the same drawbacks pertaining to limited indications, and questionable efficacy and durability persist [97, 98].

Conclusion

As life expectancy of the general population increases, the medical community can inevitably expect to see a higher number of patients with disc disease, and a longer duration of disc disease in individual patients. Therefore, a long-term treatment plan is necessary, preferably one that prevents or reverses the degenerative process itself and improves the quality of life for patients. In parallel, surgical tools and technique must continue to be refined with the goal of providing the least invasive and least disruptive, but robust and durable surgery. In these efforts, it is the responsibility of the physician to scrutinize and study each emerging therapy with proper due diligence, keeping the best interest of the patient always at the forefront.

References

[1] Ball, J. R., Hurlbert, R. J., *Concepts of Disk Degeneration and Regeneration*, in *Youmans Neurological Surgery*, H. R. Winn, Editor. 2011, Saunders: Philadelphia, PA. p. 2752-2762.

[2] Manchikanti, L., et al., *Comprehensive review of epidemiology, scope, and impact of spinal pain.* Pain Physician, 2009. 12(4): p. E35-70.

[3] Kepler, C. K., et al., *Intervertebral disk degeneration and emerging biologic treatments.* J Am Acad Orthop Surg, 2011. 19(9): p. 543-53.

[4] Surkitt, L. D., et al., *Efficacy of directional preference management for low back pain: a systematic review.* Phys Ther, 2012. 92(5): p. 652-65.

[5] Garcia, A. N., et al., *Identifying Patients With Chronic Low Back Pain Who Respond Best to Mechanical Diagnosis and Therapy: Secondary Analysis of a Randomized Controlled Trial.* Phys Ther, 2015.

[6] Clare, H. A., R. Adams, and C. G. Maher, *Reliability of McKenzie classification of patients with cervical or lumbar pain.* J Manipulative Physiol Ther, 2005. 28(2): p. 122-7.

[7] Meile, V., Bhalla T, Jones GA, Benzel EC., *Concepts and Mechanisms of Spinal Biomechanics*, in *Youmans Neurological Surgery*, H. R. Winn, Editor. 2011, Saunders: Philadelphia. p. 2700-2710.

[8] Maidhof, R., et al., *Emerging trends in biological therapy for intervertebral disc degeneration.* Discov Med, 2012. 14(79): p. 401-11.

[9] Sakai, D., *Future perspectives of cell-based therapy for intervertebral disc disease.* Eur Spine J, 2008. 17 Suppl 4: p. 452-8.

[10] Meisel, H. J., et al., *Clinical experience in cell-based therapeutics: disc chondrocyte transplantation A treatment for degenerated or damaged intervertebral disc.* Biomol Eng, 2007. 24(1): p. 5-21.

[11] Pak, J., et al., *Cartilage Regeneration in Human with Adipose Tissue-Derived Stem Cells: Current Status in Clinical Implications.* Biomed Res Int, 2016. 2016: p. 4702674.

[12] Rizvi, M., *Novel treatment strategies for intervertebral disc degeneration.* Saudi J Health Sci, 2015. 4: p. 5-15.

[13] Sun, Z., et al., *Molecular immunotherapy might shed a light on the treatment strategies for disc degeneration and herniation.* Med Hypotheses, 2013. 81(3): p. 477-80.

[14] Kaneyama S, N.K., Takada T, Suzuki T, Shimomura T, Maeno K, *Fas ligand expression on human nucleus pulposus cells decreases with disc degeneration process.* 2008.

[15] Satoh, K., et al., *Presence and distribution of antigen-antibody complexes in the herniated nucleus pulposus.* Spine (Phila Pa 1976), 1999. 24(19): p. 1980-4.

[16] Tsaryk, R., et al., *Collagen-low molecular weight hyaluronic acid semi-interpenetrating network loaded with gelatin microspheres for cell and growth factor delivery for nucleus pulposus regeneration.* Acta Biomater, 2015. 20: p. 10-21.

[17] Cui, X., et al., *Electrospun scaffold containing TGF-beta1 promotes human mesenchymal stem cell differentiation towards a nucleus pulposus-like phenotype under hypoxia.* IET Nanobiotechnol, 2015. 9(2): p. 76-84.

[18] Endres, M., et al., *Augmentation and repair tissue formation of the nucleus pulposus after partial nucleotomy in a rabbit model.* Tissue Cell, 2014. 46(6): p. 505-13.

[19] Xu, H., et al., *[Fabrication and analysis of a novel tissue engineered composite biphasic scaffold for annulus fibrosus and nucleus pulposus].* Zhongguo Xiu Fu Chong Jian Wai Ke Za Zhi, 2013. 27(4): p. 475-80.

[20] Xu, B., et al., *Intervertebral Disc Tissue Engineering with Natural Extracellular Matrix-Derived Biphasic Composite Scaffolds.* PLoS One, 2015. 10(4): p. e0124774.

[21] Chen, Y., et al., *Comparison of titanium and polyetheretherketone (PEEK) cages in the surgical treatment of multilevel cervical spondylotic myelopathy: a prospective, randomized, control study with over 7-year follow-up.* Eur Spine J, 2013. 22(7): p. 1539-46.

[22] Deng, Y., et al., *Effect of surface roughness on osteogenesis in vitro and osseointegration in vivo of carbon fiber-reinforced polyetheretherketone-nanohydroxyapatite composite.* Int J Nanomedicine, 2015. 10: p. 1425-47.

[23] Dong, J., et al., *Meta-Analysis Comparing Zero-Profile Spacer and Anterior Plate in Anterior Cervical Fusion.* PLoS One, 2015. 10(6): p. e0130223.

[24] Buttermann, G. R., et al., *Interbody device endplate engagement effects on motion segment biomechanics.* Spine J, 2009. 9(7): p. 564-73.

[25] Blumenthal, S. L., D.D. Ohnmeiss, and Nass, *Intervertebral cages for degenerative spinal diseases.* Spine J, 2003. 3(4): p. 301-9.

[26] Faundez, A. A., et al., *Position of interbody spacer in transforaminal lumbar interbody fusion: effect on 3-dimensional stability and sagittal lumbar contour.* J Spinal Disord Tech, 2008. 21(3): p. 175-80.

[27] Tsitsopoulos, P. P., et al., *Would an anatomically shaped lumbar interbody cage provide better stability? An in vitro cadaveric biomechanical evaluation.* J Spinal Disord Tech, 2012. 25(8): p. E240-4.

[28] Nemoto, O., et al., *Comparison of fusion rates following transforaminal lumbar interbody fusion using polyetheretherketone cages or titanium cages with transpedicular instrumentation.* Eur Spine J, 2014. 23(10): p. 2150-5.

[29] Olivares-Navarrete, R., et al., *Osteoblasts exhibit a more differentiated phenotype and increased bone morphogenetic protein production on titanium alloy substrates than on poly-ether-ether-ketone.* Spine J, 2012. 12(3): p. 265-72.

[30] Rao, P. J., et al., *Spine interbody implants: material selection and modification, functionalization and bioactivation of surfaces to improve osseointegration.* Orthop Surg, 2014. 6(2): p. 81-9.

[31] Devine, D. M., et al., *Coating of carbon fiber-reinforced polyetheretherketone implants with titanium to improve bone apposition.* J Biomed Mater Res B Appl Biomater, 2013. 101(4): p. 591-8.

[32] Mroz, T. E., et al., *Complications related to osteobiologics use in spine surgery: a systematic review.* Spine (Phila Pa 1976), 2010. 35(9 Suppl): p. S86-104.

[33] Pimenta, L., et al., *Biomechanics of lateral interbody spacers: going wider for going stiffer.* ScientificWorldJournal, 2012. 2012: p. 381814.

[34] Phan, K., et al., *Lateral lumbar interbody fusion for sagittal balance correction and spinal deformity.* J Clin Neurosci, 2015. 22(11): p. 1714-21.

[35] Alimi, M., et al., *Radiological and clinical outcomes following extreme lateral interbody fusion.* J Neurosurg Spine, 2014. 20(6): p. 623-35.

[36] Uribe, J. S., et al., *Finite element analysis of lordosis restoration with anterior longitudinal ligament release and lateral hyperlordotic cage placement.* Eur Spine J, 2015. 24 Suppl 3: p. 420-6.

[37] Uribe, J. S., et al., *Lordosis restoration after anterior longitudinal ligament release and placement of lateral hyperlordotic interbody cages during the minimally invasive lateral transpsoas approach: a radiographic study in cadavers.* J Neurosurg Spine, 2012. 17(5): p. 476-85.

[38] Lee, Y. S., S. W. Park, and Y. B. Kim, *Direct lateral lumbar interbody fusion: clinical and radiological outcomes.* J Korean Neurosurg Soc, 2014. 55(5): p. 248-54.

[39] Uribe, J. S., *Neural anatomy, neuromonitoring and related complications in extreme lateral interbody fusion: video lecture.* Eur Spine J, 2015. 24 Suppl 3: p. 445-6.

[40] Pekmezci, M., et al., *Comparison of expandable and fixed interbody cages in a human cadaver corpectomy model, part I: endplate force characteristics.* J Neurosurg Spine, 2012. 17(4): p. 321-6.

[41] Gonzalez-Blohm, S. A., et al., *In vitro evaluation of a lateral expandable cage and its comparison with a static device for lumbar interbody fusion: a biomechanical investigation.* J Neurosurg Spine, 2014. 20(4): p. 387-95.

[42] Pekmezci, M., et al., *Comparison of Expandable and Fixed Interbody Cages in a Human Cadaver Corpectomy Model: Fatigue Characteristics.* J Spinal Disord Tech, 2012.

[43] Cannestra, A. F., et al., *MIS Expandable Interbody Spacers: A Literature Review and Biomechanical Comparison of an Expandable MIS TLIF with Conventional TLIF and ALIF.* Spine (Phila Pa 1976), 2016.

[44] Schwab, F. J., et al., *Radiographical spinopelvic parameters and disability in the setting of adult spinal deformity: a prospective multicenter analysis.* Spine (Phila Pa 1976), 2013. 38(13): p. E803-12.

[45] Diebo, B. G., et al., *Sagittal deformities of the spine: factors influencing the outcomes and complications.* Eur Spine J, 2015. 24 Suppl 1: p. S3-15.

[46] Le Huec, J. C., et al., *Evidence showing the relationship between sagittal balance and clinical outcomes in surgical treatment of degenerative spinal diseases: a literature review.* Int Orthop, 2015. 39(1): p. 87-95.

[47] Diebo, B. G., et al., *Sagittal alignment of the spine: What do you need to know?* Clin Neurol Neurosurg, 2015. 139: p. 295-301.

[48] Terran, J., et al., *The SRS-Schwab adult spinal deformity classification: assessment and clinical correlations based on a prospective operative and nonoperative cohort.* Neurosurgery, 2013. 73(4): p. 559-68.

[49] Schwab, F., et al., *Scoliosis Research Society-Schwab adult spinal deformity classification: a validation study.* Spine (Phila Pa 1976), 2012. 37(12): p. 1077-82.

[50] Hallager, D. W., et al., *A comprehensive analysis of the SRS-Schwab Adult Spinal Deformity Classification and confounding variables - a prospective, non-US cross-sectional study in 292 patients.* Spine (Phila Pa 1976), 2015.

[51] Lee, J. H., et al., *Effects of lordotic angle of a cage on sagittal alignment and clinical outcome in one level posterior lumbar interbody fusion with pedicle screw fixation.* Biomed Res Int, 2015. 2015: p. 523728.

[52] Godde, S., et al., *Influence of cage geometry on sagittal alignment in instrumented posterior lumbar interbody fusion.* Spine (Phila Pa 1976), 2003. 28(15): p. 1693-9.

[53] Yson, S. C., et al., *Segmental lumbar sagittal correction after bilateral transforaminal lumbar interbody fusion.* J Neurosurg Spine, 2012. 17(1): p. 37-42.

[54] Fernstrom, U., *Arthroplasty with intercorporal endoprothesis in herniated disc and in painful disc.* Acta Chir Scand Suppl, 1966. 357: p. 154-9.

[55] Janssen, M. E., et al., *ProDisc-C Total Disc Replacement Versus Anterior Cervical Discectomy and Fusion for Single-Level Symptomatic Cervical Disc Disease: Seven-Year Follow-up of the Prospective*

Randomized U.S. Food and Drug Administration Investigational Device Exemption Study. J Bone Joint Surg Am, 2015. 97(21): p. 1738-47.

[56] Radcliff, K., et al., *Seven-year cost-effectiveness of ProDisc-C total disc replacement: results from investigational device exemption and post-approval studies.* J Neurosurg Spine, 2016: p. 1-9.

[57] Radcliff, K., J. Zigler, and J. Zigler, *Costs of cervical disc replacement versus anterior cervical discectomy and fusion for treatment of single-level cervical disc disease: an analysis of the Blue Health Intelligence database for acute and long-term costs and complications.* Spine (Phila Pa 1976), 2015. 40(8): p. 521-9.

[58] Davis, R. J., et al., *Two-level total disc replacement with Mobi-C cervical artificial disc versus anterior discectomy and fusion: a prospective, randomized, controlled multicenter clinical trial with 4-year follow-up results.* J Neurosurg Spine, 2015. 22(1): p. 15-25.

[59] Ament, J. D., et al., *Cost-effectiveness of cervical total disc replacement vs fusion for the treatment of 2-level symptomatic degenerative disc disease.* JAMA Surg, 2014. 149(12): p. 1231-9.

[60] Ament, J. D., et al., *Cost Utility Analysis of the Cervical Artificial Disc vs Fusion for the Treatment of 2-Level Symptomatic Degenerative Disc Disease: 5-Year Follow-up.* Neurosurgery, 2016.

[61] Ding, D. and M. E. Shaffrey, *Cervical disk arthroplasty: patient selection.* Clin Neurosurg, 2012. 59: p. 91-7.

[62] Alvin, M. D., et al., *Cervical arthroplasty: a critical review of the literature.* Spine J, 2014. 14(9): p. 2231-45.

[63] Rousseau, M. A., et al., *Disc arthroplasty design influences intervertebral kinematics and facet forces.* Spine J, 2006. 6(3): p. 258-66.

[64] Eliasberg, C. D., et al., *Complications and Rates of Subsequent Lumbar Surgery Following Lumbar Total Disc Arthroplasty and Lumbar Fusion.* Spine (Phila Pa 1976), 2016. 41(2): p. 173-81.

[65] Jacobs, W., et al., *Total disc replacement for chronic back pain in the presence of disc degeneration.* Cochrane Database Syst Rev, 2012. 9: p. CD008326.

[66] Siepe, C. J., et al., *Mid- to long-term results of total lumbar disc replacement: a prospective analysis with 5- to 10-year follow-up.* Spine J, 2014. 14(8): p. 1417-31.

[67] Dasenbrock, H. H., et al., *The efficacy of minimally invasive discectomy compared with open discectomy: a meta-analysis of prospective randomized controlled trials.* J Neurosurg Spine, 2012. 16(5): p. 452-62.

[68] Phan, K., et al., *Minimally invasive versus open transforaminal lumbar interbody fusion for treatment of degenerative lumbar disease: systematic review and meta-analysis.* Eur Spine J, 2015. 24(5): p. 1017-30.

[69] Telfeian, A.E., et al., *A brief history of endoscopic spine surgery.* Neurosurg Focus, 2016. 40(2): p. E2.

[70] Ahn, S. S., S. H. Kim, and D. W. Kim, *Learning Curve of Percutaneous Endoscopic Lumbar Discectomy Based on the Period (Early vs. Late) and Technique (in-and-out vs. in-and-out-and-in): A Retrospective Comparative Study.* J Korean Neurosurg Soc, 2015. 58(6): p. 539-46.

[71] Tzaan, W. C., *Anterior percutaneous endoscopic cervical discectomy for cervical intervertebral disc herniation: outcome, complications, and technique.* J Spinal Disord Tech, 2011. 24(7): p. 421-31.

[72] Lee, J. H. and S. H. Lee, *Clinical and radiographic changes after percutaneous endoscopic cervical discectomy: a long-term follow-up.* Photomed Laser Surg, 2014. 32(12): p. 663-8.

[73] Ahn, Y., et al., *Factors predicting excellent outcome of percutaneous cervical discectomy: analysis of 111 consecutive cases.* Neuroradiology, 2004. 46(5): p. 378-84.

[74] Deng, Z. L., et al., *Anterior transcorporeal approach of percutaneous endoscopic cervical discectomy for disc herniation at the c4-5 level: a technical note.* Spine J, 2016.

[75] Yao, N., et al., *Full-endoscopic technique for anterior cervical discectomy and interbody fusion: 5-year follow-up results of 67 cases.* Eur Spine J, 2011. 20(6): p. 899-904.

[76] Soliman, H. M., *Cervical microendoscopic discectomy and fusion: does it affect the postoperative course and the complication rate? A blinded randomized controlled trial.* Spine (Phila Pa 1976), 2013. 38(24): p. 2064-70.

[77] Ruetten, S., et al., *Full-endoscopic cervical posterior foraminotomy for the operation of lateral disc herniations using 5.9-mm endoscopes: a prospective, randomized, controlled study.* Spine (Phila Pa 1976), 2008. 33(9): p. 940-8.

[78] Kim, C. H., et al., *Changes in cervical sagittal alignment after single-level posterior percutaneous endoscopic cervical diskectomy.* Global Spine J, 2015. 5(1): p. 31-8.

[79] Hardenbrook, M., et al., *The anatomic rationale for transforaminal endoscopic interbody fusion: a cadaveric analysis.* Neurosurg Focus, 2016. 40(2): p. E12.

[80] Li, X., et al., *Percutaneous endoscopic lumbar discectomy for recurrent lumbar disc herniation.* Int J Surg, 2016. 27: p. 8-16.

[81] Teli, M., et al., *Higher risk of dural tears and recurrent herniation with lumbar micro-endoscopic discectomy.* Eur Spine J, 2010. 19(3): p. 443-50.

[82] Li, Z. Z., et al., *Percutaneous lumbar foraminoplasty and percutaneous endoscopic lumbar decompression for lateral recess stenosis through transforaminal approach: Technique notes and 2 years follow-up.* Clin Neurol Neurosurg, 2016. 143: p. 90-94.

[83] Sanusi, T., et al., *Endoscopic lumbar discectomy under local anesthesia may be an alternative to microdiscectomy: A single centre's experience using the far lateral approach.* Clin Neurol Neurosurg, 2015. 139: p. 324-7.

[84] Smith, N., et al., *Systematic review of microendoscopic discectomy for lumbar disc herniation.* Eur Spine J, 2013. 22(11): p. 2458-65.

[85] Gadjradj, P. S., et al., *Clinical outcomes after percutaneous transforaminal endoscopic discectomy for lumbar disc herniation: a prospective case series.* Neurosurg Focus, 2016. 40(2): p. E3.

[86] Sinkemani, A., et al., *Outcomes of Microendoscopic Discectomy and Percutaneous Transforaminal Endoscopic Discectomy for the Treatment of Lumbar Disc Herniation: A Comparative Retrospective Study.* Asian Spine J, 2015. 9(6): p. 833-40.

[87] Belykh, E., et al., *Prospective comparison of microsurgical, endoscopic, and endoscopically assisted discectomies: Clinical effectiveness and complications in railway workers.* World Neurosurg, 2016.

[88] Rasouli, M. R., et al., *Minimally invasive discectomy versus microdiscectomy/open discectomy for symptomatic lumbar disc herniation.* Cochrane Database Syst Rev, 2014. 9: p. CD010328.

[89] Sairyo, K., et al., *Surgery related complications in percutaneous endoscopic lumbar discectomy under local anesthesia.* J Med Invest, 2014. 61(3-4): p. 264-9.

[90] Wang, M. Y. and J. Grossman, *Endoscopic minimally invasive transforaminal interbody fusion without general anesthesia: initial clinical experience with 1-year follow-up.* Neurosurg Focus, 2016. 40(2): p. E13.

[91] Yang, B., et al., *Treatment of cervical disc herniation through percutaneous minimally invasive techniques.* Eur Spine J, 2014. 23(2): p. 382-8.

[92] Buy, X. and A. Gangi, *Percutaneous treatment of intervertebral disc herniation.* Semin Intervent Radiol, 2010. 27(2): p. 148-59.

[93] Stagni, S., et al., *A minimally invasive treatment for lumbar disc herniation: DiscoGel(R) chemonucleolysis in patients unresponsive to chemonucleolysis with oxygen-ozone.* Interv Neuroradiol, 2012. 18(1): p. 97-104.

[94] Brouwer, P. A., et al., *Percutaneous laser disc decompression versus conventional microdiscectomy in sciatica: a randomized controlled trial.* Spine J, 2015. 15(5): p. 857-65.

[95] Manchikanti, L., et al., *An update of the systematic assessment of mechanical lumbar disc decompression with nucleoplasty.* Pain Physician, 2013. 16(2 Suppl): p. SE25-54.

[96] Crockett, M. T., et al., *Ozone-augmented percutaneous discectomy: a novel treatment option for refractory discogenic sciatica.* Clin Radiol, 2014. 69(12): p. 1280-6.

[97] Manchikanti, L., et al., *Percutaneous lumbar mechanical disc decompression utilizing Dekompressor(R): an update of current evidence.* Pain Physician, 2013. 16(2 Suppl): p. SE1-24.

[98] Manchikanti, L., et al., *An updated review of automated percutaneous mechanical lumbar discectomy for the contained herniated lumbar disc.* Pain Physician, 2013. 16(2 Suppl): p. SE151-84.

EDITOR'S CONTACT INFORMATION

Dr. Allen Ho
Stanford University School of Medicine
300 Pasteur Drive, R281,
Stanford, CA 94303-5327
aho@stanford.edu

INDEX

A

B

C

D

E

F

I

N

O

P

Q

R

S

T

U

V

W

X